AF807319

Intraoperative Cranial Nerve Monitoring in Otolaryngology-Head and Neck Surgery

Joseph Scharpf • Gregory W. Randolph
Editors

Intraoperative Cranial Nerve Monitoring in Otolaryngology-Head and Neck Surgery

Springer

Editors
Joseph Scharpf
Head and Neck Institute
Cleveland Clinic
Cleveland, OH
USA

Gregory W. Randolph
Otolaryngology-Head and Neck Surgery
Massachusetts Eye and Ear Infirmary
Boston, MA
USA

ISBN 978-3-030-84915-3 ISBN 978-3-030-84916-0 (eBook)
https://doi.org/10.1007/978-3-030-84916-0

© The Editor(s) (if applicable) and The Author(s), under exclusive license to Springer Nature Switzerland AG 2022
This work is subject to copyright. All rights are solely and exclusively licensed by the Publisher, whether the whole or part of the material is concerned, specifically the rights of translation, reprinting, reuse of illustrations, recitation, broadcasting, reproduction on microfilms or in any other physical way, and transmission or information storage and retrieval, electronic adaptation, computer software, or by similar or dissimilar methodology now known or hereafter developed.
The use of general descriptive names, registered names, trademarks, service marks, etc. in this publication does not imply, even in the absence of a specific statement, that such names are exempt from the relevant protective laws and regulations and therefore free for general use.
The publisher, the authors, and the editors are safe to assume that the advice and information in this book are believed to be true and accurate at the date of publication. Neither the publisher nor the authors or the editors give a warranty, expressed or implied, with respect to the material contained herein or for any errors or omissions that may have been made. The publisher remains neutral with regard to jurisdictional claims in published maps and institutional affiliations.

This Springer imprint is published by the registered company Springer Nature Switzerland AG
The registered company address is: Gewerbestrasse 11, 6330 Cham, Switzerland

I would like to dedicate this book to my wife Tanya P Scharpf for her enduring love and support in my career and life. Her faith and selfless devotion to our family have made all things possible.

I am also so grateful for my children Joseph and Alexandra, whose love, compassion, and understanding inspire me each day and are a blessing to me.

I finally want to thank my parents Joseph and Teresa Scharpf for all their love and sacrifices to provide opportunities for me and encourage me to pursue a career in medicine.

—Joseph Scharpf

To my wife, Lorraine, your living faith and love has given me strength. Your faith, hard work, and selfless devotion to others has been my guiding light on this our path together.

To my children, Gregory, your artistic lens on the world has taught me. Benjamin, I'm proud of the man you have become and your abiding concern for others. Madeline, your intelligence, accomplishments, and grace through all inspire me.

To my mother, Frances, you have fostered a hopeful strength and a desire to learn.

—Gregory W. Randolph

Preface

Advances in intraoperative cranial nerve monitoring in Otolaryngology-Head and Neck Surgery have resulted in the optimization of patient outcomes and have improved the safety profile for our surgeries in the head and neck. There has been an expansion in both clinical applications and indications for nerve monitoring in the head and neck. Continuous innovation in the field has been led by many dedicated specialists contributing to this book including members of the International Neuromonitoring Study Group, founded by Dr. Gregory Randolph and Professor Henning Dralle. The Task Force on Cranial Nerve Monitoring of the American Academy of Otolaryngology-Head and Neck Surgery (AAOHNS) has provided further support for nerve monitoring with its position statement and task force report.

This book was conceived to fill the void that existed in having one source accessible to practitioners and trainees dedicated to intraoperative nerve monitoring. The book draws upon internationally recognized experts to elucidate the values, techniques, and limitations of intraoperative cranial nerve monitoring in head and neck surgery. It is our hope that this book will serve to further the knowledge of surgeons and multidisciplinary teams in their pursuit of providing their patients with the best care possible. We also hope that it will inspire future research and efforts to improve upon our existing knowledge to help the patients of tomorrow.

Finally, we would like to thank our students, residents, and fellows, whom we have been privileged to mentor and train over the courses of our careers, and to our patients who have been so appreciative of the value that intraoperative nerve monitoring brings to their care. We would also like to thank Samantha Lonuzzi from Springer for her support in bringing this work to fruition.

Cleveland, OH, USA — Joseph Scharpf
Boston, MA, USA — Gregory W. Randolph

Contents

Contributors

Amr H. Abdelhamid Ahmed Division of Thyroid and Parathyroid Endocrine Surgery, Department of Otolaryngology-Head & Neck Surgery, Massachusetts Eye and Ear Infirmary, Harvard Medical School, Boston, MA, USA

Peter Angelos Department of Surgery and MacLean Center for Clinical Medical Ethics, The University of Chicago, Chicago, IL, USA

Marcin Barczynski Department of Endocrine Surgery, Third Chair of General Surgery, Jagiellonian University Medical College, Krakow, Poland

Douglas M. Bennion Department of Otolaryngology – Head and Neck Surgery, University of Iowa, Iowa City, IA, USA

Antonio Bertelli Department of Surgery, Head and Neck Surgery Division, Santa Casa de Sao Paulo Medical School, Sao Paulo, Sao Paulo, Brazil

Juliana Bonilla-Velez Department of Otolaryngology–Head and Neck Surgery, University of Washington School of Medicine, Seattle, WA, USA

Division of Pediatric Otolaryngology, Seattle Children's Hospital, Seattle, WA, USA

Center for Clinical and Translational Research, Seattle Children's Research Institute, Seattle, WA, USA

Claudio R. Cernea Department of Surgery, University of São Paulo School of Medicine, São Paulo, Sao Paulo, Brazil

Betty Y. Chen Department of Otolaryngology-Head and Neck Surgery, Southern Illinois University School of Medicine, Springfield, IL, USA

Feng-Yu Chiang Department of Otolaryngology, E-Da Hospital, School of Medicine, College of Medicine, I-Shou University, Kaohsiung, Taiwan

Kevin J. Contrera Head and Neck Institute, Cleveland Clinic, Cleveland, OH, USA

Kirsten F.A.A. Dabekaussen Department of Surgery, Brigham and Women's Hospital, Harvard Medical School, Boston, MA, USA

Vaninder K. Dhillon Division of Laryngology and Endocrine Head and Neck Surgery, Johns Hopkins University, Department of Otolaryngology-Head and Neck Surgery, Bethesda, MD, USA

David Goldenberg The Department of Otolaryngology-Head and Neck Surgery, The Pennsylvania State University, The Milton S. Hershey Medical Center, Hershey, PA, USA

Simon A. Holoubek Department of Otolaryngology – Head and Neck Surgery, Augusta University, Augusta, GA, USA

Ayaka J. Iwata Department of Otolaryngology-Head and Neck Surgery, Kaiser Permanente, Santa Clara, CA, USA

Emad Kandil Department of Surgery, Tulane University School of Medicine, New Orleans, LA, USA

Amanda Silver Karcioglu Division of Thyroid and Parathyroid Endocrine Surgery, Department of Otolaryngology-Head & Neck Surgery, Massachusetts Eye and Ear Infirmary, Harvard Medical School, Boston, MA, USA

Navkiranjot Kaur Cleveland Clinic Lerner College of Medicine of Case Western Reserve University, Education Institute, Cleveland Clinic, Cleveland, OH, USA

Allison Keane The Department of Otolaryngology-Head and Neck Surgery, The Pennsylvania State University, The Milton S. Hershey Medical Center, Hershey, PA, USA

Maxwell Y. Lee Cleveland Clinic Lerner College of Medicine of Case Western Reserve University, Education Institute, Cleveland Clinic, Cleveland, OH, USA

Whitney Liddy Department of Otolaryngology – Head and Neck Surgery, Northwestern University Feinberg School of Medicine, Chicago, IL, USA

Jeffrey C. Liu Department of Otolaryngology Head and Neck Surgery, Lewis Katz School of Medicine at Temple University, Philadelphia, PA, USA

Department of Surgical Oncology, Fox Chase Cancer Center, Philadelphia, PA, USA

Garren M.I. Low Department of Otorhinolaryngology-Head and Neck Surgery, University of Texas Health Sciences Center at Houston, Houston, TX, USA

Pavan Mallur Department of Otolaryngology, Harvard Medical School, Boston, MA, USA

Jeffrey Mella University of Virginia, Department of Otolaryngology, Head and Neck Surgery, Charlottesville, VA, USA

Nicole Molin Department of Otolaryngology Head and Neck Surgery, Lewis Katz School of Medicine at Temple University, Philadelphia, PA, USA

Arbaz A. Momin Cleveland Clinic Lerner College of Medicine of Case Western Reserve University, Education Institute, Cleveland Clinic, Cleveland, OH, USA

Anisha Rhea Noble Department of Otolaryngology–Head and Neck Surgery, University of Washington School of Medicine, Seattle, WA, USA

Julia E. Noel Department of Otolaryngology Head & Neck Surgery, Stanford University School of Medicine, Stanford, CA, USA

Tomislav Novosel Thyroid and Parathyroid Center, Klinikum Bad Salzungen GmbH, Bad Salzungen, Germany

Lisa A. Orloff Department of Otolaryngology Head & Neck Surgery, Stanford University School of Medicine, Stanford, CA, USA

Nitin A. Pagedar Department of Otolaryngology – Head and Neck Surgery, University of Iowa, Iowa City, IA, USA

Phillip K. Pellitteri Department of Otolaryngology/HNS, Geisinger Commonwealth School of Medicine, Geisinger Wyoming Valley Medical Center, Wilkes Barre, PA, USA

Nicholas C. Purdy Geisinger Commonwealth School of Medicine, Danville, PA, USA

Gregory W. Randolph Thyroid and Parathyroid Endocrine Surgery Division, Department of Otolaryngology, Massachusetts Eye and Ear Infirmary, Boston, MA, USA

Division of Surgical Oncology, Endocrine Surgery Service, Department of Surgery, Massachusetts General Hospital, Boston, MA, USA

Otolaryngology-Head and Neck Surgery, Claire and John Bertucci Endowed Chair in Thyroid Surgical Oncology, Harvard Medical School, Boston, MA, USA

Leonardo Rangel State University of Rio de Janeiro, Rio de Janeiro, Brazil

Jonathon O. Russell Department of Otolaryngology, Head and Neck Surgery, Johns Hopkins University, Baltimore, MD, USA

Joseph Scharpf Head and Neck Institute, Cleveland Clinic, Cleveland, OH, USA

Rick Schneider Department of Visceral, Vascular and Endocrine Surgery, Martin Luther University Halle-Wittenberg, Halle (Saale), Germany

Nicholas R. Scott-Wittenborn Department of Otolaryngology, Head and Neck Surgery, Johns Hopkins University, Baltimore, MD, USA

Areej Shihabi Department of Surgery, Tulane University School of Medicine, New Orleans, LA, USA

Jennifer J. Shin Department of Otolaryngology-Head and Neck Surgery, Department of Surgery, Brigham and Women's Hospital, Harvard Medical School, Boston, MA, USA

David C. Shonka Jr University of Virginia, Department of Otolaryngology, Head and Neck Surgery, Charlottesville, VA, USA

Catherine F. Sinclair Department of Otolaryngology-Head and Neck Surgery, Icahn School of Medicine at Mount Sinai, New York, NY, USA

Division of Head and Neck Surgery, Mt. Sinai West Hospital, New York, NY, USA

Michael C. Singer Department of Otolaryngology–Head and Neck Surgery, Henry Ford Hospital, Detroit, MI, USA

Brendan C. Stack Department of Otolaryngology-Head and Neck Surgery, Southern Illinois University School of Medicine, Springfield, IL, USA

Michael P. Steinmetz Center for Spine Health, Department of Neurosurgery, Neurological Institute, Cleveland Clinic Foundation, Cleveland, OH, USA

David L. Steward Department of Otolaryngology-Head and Neck Surgery, University of Cincinnati, College of Medicine, Cincinnati, OH, USA

Maria V. Suurna Department of Otolaryngology-Head and Neck Surgery, Weill Cornell Medicine, New York, NY, USA

David J. Terris Department of Otolaryngology – Head and Neck Surgery, Augusta University, Augusta, GA, USA

Ralph Tufano Department of Otolaryngology, Head and Neck Surgery, Johns Hopkins University, Baltimore, MD, USA

Erivelto M. Volpi CETRUS Medical Education Center, Sao Paulo, Sao Paulo, Brazil

Richard J. Wong Department of Surgery, Memorial Sloan-Kettering Cancer Center, New York, NY, USA

Che-Wei Wu Department of Otorhinolaryngology-Head and Neck Surgery, Kaohsiung Municipal Siaogang Hospital, Faculty of Medicine, College of Medicine, Kaohsiung Medical University, Kaohsiung, Taiwan

Mark Zafereo Department of Head and Neck Surgery, University of Texas MD Anderson Cancer Center, Houston, TX, USA

Part I

Nerve Monitoring Principles

Joe Scharpf

Historical Perspective on Nerve Monitoring During Head and Neck Surgery

1

Jeffrey Mella and David C. Shonka Jr.

The Cranial Nerves

The use of intraoperative neuromonitoring in head and neck surgery evolved from the pursuit of identification and safe preservation of the cranial nerves. Thus, the history of intraoperative neuromonitoring in head and neck surgery begins in antiquity with the discovery of the cranial nerves.

The cranial nerves were a source of great intrigue to the earliest anatomists and physiologists. Herophilus (335–280 BC) and Erasistratus (204–250 BC), members of the Alexandrian school, provided the first reference to cranial nerves, identifying seven pairs of nerves originating in the brain [1]. However, details of their work were lost, likely in the burning of the Alexandrian library [2]. Most of our knowledge of these Alexandrian anatomists are derived piecemeal from references made to their work by successors such as Galen and Caelius Aurelianus (fifth century) [2].

Claudius Galenus, better known as Galen (129–200 AD), brought anatomy and physiology into the service of medicine. Human dissections were forbidden during his time, so he gained his vast knowledge of anatomy through animal dissection and vivisection of fish, birds, pigs, mice, goats, sheep, apes, horses, mules, lynxes, bears, weasels, and elephants [2]. Following the example of Erasistratus, Galen based most of his anatomical experiments on the principle of ablation, ligating, or severing structures to identify their function. This provided an effective means for studying the cranial nerves. Indeed, one of Galen's proudest moments came shortly after his discovery of aphonia in a squealing pig after cutting a pair of nerves in the neck. He gathered the foremost philosophers in Rome to demonstrate his discovery. He further went on to describe the two nerves that descended from the brain on each side of the neck toward the heart before reversing course and ascending toward the larynx. He named the nerves, the recurrent nerves, or reversivi [3]. Through similar ablative experiments, Galen identified and described seven cranial nerves that he ordered anterior to posterior [4]. His description of the cranial nerves remained valid for more than 1200 years until the Italian Renaissance when human cadaver dissections revealed errors in Galen's animal analogies [4] (Fig. 1.1).

Andreas Vesalius, named by many as the father of modern anatomy (1514–1464), and Bartolomeo Eustachius (1564) corrected some of these errors but maintained the classification of seven pairs of nerves [5, 6]. Notable anatomists like Fallopius and Thomas Willis formulated new classifications of eight and nine cranial nerves,

J. Mella · D. C. Shonka Jr. (✉)
University of Virginia, Department of Otolaryngology, Head and Neck Surgery, Charlottesville, VA, USA
e-mail: jm3jq@hscmail.mcc.virginia.edu; DCS5Z@hscmail.mcc.virginia.edu

© The Author(s), under exclusive license to Springer Nature Switzerland AG 2022

J. Scharpf, G. W. Randolph (eds.), *Intraoperative Cranial Nerve Monitoring in Otolaryngology-Head and Neck Surgery*, https://doi.org/10.1007/978-3-030-84916-0_1

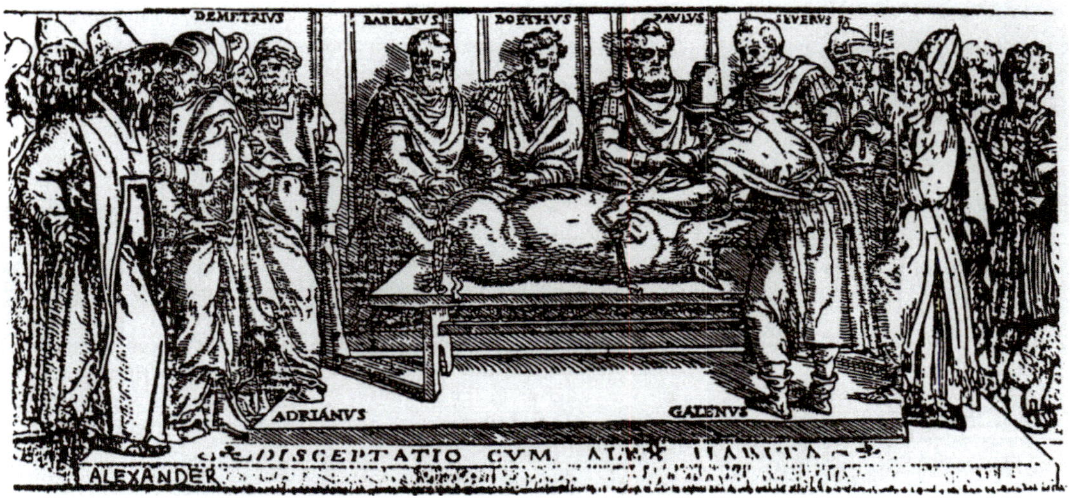

Fig. 1.1 Galen demonstrating aphonia after dividing the recurrent laryngeal nerve of a squealing pig. (From Galeni Librorum Quarte Classis. Venetijs Apud Iuntas, 1586. https://urldefense.proofpoint.com/v2/url?u=https-3A__commons.wikimedia.org_wiki_File-3AGalen-2DPig-2DVivisection.jpg&d=DwIFAw&c=vh6FgFndue jNhPPD0fl_yRaSfZy8CWbWnIf4XJhSqx8&r=JduzatgI bQjzhEN2FZse0xwASdG1pgE8zp5vGgbMjQg&m=Ov IgSWfJb5cytrkXwEhmvbv6r88-12PzxxKURD_dFWo&s=POHBYVq_yIODXVq8gW7PDLwUnclSSHWb-Gq-cyM8dQc&e=)

respectively [1]. It wasn't until 1778 that Sommerring described the modern classification of 12 pairs of cranial nerves in his doctoral dissertation which remains valid today [1, 7]. With accurate understanding of the form and function of the cranial nerves, surgeons were armed with the knowledge of their location and the importance of preserving them.

The Birth of Electrophysiology

Arguably the most notable figure in the history of electrophysiology is Luigi Galvani. Around the same time that Sommerring established our knowledge of the 12 pairs of cranial nerves, Galvani sent shockwaves through the scientific and medical communities with his discovery of bioelectricity. Galvani was born in 1737 to Domenico and Barbara Foschi. As the son of a goldsmith, with no strong scholarly tradition in their family, Galvani enrolled at the University of Bologna where he attended a 4-year course in medicine [8]. It was there that he was introduced to the Academy of Sciences, an institution designed to introduce modern disciplines into the training of scientists and physicians as a complement to their university studies. Galvani learned the disciplines of physics and chemistry and was introduced to the inventions of the electrostatic machine and Leyden jar that would later be used in his famous experiments [8]. Despite his primary focus on his training in medicine and surgery, Galvani maintained a particular interest in electricity. After graduating in medicine and philosophy in 1759, he took up appointments as a lecturer at both the University of Bologna and the Institute of Sciences where he began his illustrious academic career. By 1770, Galvani was elected to the President of Academy of Sciences, an appointment that brought prestige and attention to his work [8].

To understand Galvani's interests, it is helpful to briefly examine the scientific environment that characterized his early career. The source of muscular contraction or animation of life was a heavily debated topic during the late eighteenth century, particularly in Bologna. A century earlier, Thomas Willis published his classical work Cerebri Anatome (1664) in which he proposed the theory of Animal Spirit [9, 10]. He postulated that nerves were conduits between the brain and the periphery along which Animal Spirit flowed. This was largely accepted until Albrecht von Haller published his theory of irritability and sensibility in which he denied the role of nerves in muscular contraction, stating that muscles contract in response to a variety of mechanical stimuli [11]. The Hallerian theory gained great interest throughout Europe. However, a notable anatomist Tommaso Laghi (1709–1764) was critical of Haller's ideas [12]. He postulated that nerves were integral to animation through an electrical fluid that flowed through the nervous system [13]. His ideas could be characterized as a primitive form of neuroelectric theory of muscular contraction.

Concurrent to Laghi's work, Giuseppe Gardini and Pierre Bertholon publicized their observations on the effects of electricity on living beings, namely, commotion of limbs and increase in perspiration [8, 14]. Inspired by their work, Galvani focused his research efforts on the medical application of electricity. From 1780 to 1782, Galvani performed a series of experiments, which led to his famous discovery that muscles contract in response to electrical stimuli via the nervous system [8, 15]. In the first experiment, Galvani dissected a frog, removing the thighs entirely and leaving the legs attached to the spinal column by the sciatic nerves alone. He discovered that when the frog was placed on a static electrical machine, the frogs' legs contracted in response to the touch of the sciatic nerve with a metal scalpel [15, 16]. Through repeated experiments, he proved that contraction occurred in response to direct stimuli or sparks jumping over a distance and to stimuli applied through a large variety of electrical conductors. He hypothesized that nerves were like Leyden jars with a variable charge between the inner core and insulating outer membrane [17]. He then set out to test a theory that contraction would occur in response to atmospheric electricity. He described an experiment in which he hung a frog attached by a brass hook connected to a long wire circuit designed to capture atmospheric electricity during a thunderstorm. He noted that contraction occurred not only in response to the storm but every time the circuit was completed by an iron plate. He repeated the experiment indoors and again noted contraction whenever a copper hook connected to the spinal column was brought into contact with an iron plate [16, 17]. The observation was repeated with circuit between a variety of conductive metals. This led to his proposal that there was an inherent electricity within the animal itself [17, 18]. He coined the term animal electricity in a published summary of his work and laid out the theory of neuroelectric muscle contraction in 1791 in his most cited publication "De Viribus Electricitatis in motu musculari commentarius" ("Commentary on the Effect of Electricity on Muscular Motion") [15]. The discovery of electricity's role in muscular animation laid a scientific foundation on which neuromonitoring was built (Figs. 1.2, 1.3, and 1.4).

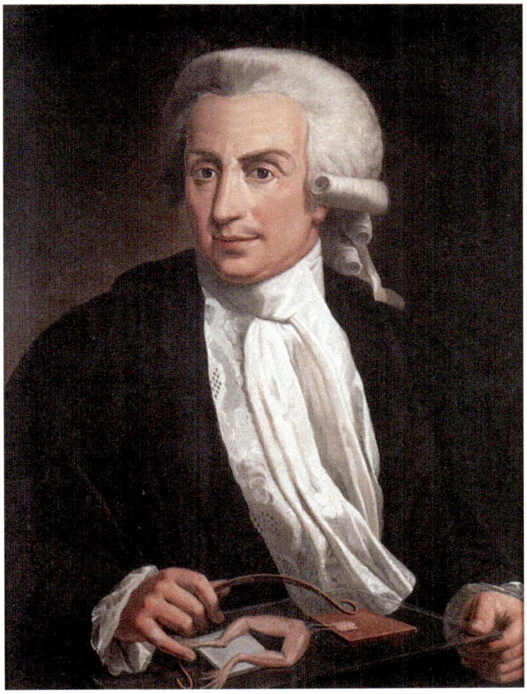

Fig. 1.2 Portrait of Luigi Galvani holding his frog galvanoscope, the instrument he used to discover "animal electricity." (Portrait displayed at the Museum of Palazzo Poggi. https://urldefense.proofpoint.com/v2/url?u=https-3A__commons.wikimedia.org_wiki_File-3ALuigi-5FGalvani-2C-5Foil-2Dpainting.jpg&d=DwIFAw&c=vh6FgFnduejNhPPD0fl_yRaSfZy8CWbWnIf4XJhSqx8&r=JduzatgIbQjzhEN2FZse0xwASdG1pgE8zp5vGgbMjQg&m=OvIgSWfJb5cytrkXwEhmvbv6r88-12PzxxKURD_dFWo&s=LDJXrdIQHMq7cuTmYDY8psJ3DogH87EABwUxOG_mts0&e=)

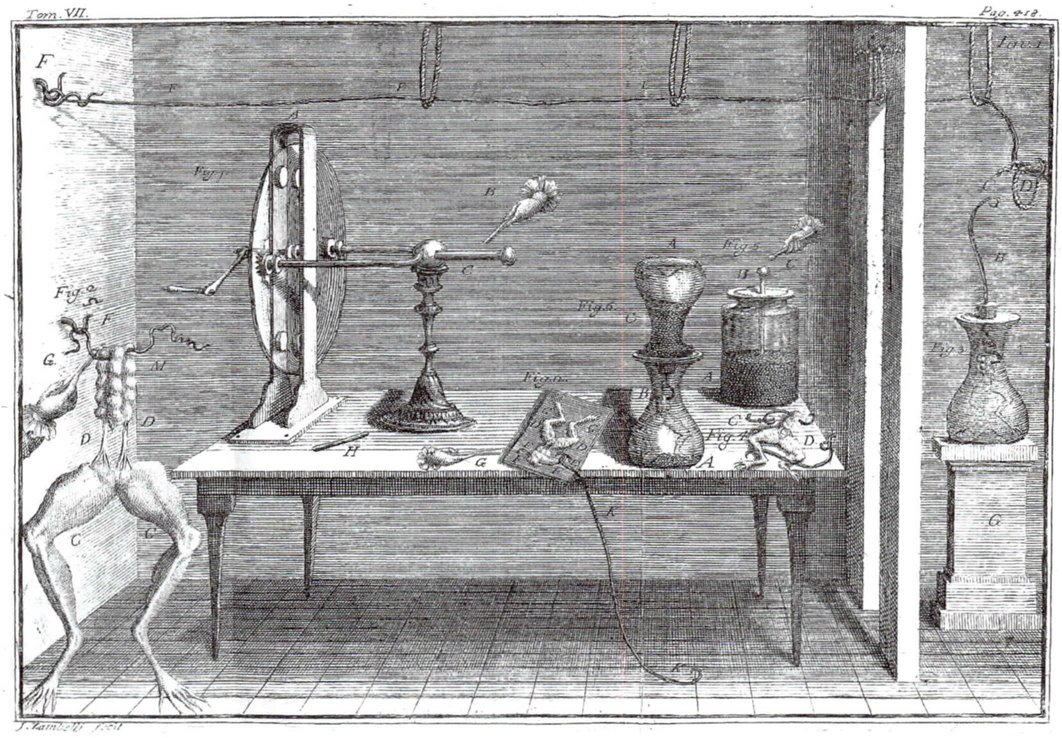

Fig. 1.3 Illustration of Galvani's dissections and experiments with frog legs. (From De Vibrus Electricitatis in Motu Musculari, Commenatrius, 1791. https://urldefense.proofpoint.com/v2/url?u=https-3A__commons.wikimedia.org_wiki_File-3ALuigi-5FGalvani-5FExperiment.jpeg&d=DwIFAw&c=vh6FgFnduejNhPPD0fl_yRaSfZy8CWbWnlf4XJhSqx8&r=JduzatgIbQjzhEN2FZse0xwASdG1pgE8zp5vGgbMjQg&m=OvIgSWfJb5cytrkXwEhmvbv6r88-12PzxxKURD_dFWo&s=6P67Gd-tQXa0vmpSRBMBde909fzBspAkbRcf8aO4tLA&e=)

The Discovery of the Nerve Action Potential: A Triumph of Technology

Over the next half century, physicists and physiologists worked to build on Galvani's discovery of animal electricity. Prior to 1820, for an electric phenomenon to be appreciated, the voltage or current had to be large enough to produce a spark or other physical effects [19]. In order to study the minute currents that run through muscles and nerves, more sensitive instruments were needed. Hans Christian Ørsted, a Danish physicist, made possible the invention of such an instrument with his discovery of electromagnetism – specifically that of a compass needle deflecting when brought into proximity with an electrical current running through a coiled wire [19, 20]. Johann Schweigger and Andre-Marie Ampere used Ørsted's discovery to develop an instrument for measuring current. They wrapped a coiled wire around a suspended magnetic needle that was free to rotate and noted that they could detect the current in the wire by measuring the movement of the needle. Schweigger reported their work at the University of Halle in 1820 and named the invention the galvanometer, after the already famed Luigi Galvani [21]. The original galvanometer relied on the Earth's magnetic pole which limited the ability to detect small currents. Leopoldo Nobili unlocked the ability to measure feeble currents by inventing the astatic galvanometer using a figure of eight coil wrapped around two needles with opposing orientation. He presented his instrument to the Academy of Sciences in 1825 [22]. Nobili's astatic galvanoscope proved to be instrumental in the earliest detection of muscular current.

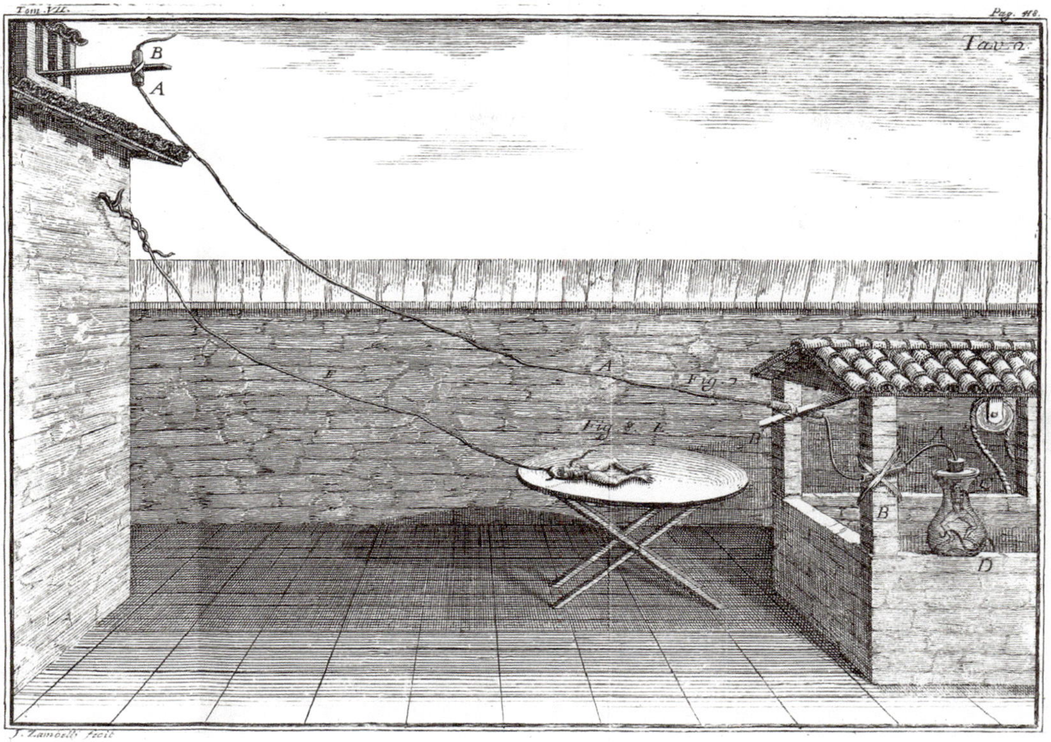

Fig. 1.4 Illustration of Galvani's experimental design to test frog leg contraction in response to atmospheric electricity. (From De Vibrus Electricitatis in Motu Musculari, Commenatrius, 1791. https://urldefense.proofpoint.com/v2/url?u=https-3A__commons.wikimedia.org_wiki_File-3AGalvani-5Ffrog-5Flegs-5Fexperiment-5Fsetup.png&d=DwIFAw&c=vh6FgFnduejNhPPD0fl_yRaSfZy8CWbWnIf4XJhSqx8&r=JduzatgIbQjzhEN2FZse0xwASdG1pgE8zp5vGgbMjQg&m=OvIgSWfJb5cytrkXwEhmvbv6r88-12PzxxKURD_dFWo&s=sUMwS_VaZUzjoT-VldBACDy9RSuYtGyKKyTWSJ9Mvd8&e=)

Carlo Matteucci, born in 1811, studied mathematics at the University of Bologna and dedicated his work to the study of bioelectricity. Inspired by the works of Galvani, Matteucci developed an instrument for detecting extremely small voltages using a dissected frog leg attached to its nerve. He referred to it as the rheoscopic frog, or frog galvanoscope [38]. Using both the frog galvanosope and Nobili's astatic galvanometer, he detected a current on the injured surface of a muscle and proved that muscle tissue had inherent electrical current. He also discovered that muscle current decreased during tetany, which led to his postulating the existence of a resting membrane potential of a muscle [23]. His published work directly inspired the discovery of the nerve action potential [19].

Emil du Bois-Reymond was a student of renowned Berlin physiologist, Johannes Mueller. In 1841, Mueller asked du Bois-Reymond to repeat the experiments of Matteucci. As an excellent experimentalist and with superior instruments, du Bois-Reymond built on Matteucci's work. He hypothesized and later proved that nerve and muscle tissues were similar to a Leyden jar, with opposing polarities across the surface membrane [19, 21]. He also demonstrate that nerve current, like muscle current, also decreases during repeated stimulation. He named this decrease, "negative variation." He and his student Julius Bernstein then went on to measure conduction velocities of both the excitatory and negative variation phases of a nerve conduction with a machine called a differential rheotome. The machine, devised by du Bois-Reymond but completed by Bernstein, connected the galvanometer to recording electrodes for less than a millisecond. By shortening the interval between stimulus and measurement, Bernstein could detect the various phases of the action potential. He used this method to prove his theory that an action potential had both a positive excitatory phase and negative refractory phase and their respective conduction velocities were equivalent [19, 21].

Electroencephalography (EEG), Peripheral Nerve Stimulation, Electromyography (EMG), and the Birth of Neuromonitoring

A landmark discovery in the history of neuromonitoring came in 1875 when a British physician named Richard Caton reported to the British Medical Association that he had successfully used a galvanometer to measure the electrical impulses on the surface of live rabbits and monkeys [24, 25]. Caton also went on to show that the electrical activity within the brain changes in response to sleep, anesthesia, and light shining in the eyes and ceases with the death of the animal. It wasn't until 50 years later when in 1929 a German psychiatrist named Hans Berger successfully reported recording the electrical activity of the human brain and named his method of detection the electroencephalograph (EEG) [25]. Early in Berger's life, his sister sent him a telegram after sensing he was in danger. This experience convinced him of the reality of telepathy, and he directed his early career to proving the existence of a psychic energy. This fueled his study of both psychiatry and neurology. In 1897, he obtained a medical degree from the Friedrich Schiller University of Jena where he was hired as an assistant professor in the psychiatry department to which he later served as chairman. He used his children Klaus and Ilse as his subjects for much of his early work surrounding EEG. Berger developed multiple methods for placing electrodes including directly onto the skull under the periosteum and noninvasive measures over the skin of the scalp. Using his newly invented EEG, Berger identified and characterized both alpha and beta brain waves and was later nominated for a Nobel Prize for his work.

Concurrent to Berger's discovery of electroencephalography (EEG), and perhaps more notable to our discussion, was the rise of peripheral nerve stimulators. Guillaume-Benjamin Duchenne is among the most influential neurologists in history and an integral figure in the history of neuromonitoring. As a French physician in 1835, Duchenne revived Galvani's work on the electric stimulation of muscles. He experimented with a technique called electropuncture in which muscles were stimulated by an electric pulse administered subcutaneously with sharp electrodes. He also developed a noninvasive technique for transcutaneous administration of electrical stimulation. He went on to describe multiple diagnostic and therapeutic applications of electrically stimulated muscle contraction and published his work in 1855 [27]. His techniques allowed him to characterize multiple neurologic disorders that now bear his name including Duchenne muscular dystrophy. Duchenne was fascinated with the mechanisms of facial animation. In one of most notable works, *e la physionomie Humaine* (*The Mechanism of Human Facial Expression*) [28], he describes the use of faraday shocks delivered with an electric probe to isolate the muscles of facial expression. His work included original photographs of Duchenne inducing the array of facial expressions and emotion on his subjects in this manner [28]. In 1861, Wilhelm Erb, a contemporary of Duchenne's whose name he shares the eponymous disease of Erb-Duchenne palsy, used a similar technique to discover the notable surgical landmark in head and neck surgery, Erb's point [29]. Duchenne and Erb's primitive work with electrical stimulation of muscles bears notable resemblance to modern techniques of nerve stimulation during head and neck surgery (Fig. 1.5).

Peripheral nerve stimulation gained wide acceptance as a modulator for pain, and Julius Althaus reported the routine use of electrical stimulation to relieve pain after extremity surgery [30]. In 1919, Charles Kent patented an electric-massage machine which has been described as

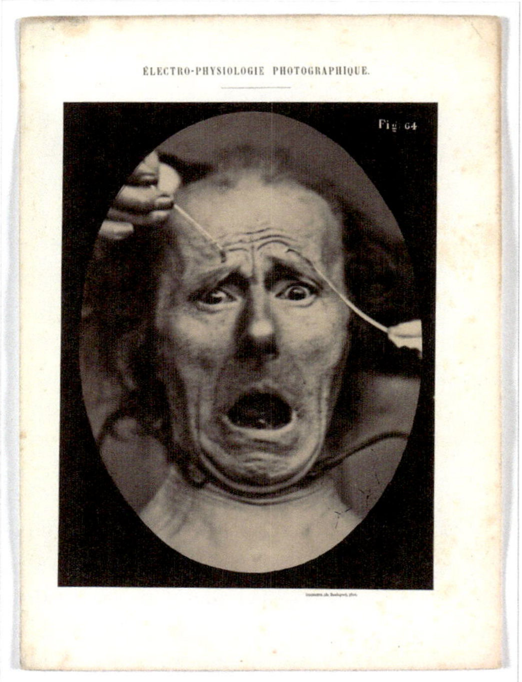

Fig. 1.5 Duchenne and an assistant produce facial expression through faraday shocks with a peripheral nerve stimulator. (Electro–Physiologie, 1862. https://urldefense.proofpoint.com/v2/url?u=https-3A__www.metmuseum.org_art_collection_search_302241&d=DwIFAw&c=vh6FgFnduejNhPPD0fl_yRaSfZy8CWbWnIf4XJhSqx8&r=JduzatgIbQjzhEN2FZse0xwASdG1pgE8zp5vGgbMjQg&m=OvIgSWfJb5cytrkXwEhmvbv6r88-12PzxxKURD_dFWo&s=xfgwHQoGG2jAJ1XMdHiMnkd3YS7OaUoJprGCb11v1Vw&e=)

the first transcutaneous electrical nerve stimulation (TENS) unit ever sold commercially [30]. With EEG, and peripheral nerve stimulation now commonplace, EMG was the final needed breakthrough to make intraoperative neuromonitoring a possibility.

Edgar Douglas Adrian and Detlev Bronk used the recently invented capillary electrometer and a cathode-ray tube to perform an experiment measuring the action potential generated by a single nerve fiber [26, 31]. Adrian describes using needle electrodes connected directly to a single nerve fiber and recording electrical activity via an amplified loud speaker [31]. They successfully measured the electrical activity of the muscle fibers innervated by a single motor neuron fiber.

Joseph Erlanger influenced early development of EMG with his studies on nerve conduction. As a graduate from the Johns Hopkins School of Medicine in 1899, Erlanger took a position as chair of physiology at the University of Madison Wisconsin. There, he and his student Herbert Gasser developed a modified western electric oscilloscope to graph the action potential of a frog's sciatic nerve [32]. They went on to discover that the conduction velocity of nerves varied by their diameter and were awarded the Nobel Prize in medicine in 1944 for their discoveries.

Edward Lambert, considered by many to be the father of EMG, was born in Minneapolis in 1915. After completing his doctorate in medicine at the University of Illinois, he joined the Mayo Clinic in 1943 where he began his clinical studies on electrophysiology. While the technology behind EMG existed prior to his time, Lambert first envisioned and realized EMG's clinical utility in medicine. He set up the first clinical EMG laboratory where he went on to discover the neuromuscular disorder that now bears his name, Lambert-Eaton myasthenic syndrome [26, 33].

From 1940 to 1970, EMG was commonly used as an experimental diagnostic tool. It wasn't until the additional discovery of "evoked potentials" that its role in surgery became evident. In 1951, George Dawson discovered that consistent patterned responses to stimulation of the brain, spinal cord, or peripheral nerves could be recorded independent of the background electrical activity of muscle or nervous tissue. He used an oscilloscope superimposed on photographic film. With repeated stimulation, the electrical response produced an overexposure on one area of the film, whereas the background electrical activity diffusely exposed the whole film. He used this method to record low-amplitude potentials and discovered a consistent response to auditory, tactile, and visual stimuli [34].

In 1944, Weddel first introduced EMG to the world of otolaryngology when he described EMG characteristics of both facial and intrinsic laryngeal muscle in normal and paralyzed states [35]. In 1956, Faaborg-Andersen published an article in *Nature* in 1956 describing his use of EMG on internal laryngeal musculature during phonation. He set out to prove the hypothesized myoelastic theory of phonation by the study of electrical impulses delivered to the larynx by the recurrent laryngeal nerve. He successfully disproved the belief that the vocal cords vibrated at the same rate as the frequency of electrical impulses delivered from the recurrent laryngeal nerve [36].

In 1963, Sir Terence Cawthorne, a British trained neurotologist described the use of bipolar electric stimulation to assess facial nerve function before and after acoustic neuroma surgery. His methods of detecting a response to stimulation included both visual inspection of muscle contraction by his surgical assistants and EMG. He successfully demonstrated a relationship between ability of the facial nerve to conduct a delivered electrical impulse to prognosis and degree of recovery from paralysis [37].

The Rise of Intraoperative Neuromonitoring

With the discoveries of EEG, nerve stimulation, EMG, and evoked potentials, intraoperative neuromonitoring was now technologically possible. In 1937, the worlds of surgery and electrophysiology collided. Wilder Penfield, a Canadian neurosurgeon, was the first to describe the use of intraoperative monopolar electrical stimulation of the cerebral cortex as a test of cortical function during surgery for epilepsy [38, 39]. In so doing, he mapped the patient's cortex and coined the term electrocorticography. This is considered by many as the first description of intraoperative neuromonitoring in history. Since Penfield, neurophysiologic monitoring has branched, evolved, and adapted to include an amazing breadth of neurophysiologic technological modalities including EEG, EMG, and motor and sensory evoked potentials utilized by a variety of fields including neurosurgery, orthopedic surgery, cardiac surgery, interventional radiology, and plastic and reconstructive surgery. We will narrow our focus to include only the historical perspective of intraoperative neuromonitoring within head and neck surgery.

Intraoperative Facial Nerve Monitoring

With EMG and nerve stimulation gaining traction in the clinic setting, the stage was set for the introduction of intraoperative facial nerve monitoring. It should be noted that in 1898, Krauze first noted the use of electrical stimulation of the facial nerve during acoustic neuroma surgery [40]. However, the use of nerve monitoring in head and neck surgery did not gain traction until the 1960s. Parsons first recognized the utility of electrical stimulation in identifying the peripheral facial nerve from surrounding fascia during parotidectomy. He built his own portable transistorized stimulator powered by ordinary flashlight cells. He described increasing or decreasing the voltage of electrical stimulation to assess the integrity of the nerve. He found an association between the ability of the main trunk of the facial nerve to stimulate appropriately at a low setting with full facial nerve function immediately postoperatively [41]. Likewise, Hilger created "the Hilger nerve stimulator" which he described in 1963. He reported use of the Hilger nerve stimulator both in the clinical and surgical settings. He recommended using a lower setting (0–5 milliamperes) when stimulating a surgically exposed facial nerve [41] (Fig. 1.6).

Although both Parsons and Hilger could reliably activate the facial nerve with their electric stimulators, they relied on surgical assistants or their own visual inspection of muscle twitch to

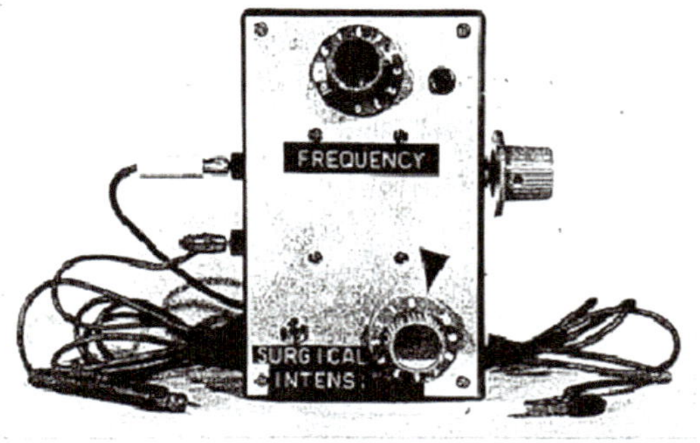

Fig. 1.6 Parsons' home-built nerve stimulator. (From Electrical Nerve Stimulation at Surgery, 1968)

detect a response. Jako improved the reliability of detection of facial muscle activation by incorporating a photoelectric device applied to the cheek [42]. Jako's device detected facial muscle contraction and alerted the surgeon with an audible alarm. By substituting the human aspect of detecting facial muscle activation with an objective measure that created an alarm to the surgeon, Jako's technique provided a large step forward in the sensitivity and progression of neuromonitoring. Several variations of this technique were refined and improved [43, 44]. Sugita and Kobayashi described a method using disc accelerometers as motion detectors applied to the face that converted facial motion into a quantifiable electric signal. Notably, they reported lower rates of facial nerve injury with this method. While these methods improved sensitivity of response when compared with human observation, they lacked specificity for facial nerve activity and could be activated by movements of the surgeon or other muscle groups like those of mastication [43].

Delgado added improved sensitivity and specificity of neurophysiologic facial nerve monitoring by introducing intraoperative EMG. He used a nerve stimulator to activate the intracranial facial nerve and used surface EMG electrodes on the face to assess response to facial nerve stimulation. He published a study of 14 patients with acoustic tumors. Each patient underwent extensive preoperative EMG. The leads with greatest sensitivity to proximal nerve stimulation were then chosen for intraoperative use. Adding the ability to deliver a variable stimulus and record varying strengths of response greatly improved the sensitivity and clinical utility of intraoperative neuromonitoring of the facial nerve [45]. Delgado's method notably lacked an audible alarm and relied on a technician to read the EMG and alert the surgeon of facial nerve activation.

Moller ushered in the modern era of facial nerve monitoring when in 1984, he published his technique for nerve monitoring that closely resembles the nerve monitoring setup still in use today. He refined Delgado's technique with use of intramuscular EMG electrodes placed into the orbicularis oculi and orbicularis oris. The potentials were displayed on an oscilloscope and made audible through a loudspeaker alerting the surgeon of mechanical activation by dissection or intentional stimulation when identifying the nerve. In this way, he argued that the facial nerve was under continuous neuromonitoring [46]. The nerve stimulator he used was a low-impedance, constant-voltage, monopolar stimulator as opposed to the commonly used bipolar constant-current stimulator. He argued that using this method allowed for more consistent stimulation of the facial nerve and required fewer intraoperative adjustments of stimulation voltage. He noted the presence of CSF that could cause a variable degree of shunting of current and require fewer adjustments of stimulation voltage intraoperative. He also described using nerve monitoring not only for identifying the nerve but for assessing areas of acoustic tumors involved with the nerve to guide resection [46, 47].

Daube used a similar system with intramuscular electrodes placed and checked prior to induction of anesthesia. Unlike Moller, he advocated for a bipolar nerve stimulator arguing that it provided less spread of current and increased accuracy. He showed that in a large series of patients undergoing acoustic neuroma operations, facial nerve function was preserved in 92% of those nerves that were monitored compared to 84% of the unmonitored cohort. Additionally, cochlear nerve preservation improved from 37% in the unmonitored group to 47% in the monitoring group. He noted that nerve monitoring provided better results with increasing size of tumors [48]. Likewise, Harner reported better preservation of facial nerve in patients undergoing large (>4 cm) acoustic neuroma excision via sub-occipital approach with 67% preservation of monitored nerves versus 33% in the unmonitored cohort [49].

Prass and Luders made a lasting contribution to nerve stimulator design when they described the advantage of a flush-tip monopolar stimulus probe. They noted accurate stimulation of the nerve with both constant current and constant voltage settings negating the shunting effect of CSF or other surrounding fluid. Prass went on to file a patent for the design in 1990. His design remains the most popular nerve stimulator in head and neck surgery (Prass Standard Flush-Tip Probe, Medtronic, Xomed, Jacksonville, FL). Prass and Luders went on to publish findings of specific EMG patterns related to various surgical manipulations of the nerve to better interpret EMG-based neuromonitoring alarms [44].

Below is an original photograph of a flush-tipped stimulus probe described by Prass. The flushed tip allowed consistent stimulation regardless of presence of CSF or other fluid that may otherwise shunt current away from the nerve in question.

In 1988, Xomed-Treace, a company based in Jacksonville, Florida, introduced the Nerve Integrity Monitoring System (NIM-2). Due to its user-friendly hardware, commercial availability, and reliability, the NIM-2 system became widely accepted and remains the most common system for nerve monitoring in head and neck surgery today.

Silverstein advocated for routine use of the facial nerve monitoring in all otologic procedures involving the facial nerve. He noted a relationship between the depth of bone covering the facial nerve within the bony canal and the threshold of current needed for stimulation [50]. In 1991 at the NIH Consensus Development Conference on Acoustic neuroma, it was strongly recommended that intraoperative monitoring of the facial nerve be included in surgical therapy for vestibular schwannoma [51].

Since the development of intraoperative neuromonitoring, controversy has ensued about its routine use in parotid and skull base surgery. In 1994, Roland criticized nerve monitoring for being too expensive and warned about substituting nerve monitoring for sound anatomic and surgical knowledge of the facial nerve.

Over the last 30 years, intraoperative facial nerve monitoring has been extensively studied and shown to improve nerve preservation in a wide variety of head and neck procedures including parotidectomy [52], acoustic neuroma surgery [46, 53], skull base surgery [54, 55], cochlear implantation [56], chronic ear surgery [57], and cholesteatoma [58]. Its popularity and routine use has followed suit and has continued to grow in response as more data prove its benefit. In 2018, Gidley published a cross-sectional study performed by the AAO-HNS intraoperative neuromonitoring task force which showed that a majority of surgeons use intraoperative neuromonitoring for almost all otologic procedures with tympanoplasty and stapedectomy being the exceptions. They also showed universal exposure to intraoperative neuromonitoring among otolaryngology resident training [59].

Intraoperative Recurrent Laryngeal Nerve Monitoring

The rapid evolution and adoption of intraoperative neuromonitoring of the recurrent laryngeal nerve paralleled that of facial nerve monitoring. The last 50 years has seen an explosion in methodologies and technologies for monitoring the recurrent laryngeal nerve.

Lahey ushered in a new era of thyroid surgery in 1938 when he advocated for the routine dissection of the RLN in every case. He published a method for locating the nerve by first identifying the inferior thyroid artery [60]. Riddell was among the first surgeons to adopt this philosophy and proved with a large study of 2507 nerves at risk that routine dissection and visualization of the recurrent laryngeal nerve was associated with a lower rate of injury than leaving the nerve unidentified. He argued that in total thyroidectomy procedures, the recurrent laryngeal nerve should be identified with electrical stimulation and direct glottis observation with laryngoscopy following the first lobe resection prior to advancing to the contralateral side. This glottis observation method was the earliest version of recurrent laryngeal nerve monitoring recorded [61]. In 1971, Kratz advocated for direct observation of the vocal cords through a self-retaining laryngoscope. He used a 3-volt "concept" nerve stimulator to activate the recurrent laryngeal nerve and noted gross laryngeal elevation as well as vocal fold abduction via direct laryngoscopy [62].

In 1966, Shedd demonstrated in a study of the canine larynx that stimulation of the recurrent laryngeal nerve could be reliably identified by monitoring the pressure within an endotracheal tube balloon positioned between the vocal cords [63]. Zinni and Gandolfi developed pressure-sensing balloons designed to monitor both the facial and recurrent laryngeal nerves. The balloons were placed under the upper lip or between the vocal cords when monitoring the facial or recurrent laryngeal nerves respectively [64]. Engel translated this idea to humans and designed a double-cuff endotracheal tube to be used in thyroid surgery so the trachea could be occluded, and at the same time pressure recordings were taken from the glottis [65]. However, Engel's design was limited by high cuff pressure requirements. Woltering refined this design with a high-volume, low-pressure double-cuff endotracheal tube. Cuff pressures were recorded using standard arterial pressure monitor. He argued that cuff pressure was a superior technique to EMG due to surgeon unfamiliarity with EMG.

Gavilan proposed a simplified method for laryngeal nerve monitoring with direct palpation of the posterior cricoarytenoid muscle during nerve stimulation. He argued that the expense and time-intensive nature of other forms of monitoring made them impractical for routine use [66]. James also advocated for ipsilateral laryngeal palpation during RLN stimulation [67]. The importance of this method is underscored by the fact that it is still in use today as a simple method for assessing the integrity of the neuromonitoring system [68].

In 1970, Flisberg and Lindholm et al. reported 15 successful cases of intraoperative RLN identification using EMG and evoked potentials with a concentric needle electrode inserted into the vocalis muscle through the cricothyroid membrane. Using DISA bipolar needle electrodes placed cranially and caudally along the ascending recurrent laryngeal nerve, they were able to calculate nerve conduction velocities for each nerve identified [69].

Davis and Rhea noted the disadvantage to placing electrodes within the surgical field and advocated for endoscopic placement of needle electrodes transorally. They described the difficulty in both placing single needle electrodes into the vocalis without inadvertently dislodging them upon removal of the laryngoscope. In 1979, they reported new method for EMG laryngeal nerve monitoring by endoscopically placing a two-needle electrode tack via direct laryngoscopy into the vocalis muscle prior to laryngectomy or thyroidectomy procedures. Interestingly, they commented that their first work included the use of gold foil secured around an endotracheal tube as a surface electrode but had abandoned this method after noted difficulty in maintaining position within the glottis [70].

Lipton also favored the use of endoscopically placed electrodes but instead used hooked electrodes inserted into the vocal cords. They described superior monitoring with this method to surface electrodes and published findings of background EMG activity with spontaneous respirations as well as neurotonic changes during nerve dissection or intentional stimulation [71].

In 1991, Rice and Cone-Wesson were the first to report using the Nerve Integrity Monitor (NIMS-2) in conjunction with a Prass monopolar nerve stimulator probe for recurrent laryngeal nerve monitoring. This system provided the capability of both auditory and visual feedback via background and evoked EMG [72]. While the technology they used has been refined over the last 29 years, this system remains the most commonly used method for recurrent laryngeal nerve monitoring today with one notable exception. Rice and Cone-Wesson's method for EMG also used endoscopically placed hook wires in the vocalis muscle.

Maloney also used the NIM-2 monitoring system with endoscopic placement of needle electrodes but used standard subdermal needles placed into the posterior cricoarytenoid muscles. While endoscopically placed EMG electrodes were drawing critiques for being time cumbersome, they noted the average placement for the electrodes to be 1 minute [73].

Goldstone and Schettino were inspired by Rea and Davis' earlier mention of a gold foil surface electrode wrapped around an endotracheal tube. In 1990, they designed an endotracheal tube with surface electrode wires attached to the endotracheal tube at the level of the vocal cords. They reported successful identification and monitoring of recurrent laryngeal nerves using the NIM-2 monitor in dogs [74].

Rea revisited the idea of a surface electrode in 1992 and designed a postcricoid laryngeal plate surface electrode. This electrode design was capable of functioning with three different nerve monitoring systems. Advantages of this system included the ease and noninvasive nature of placement. However, the postcricoid electrode plate was only available in one size and was reported to occasionally become dislodged intraoperatively undermining confidence in the system [75]. Nevertheless, the postcricoid paddle electrode gained some acceptance, and its use has been reported in modern nerve monitoring [76].

The invention of the NIM-2 EMG endotracheal tube proved to be a critical piece in the evolution of recurrent laryngeal nerve monitoring. Eisle reported in 1996 that he successfully monitored ten patients with the NIM-2 tube design after which he gained FDA approval for broader use. The design consisted of a pair of 0.16-inch diameter stainless-steel wire electrodes incorporated into the silicone tube that spanned 3 centimeters on both sides of the glottis. Ground wire and the Prass nerve stimulator probe were then connected to the NIM-2 nerve monitor and set to a setting of 100 μs at a rate of 4 bursts/second. Stimulating current was started to 0.1 mA and increased by 0.05 mA until an evoked potential was seen. Eisle's study included the average stimulation thresholds for this system and found them to be comparable to intramuscular EMG electrodes. He also warned about the potential for false negatives from malposition of the endotracheal tube and highlighted the need for objective data proving the benefit to nerve monitoring given the added time and cost of its routine use [76].

The system described by Eisle over 20 years ago remains the most common neuromonitoring system for recurrent laryngeal nerve monitoring today. The hardware, software, and design have undergone many refinements over the last two decades with the third generation device in use today, NIM-3 Response (Medtronic, Xomed, Jacksonville, FL)

Over the last 30 years, widespread use of recurrent laryngeal nerve monitoring yielded an impressive amount of data surrounding its benefit and use. Retrospective studies demonstrate that nerve monitoring in thyroid or parathyroid surgery aids in identification of the RLN [77, 78], particularly in reoperative cases [79]. However, its benefit relating to recurrent laryngeal nerve injury remains controversial even today. Barczyński is the only author to have published a prospective randomized controlled trial comparing neuromonitoring to direct visualization. This group performed a randomized trial of 1000 nerves at risk. The Neurosign® 100 system (Inomed, Teningen, Germany) was utilized in half of the patients, while the other half underwent visualization alone without neuromonitoring. Notably, this system involved an intramuscular electrode placed into the vocalis through the cricothyroid ligament. Barczyński found that that nerve monitoring decreased the rate of transient RLN paresis by 2.9%. No significant difference was identified in rates of permanent paralysis. Given the controversy surrounding the benefit of nerve monitoring in RLN injury, Higgins performed a large meta-analysis including 64,699 nerves at risk. He found no difference in rates of injury or transient or persistent paralysis [80]. Notably, Dralle calculated how many patients would need to be studied to show a statistical difference in rates of injury and concluded that 9 million patients per arm would be required to show a statistically significant benefit due to the low rate of recurrent laryngeal nerve injury. This astronomic number may explain why controversy persists despite years of available data [81].

Several consensus statements regarding the use of electrophysiologic monitoring of the recurrent laryngeal nerve have been published in recent years [82, 83]. In an international guideline, Randolph summarized the various iterations and forms of neuromonitoring that remain in use today arguing that the process of evolution and refinement is still very much active in the field. Our ability to interpret and react to neuromonitoring data has also grown substantially into new algorithms and methods for approaching situations like a "loss of signal" during surgery [83].

A Look into the Future

The recent introduction of continuous intraoperative recurrent laryngeal nerve monitoring has been described as a quantum leap forward in technology [84]. Lamadé first introduced the idea of an implantable cuff tripolar vagal electrode designed to provide automatic periodic vagal nerve stimulation [85]. Since introduction, continuous vagal nerve monitoring systems have been refined and are currently offered at many premier institutions across the world. With automatic periodic vagal nerve stimulation at short intervals and continuous EMG monitoring, the technology detects real-time changes in nerve signal integrity and alerts the surgeon to impending injury. More recently, an endotracheal tube-based method for achieving continuous vagal nerve monitoring has been proposed using the laryngeal adductor reflex. Without the need for a cuff electrode placed directly on the vagus nerve, an endotracheal tube-based method provides a measure of safety and simplicity to real-time vagus nerve monitoring [86]. These and other recent innovations will be discussed throughout the rest of the book.

Conclusion

From the birth of electrophysiology with Luigi Galvani to the remarkable technique of continuous vagal nerve monitoring available today, the story of neurophysiological monitoring in head and neck surgery is one of landmark scientific discoveries by famed physicians and scientists throughout the world. Intraoperative neuromonitoring in head and neck surgery continues to adapt to provide the surgeon and patient a path toward consistent identification, reliable protection, and ultimate preservation of the cranial nerves.

References

1. Porras-Gallo MI, Peña-Meliáan Á, Viejo F, Hernáandez T, Puelles E, Echevarria D, Ramón Sañudo J. Overview of the history of the cranial nerves: from Galen to the 21st century. Anat Rec. 2019;302(3):381–93.
2. Keele KD. Three early masters of experimental medicine-Erasistratus, Galen and Leonardo da Vinci. Proc R Soc Med. 1961;54:577–88.
3. Randolph GW. Surgery of the thyroid and parathyroid glands: expert consult premium edition-enhanced online features and print. Elsevier Health Sciences; 2012.
4. Smith ES. Galen's account of the cranial nerves and the autonomic nervous system. Clio medica (Amsterdam, Netherlands). 1971;6(2):77.
5. Siraisi NG. Vesalius and human diversity in De humani corporis fabrica. J Warburg Courtauld Inst. 1994;57:60–88.
6. Eustachi B. Opuscula anatomica. 1726.
7. Corrales CE, Mudry A, Jackler RK. Perpetuation of errors in illustrations of cranial nerve anatomy. J Neurosurg. 2016;127(1):192–8.
8. Bresadola M. Medicine and science in the life of Luigi Galvani (1737–1798). Brain Res Bull. 1998;46(5):367–80.
9. Willis T, Wren C. Cerebri anatome: cui accessit nervorum descriptio et usus. Typis Tho. Roycroft, Impensis Jo. Martyn & Ja. Allestry; 1978.
10. O'Connor JP. Thomas Willis and the background to Cerebri Anatome. J R Soc Med. 2003;96(3):139–43.
11. Frixione E. Irritable glue: the Haller–Whytt controversy on the mechanism of muscle contraction. In: Brain, mind and medicine: essays in eighteenth-century neuroscience. Boston: Springer; 2007. p. 115–24.
12. Bernardi W. The controversy on animal electricity in eighteenth-century Italy: Galvani, Volta and others. Bevilacqua and Fregonese Eds. Nuova Voltiana. 2000;1:101–4.
13. Laghi T. De sensitivitate atque irritabilitate Halleriana. In: Fabri GB, editor. Sulla insensitività ed irritabilità Halleriana. Opuscoli di vari autori, vol. 2. Corciolani ed. Bologna: Eredi Colli; 1757. p. 326–45.
14. Smith CU. Brain and mind in the 'long' eighteenth century. In: Brain, mind and medicine: essays in eighteenth-century neuroscience. Boston: Springer; 2007. p. 15–28.
15. Galvani L. De viribus electricitatis in motu musculari. Commentarius. De Bonoiensi Scientiarum et Artium Intituo atque Academie Commentarii. 1791;7:363–418.
16. Hoff HE. Galvani and the pre-Galvanian electrophysiologists. Ann Sci. 1936;1(2):157–72.
17. Piccolino M. Luigi Galvani and animal electricity: two centuries after the foundation of electrophysiology. Trends Neurosci. 1997;20(10):443–8.
18. Kipnis N. Luigi Galvani and the debate on animal electricity, 1791–1800. Ann Sci. 1987;44(2):107–42.
19. Schuetze SM. The discovery of the action potential. Trends Neurosci. 1983;6:164–8.
20. Oersted HC. Experiments on the effect of a current of electricity on the magnetic needle. Ann Philos. 1820;16(4):273–6.

21. Keithley JF. The story of electrical and magnetic measurements: from 500 BC to the 1940s. Hoboken: Wiley; 1999.
22. Nobili L. "Sur un nouveau galvanomètre". Bibliothèque Universelle. Sci Arts. 1825;29:119–25.
23. Hoff HE, Geddes LA. The rheotome and its prehistory: a study in the historical interrelation of electrophysiology and electromechanics. Bull Hist Med. 1957;31(3):212–34.
24. Berger H. Über das elektrenkephalogramm des menschen. DMW-Deutsche Medizinische Wochenschrift. 1934;60(51):1947–9.
25. İnce R, Adanır SS, Sevmez F. The inventor of electroencephalography (EEG): Hans Berger (1873–1941). Childs Nerv Syst. 2020;5:1–2.
26. Kazamel M, Warren PP. History of electromyography and nerve conduction studies: a tribute to the founding fathers. J Clin Neurosci. 2017;43:54–60.
27. Duchenne GB. De l''électrisation localisée et de son application à la physiologie, à la pathologie et à la thérapeutique. Baillière; 1855.
28. Duchenne GB. Mécanisme de la physionomie humaine: où, Analyse électro-physiologique de l'expression des passions. J.-B. Baillière; 1876.
29. Erb WH. Handbuch der Elektrotherapie. FCW Vogel; 1886.
30. Althaus J. A treatise on medical electricity, theoretical and practical: and its uses in the treatment of paralysis, neuralgia and other diseases. Longmans, Green; 1873.
31. Adrian ED, Bronk DW. The discharge of impulses in motor nerve fibres: part I. Impulses in single fibres of the phrenic nerve. J Physiol. 1928;66(1):81.
32. Gasser HS, Erlanger J. A study of the action currents of nerve with the cathode ray oscillograph. Am J Physiol Legacy Content. 1922;62(3):496–524.
33. Eaton LM, Lambert EH. Electromyography and electric stimulation of nerves in diseases of motor unit: observations on myasthenic syndrome associated with malignant tumors. J Am Med Assoc. 1957;163(13):1117–24.
34. Dawson GD. A summation technique for the detection of small evoked potentials. Electroencephalogr Clin Neurophysiol. 1954;6:65–84.
35. Weddell G, Feinstein B, Pattle RE. The electrical activity of voluntary muscle in man under normal and pathological conditions. Brain J Neurol. 1944;67:178–257.
36. Faaborg-Andersen K, Buchthal F. Action potentials from internal laryngeal muscles during phonation. Nature. 1956;177(4503):340–1.
37. Cawthorne T, Wilson T. Indications for intratemporal facial nerve surgery. Arch Otolaryngol. 1963;78(4):43–8.
38. Jasper H. Electrocorticograms in man. Electroencephalogr Clin Neurophysiol. 1949;2(Suppl):16–29.
39. Penfield W, Boldrey E. Somatic motor and sensory representation in the cerebral cortex of man as studied by electrical stimulation. Brain. 1937;60(4):389–443.
40. Krause F. Surgery of the brain and spinal cord: based on personal experiences. New York: Rebman; 1912.
41. Parsons EC. Electrical stimulation of the facial nerve. Laryngoscope. 1966;76(3):391–406.
42. Jako GJ. Facial nerve monitor. Trans Am Acad Ophthalmol Otolaryngol. 1965;69:340–2.
43. Sugita K, Kobayashi S. Technical and instrumental improvements in the surgical treatment of acoustic neurinomas. J Neurosurg. 1982;57(6):747–52.
44. Prass RL, Lüders H. Acoustic (loudspeaker) facial electromyographic monitoring: part 1. Evoked electromyographic activity during acoustic neuroma resection. Neurosurgery. 1986;19(3):392.
45. Delgado TE, Buchheit WA, Rosenholtz HR, Chrissian S. Intraoperative monitoring of facial muscle evoked responses obtained by intracranial stimulation of the facial nerve: a more accurate technique for facial nerve dissection. Neurosurgery. 1979;4(5):418–21.
46. Møller AR, Jannetta PJ. Preservation of facial function during removal of acoustic neuromas: use of monopolar constant-voltage stimulation and EMG. J Neurosurg. 1984;61(4):757–60.
47. Møller MB, Møller AR. Loss of auditory function in microvascular decompression for hemifacial spasm: results in 143 consecutive cases. J Neurosurg. 1985;63(1):17–20.
48. Harner SG, Daube JR, Ebersold, MJ, Beatty CW Improved preservation of facial nerve function with use of electrical monitoring during removal of acoustic neuromas. In: Mayo Clinic proceedings, vol. 62, no. 2. Elsevier; 1987 Feb 1. p. 92–102.
49. Harner SG, Daube JR, Beatty CW, Ebersold MJ. Intraoperative monitoring of the facial nerve. Laryngoscope. 1988;98(2):209–12.
50. Silverstein H, Smouha E, Jones R. Routine identification of the facial nerve using electrical stimulation during otological and neurotological surgery. Laryngoscope. 1988;98(7):726–30.
51. Neuroma A. Consensus statement/NIH consensus development conference. Natl Inst Health Consens Dev Conf. 1991;9:1–24.
52. Sood AJ, Houlton JJ, Nguyen SA, Gillespie MB. Facial nerve monitoring during parotidectomy: a systematic review and meta-analysis. Otolaryngol Head Neck Surg. 2015;152(4):631–7.
53. Sampath P, Holliday MJ, Brem H, Niparko JK, Long DM. Facial nerve injury in acoustic neuroma (vestibular schwannoma) surgery: etiology and prevention. J Neurosurg. 1997;87(1):60–6.
54. Dickins JR, Graham SS. A comparison of facial nerve monitoring systems in cerebellopontine angle surgery. Am J Otol. 1991;12(1):1–6.
55. Leonetti JP, Brackmann DE, Prass RL. Improved preservation of facial nerve function in the infratemporal approach to the skull base. Otolaryngol Head Neck Surg. 1989;101(1):74–8.

56. Hsieh HS, Wu CM, Zhuo MY, Yang CH, Hwang CF. Intraoperative facial nerve monitoring during cochlear implant surgery: an observational study. Medicine. 2015;94(4):e456.
57. Heman-Ackah SE, Gupta S, Lalwani AK. Is facial nerve integrity monitoring of value in chronic ear surgery? Laryngoscope. 2013;123(1):2–3.
58. Selesnick SH, Lynn-Macrae AG. The incidence of facial nerve dehiscence at surgery for cholesteatoma. Otol Neurotol. 2001;22(2):129–32.
59. Gidley PW, Maw J, Gantz B, Kaylie D, Lambert P, Malekzadeh S, Chandrasekhar SS. Contemporary opinions on intraoperative facial nerve monitoring. OTO Open. 2018;2(3):2473974X18791803.
60. Lahey RF. Routine dissection and demonstration of the recurrent laryngeal nerve in subtotal thyroidectomy. Surg Gynecol Obstet. 1938;66:775–7.
61. Riddell V. Thyroidectomy: prevention of bilateral recurrent nerve palsy, results of identification of the nerve over 23 consecutive years (1946-69) with a description of an additional safety measure. Br J Surg. 1970;57(1):1–1.
62. Kratz RC. The identification and protection of the laryngeal motor nerves during thyroid and laryngeal surgery: a new microsurgical technique. Laryngoscope. 1973;83(1):59–77.
63. Shedd DP, Durham C. Electrical identification of the recurrent laryngeal nerve. I. Response of the canine larynx to electrical stimulation of the recurrent laryngeal nerve. Ann Surg. 1966;163(1):47.
64. Zini C, Gandolfi A. Facial-nerve and vocal-cord monitoring during otoneurosurgical operations. Arch Otolaryngol Head Neck Surg. 1987;113(12):1291–3.
65. Engel PM, Büter HA, Page PS, Mos A. A device for the location and protection of the recurrent laryngeal nerve during operations upon the neck. Surg Gynecol Obstet. 1981;152(6):825–6.
66. Gavilán J, Gavilán C. Recurrent laryngeal nerve: identification during thyroid and parathyroid surgery. Arch Otolaryngol Head Neck Surg. 1986;112(12): 1286–8.
67. James AG, Crocker S, Woltering E, Ferrara J, Farrar W. A simple method for identifying and testing the recurrent laryngeal nerve. Surg Gynecol Obstet. 1985;161:185–6.
68. Randolph GW, Kobler JB, Wilkins J. Recurrent laryngeal nerve identification and assessment during thyroid surgery: laryngeal palpation. World J Surg. 2004;28(8):755–60.
69. Flisberg K, Lindholm T. Electrical stimulation of the human recurrent laryngeal nerve during thyroid operation. Acta Otolaryngol. 1970;69(sup263):63–7.
70. Rea JL, Davis WE, Templer JW. Recurrent nerve locating system. Ann Otol Rhinol Laryngol. 1979;88(1):92–4.
71. Lipton RJ, McCaffrey TV, Litchy WJ. Intraoperative electrophysiologic monitoring of laryngeal muscle during thyroid surgery. Laryngoscope. 1988;98(12):1292–6.
72. Rice DH, Cone-Wesson B. Intraoperative recurrent laryngeal nerve monitoring. Otolaryngol Head Neck Surg. 1991;105(3):372–5.
73. Maloney RW, Murcek BW, Steehler KW, Sibly D, Maloney RE. A new method for intraoperative recurrent laryngeal nerve monitoring. Ear Nose Throat J. 1994;73(1):30–3.
74. Goldstone AC. The electrode endotracheal tube: a state of the art method for monitoring recurrent laryngeal nerve-vocal cord muscle integrity in the intubated patient. Otolaryngol Head Neck Surg. 1990;103:249.
75. Rea JL. Postcricoid surface laryngeal electrode. Ear Nose Throat J. 1992;71(6):267–9.
76. Marcus B, Edwards B, Yoo S, Byrne A, Gupta A, Kandrevas J, Bradford C, Chepeha DB, Teknos TN. Recurrent laryngeal nerve monitoring in thyroid and parathyroid surgery: the University of Michigan experience. Laryngoscope. 2003;113(2):356–61.
77. Beck DL, Maves MD. Recurrent laryngeal nerve monitoring during thyroid surgery. Neuromonitoring in otology and head and neck surgery. Raven, New York. 1992:151–62. In the surgical treatment of acoustic neurinomas. J Neurosurg. 1982;57:747–52.
78. Barczyński M, Konturek A, Cichoń S. Value of the intraoperative neuromonitoring in surgery for thyroid cancer in identification and prognosis of function of the recurrent laryngeal nerves. Endokrynol Pol. 2006;57(4):343–56.
79. Yarbrough DE, Thompson GB, Kasperbauer JL, Harper CM, Grant CS. Intraoperative electromyographic monitoring of the recurrent laryngeal nerve in reoperative thyroid and parathyroid surgery. Surgery. 2004;136(6):1107–15.
80. Higgins TS, Gupta R, Ketcham AS, Sataloff RT, Wadsworth JT, Sinacori JT. Recurrent laryngeal nerve monitoring versus identification alone on post-thyroidectomy true vocal fold palsy: a meta-analysis. Laryngoscope. 2011;121(5):1009–17.
81. Dralle H, Sekulla C, Haerting J, Timmermann W, Neumann HJ, Kruse E, Grond S, Mühlig HP, Richter C, Voß J, Thomusch O. Risk factors of paralysis and functional outcome after recurrent laryngeal nerve monitoring in thyroid surgery. Surgery. 2004;136(6):1310–22.
82. Serpell J, Sidhu S, Vallance N, Panizza B, Randolph G. Consensus statement on intra-operative electrophysiological recurrent laryngeal nerve monitoring during thyroid surgery. ANZ J Surg. 2014;84(9):603–4.
83. Randolph GW, Dralle H, with the International Intraoperative Monitoring Study Group, Abdullah H, Barczynski M, Bellantone R, Brauckhoff M, Carnaille B, Cherenko S, Chiang FY, Dionigi G. Electrophysiologic recurrent laryngeal nerve monitoring during thyroid and parathyroid surgery: international standards guideline statement. Laryngoscope. 2011;121(S1):S1–6.
84. Schneider R, Randolph GW, Barczynski M, Dionigi G, Wu CW, Chiang FY, Machens A, Kamani D, Dralle H. Continuous intraoperative neural monitoring of the

recurrent nerves in thyroid surgery: a quantum leap in technology. Gland Surg. 2016;5(6):607.
85. Lamadé W, Ulmer C, Seimer A, Molnar V, Meyding-Lamadé U, Thon KP, Koch KP. A new system for continuous recurrent laryngeal nerve monitoring. Minim Invasive Ther Allied Technol. 2007;16(3):149–54.
86. Sinclair CF, Téllez MJ, Ulkatan S. Noninvasive, tube-based, continuous vagal nerve monitoring using the laryngeal adductor reflex: feasibility study of 134 nerves at risk. Head Neck. 2018;40(11):2498–506.

Basic and Advanced Electrophysiology, Setup, and Anesthesia

2

Kirsten F. A. A. Dabekaussen, Pavan Mallur, and Jennifer J. Shin

Introduction

Voice is the principle form of communication in humans despite the phylogenetically recent development of the larynx. The larynx is also critical to respiration, airway protection, and deglutition, and thus perceived limitations in laryngeal function may be an overall predictor of health status in patients [1]. Also fundamentally linked to quality of life, self-perceived dysphonia may result in significant limitations and restrictions in participation in voice-related activities of daily living [2]. Moreover, in professionals whose livelihood is integrally dependent on voice communication, changes or loss of voice may impede an individual's ability to work and sustain income; indeed such individuals may fall under protection of the Americans with Disabilities Act as a result of voice disorders [3]. While individual psychological and financial impact can be easily delineated, the larger socioeconomic implications of voice-related unemployment or man-hours of disability are much more difficult to discern. On a smaller scale, voice contributes to individual identity, with voice-identity recognition an accepted neuropsychological process; loss of voice may be akin to a perceived loss of identity with resultant psychosocial implications for the individual [4].

As voice is so important, a variety of metrics have been developed for quantitative assessment, forming the basis for standardized measurement of voice outcomes, which may be inherently subjective and qualitative. Quantification of vocal status promotes consistency in longitudinal evaluations and systematic study. Validated instruments such as the VHI and its abbreviated counterpart, VHI-10, quantify patients' perceived limitations in voice communication in a reliable, consistent manner [5]. Clinician-recorded auditory perceptual evaluations subjectively grade voice based on defined parameters; the most widely used scales include the Grade, Roughness, Breathiness, Asthenia, and Strain (GRBAS) scale and the Consensus Auditory-Perceptual Evaluation of Voice (CAPE-V). Objective measurements include acoustic analysis to measure pitch period and amplitude perturbations and noise-to-harmonic ratio, aerodynamic tests to measure mean phonation time and airflow, and measurement of pitch and sound pressure level. Combined, these

Kirsten F. A. A. Dabekaussen
Department of Surgery, Brigham and Women's Hospital, Harvard Medical School, Boston, MA, USA
e-mail: kdabekaussen@bwh.harvard.edu

P. Mallur
Department of Otolaryngology, Harvard Medical School, Boston, MA, USA
e-mail: pmallur@bidmc.harvard.edu

J. J. Shin (✉)
Department of Otolaryngology-Head and Neck Surgery, Department of Surgery, Brigham and Women's Hospital, Harvard Medical School, Boston, MA, USA
e-mail: jennifer_shin@meei.harvard.edu

© The Author(s), under exclusive license to Springer Nature Switzerland AG 2022
J. Scharpf, G. W. Randolph (eds.), *Intraoperative Cranial Nerve Monitoring in Otolaryngology-Head and Neck Surgery*, https://doi.org/10.1007/978-3-030-84916-0_2

metrics allow clinicians to systematically and consistently assess a subjective and sometimes nebulous facet of patient outcomes.

Surgery in the head and neck region, such as thyroid surgery, introduces risk for nerve injury due to the close proximity of critical nerves to the necessary dissection. Nerve injuries may result in vocal fold paralysis, dysphagia, hoarseness, or aphonia. Intraoperative visual identification of laryngeal nerves has served as a preventive step to nerve injury; however, an anatomically intact nerve does not directly translate into a fully functional nerve [6]. Consequently, intraoperative cranial nerve monitoring is an attractive technique for eliciting information regarding the location or functional integrity of a nerve [7]. This chapter thus addresses the electrophysiology, setup, and anesthesia considerations related to intraoperative cranial nerve monitoring in head and neck surgery. We begin with a description of basic electrophysiological concepts underlying electromyography (EMG), including the amplitude, latency, and duration of biphasic wave forms. We then describe the related setup and anesthetic considerations required to successfully apply this technique.

Electrophysiology

IONM requires an understanding of the related electrophysiology. In short, during surgery, a handheld probe is used to apply electricity to stimulate a key motor nerve and prompt nerve impulses to form. Those impulses are then transferred to the muscles producing the myoelectric signals which underlie the wave forms in the electromyography (EMG).

Figure 2.1 illustrates a biphasic wave form, which is composed of two parts. The small preceding spike on the left side represents a stimulus from the device. The wave form itself is typically described in three metrics: the amplitude, the latency, and the duration. The amplitude is defined as the height from the lowest point on the wave form to the highest point. It correlates with the number of muscle fibers responding to or polarizing during the standard EMG measurement. This amplitude can vary distinctively among and even within patients.

During awake speech, measured amplitudes may range from 100 to 800 μV.

Table 2.1 shows the normative intraoperative values, variances in amplitudes, latency, and threshold. The normative intraoperative values may range from 600 to 800 μV for the recurrent laryngeal nerve and 100–300 μV for the superior laryngeal nerve. Observed standard deviations are relatively large, likely related to multiple factors including how the probe and the electrodes make contact and the thickness, wetness, and temperature of the tissue, as well as host factors such as motor fiber patterns, age, and gender.

Latency is defined as the time between the stimulus and the occurrence of the biphasic

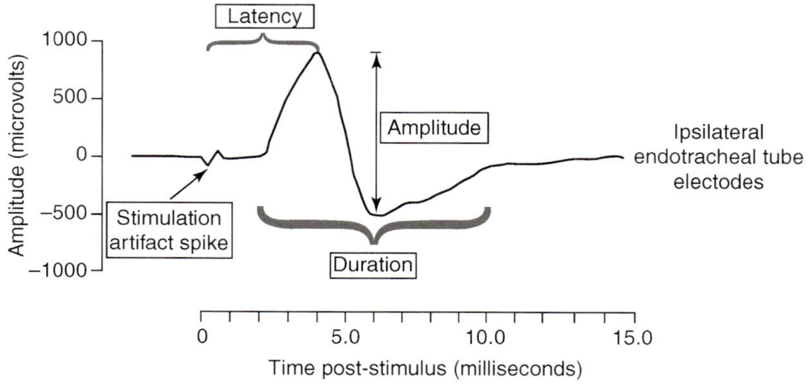

Fig. 2.1 Basic parameters of a normal biphasic electromyocardiogram wave form in intraoperative nerve monitoring. The amplitude is illustrated on the y-axis in microvolts; the x-axis represents the time post-stimulus in milliseconds. (Adapted from Randolph [11], p. 324. Copyright 2013 by Elsevier)

Table 2.1 Presenting average variances in normative intraoperative values in amplitudes, latency, and threshold in nerve monitoring[a]

	Amplitude (μV)	Latency (milliseconds)	Threshold (mA)
Right RLN	783 (±512)	3.19 (2.47–4.25)	0.51 (0.025–1.4)
Left RLN	604 (±504)	3.7 (2.5–4.34)	0.61 (0.25–1)
Right vagus	717 (±479)	6.77 (4.25–9.5)	0.41 (0.25–0.85)
Left vagus	420 (±255)	7.67 (6.1–10)	0.41 (0.1–0.8)
SLN	269 (±178.6)		0.5 (±0.1)

Adapted from Randolph [11], p. 332. Copyright 2013 by Elsevier

RLN recurrent laryngeal nerve, *SLN* superior laryngeal nerve

[a]Stimulation at 1–2 mA, ±SD or range

wave form (Fig. 2.1). Latency reflects the speed or ease of stimulation induced due to polarization. It depends on the distance from the stimulation point to the ipsilateral vocal fold. This explains a potential difference in latency length between the left and right recurrent laryngeal nerve. This difference occurs in particular if the vagus nerve is stimulated in the mid-neck during thyroidectomy. Table 2.1 shows some average latencies for the left and right recurrent laryngeal, vagus, and superior laryngeal nerve. The amplitude and latency of an observed EMG waveform are key structural elements which should be clearly seen amidst monitoring; their absence can indicate that one is viewing artifact, rather than true stimulated waveforms. Artifacts may be observed with metal-on-metal contact or cuff leakage. The other key term in nerve monitoring is the threshold. The threshold is defined as the current that first triggers a recognizable EMG activity, when applied to the nerve. The observed threshold may be 0.4 mA, and at this threshold, there is a smaller amplitude than at the maximum depolarization which typically occurs around 0.8 mA. This anticipated increase in amplitude is part of why 1.0 mA is considered a good safe suprathreshold stimulus to start a case.

Setup

Endotracheal tube-based systems record EMG data from the thyroarytenoid and/or vocalis muscles. Two types of endotracheal tubes can be employed for this procedure. The first is a manufactured endotracheal tube with paired left and right stainless-steel electrodes embedded in the tube surface. The second is a standard endotracheal tube which has been augmented with electrodes placed so that they rest 7–10 mm superior to the upper border of the tube cuff. During placement, it is critical to guarantee that there are no gaps between the electrodes and the tube, as well as no overlap between the electrodes. Regardless of the tube type selected, the tube is in place once the electrodes are seated symmetrically in the glottis after the cuff is inflated. That contact with both vocal folds allows monitoring of the thyroarytenoid and vocalis muscle depolarization. In selecting the proper tube for the case, it is also important to select a tube that will optimize contact with the vocal folds. Ideally, the largest endotracheal tube which is considered safe is used. This improves impedance and does not seem to cause any otolaryngologic effects. For most adults, a 7.0 tube is used, but pre-formed tubes are also available in 6.0 and 8.0.

In general, the monitoring system may be conceptualized as comprised of two sides. There is a recording side and a stimulation side. The recording side has the endotracheal tube, the electrodes, their ground, and their connections to the interface connector box and monitor. The stimulation side has a stimulation neural probe, its grounding electrode, and their connections to the interface box connector along with the stimulation current pulse stimulator, which is within the monitor (Fig. 2.2).

Risk of Electrical Interference

Electrocautery units, either monopolar or bipolar, may create electrical interference, which can be contained through muting cables to temporarily silence the audio and video functions of the mon-

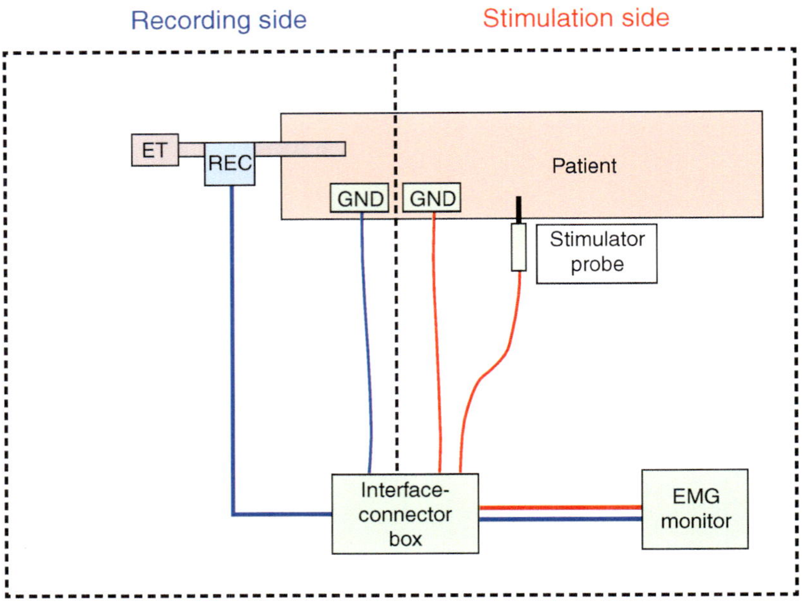

Fig. 2.2 Schematic overview of intraoperative nerve monitoring setup equipment showing the stimulation and the recording side of the system. ET endotracheal tube, REC recording electrodes, GND ground electrodes, EMG electromyography. (Adapted from Randolph [11], p. 226. Copyright 2013 by Elsevier)

itor during electrocautery unit discharge. When setting up the room, it is best to physically separate electrocautery units and the monitoring box to help keep wires apart and untangled. Electrocautery units should be placed at least 10 feet away from the neural monitoring unit. Monitoring is not affected by the activity of cardiac pacemakers and does not impact their function. It is also compatible with harmonic and LigaSure technologies.

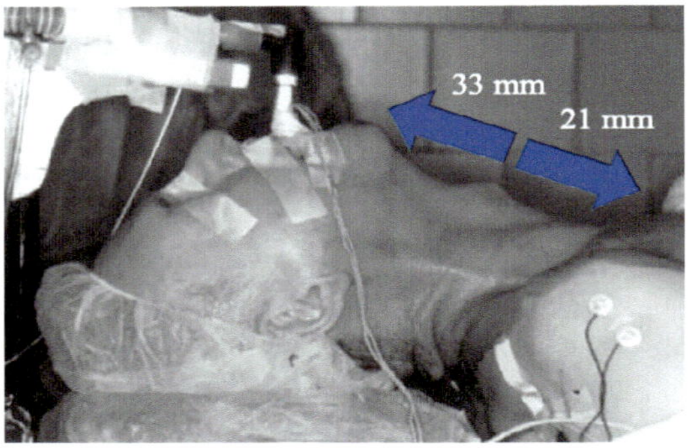

Fig. 2.3 Endotracheal tube positioning with patient in neck extended positioning for accurate electrode contact. (Adapted from Randolph [11], p. 327. Copyright 2013 by Elsevier)

Patient Positioning

Patient's position is also a key factor to consider. The endotracheal tube may be displaced up to 21 mm inward and up to 33 mm outward with the patient in a neck extended position. Thus, there is over 5 cm of potential movement from positioning alone, which emphasizes the need to confirm that the electrodes lay right in the glottis after positioning (Fig. 2.3).

Once the patient is fully positioned, there are several options to verify that positioning is correct. First, the presence of respiratory variation can be evaluated. After intubation and any paralytic given to the patient has receded, but before the inhalational plan of anesthesia is too deep, there is a window which typically occurs just before the patient would begin to move spontaneously. During this window, a coarsening of the monitor's baseline activity occurs, reflected in small wave forms, typically varying from about 30–70 mV, as shown in Fig. 2.4. This activity has been termed "respiratory variation to the baseline," and it implies good tube positioning. If it is observed, however, it also suggests that a patient may abruptly move afterward, so it is ideal to be prepared to quickly sedate with an intravenous agent (e.g., propofol).

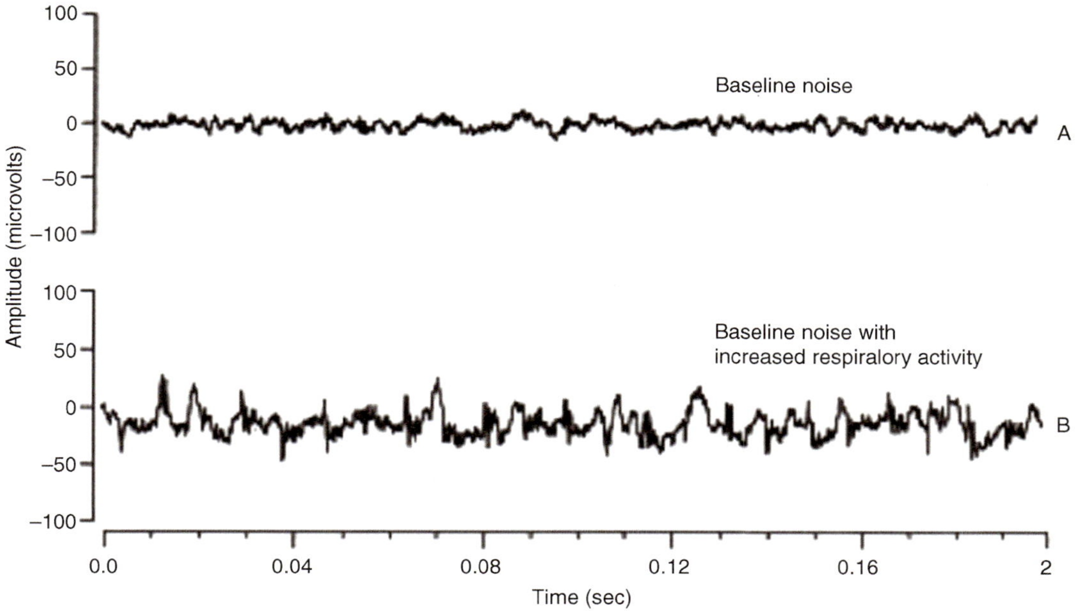

Fig. 2.4 Monitor display of references in management of the recurrent laryngeal nerve during intraoperative nerve monitoring (IONM). (Adapted from Randolph [11], p. 328. Copyright 2013 by Elsevier)

Second, laryngoscopy can be repeated either with a Mac blade, GlideScope, or fiber-optic scope. This inspection is inherently accurate but requires this additional step. A third option is the tap test, where one briskly taps the finger to the midline of the thyroid cartilage and checks for a response. However, the accuracy for the verification of endotracheal tube positioning for the tap test is unknown.

Monitor Assessment

The setup additionally includes monitor output assessment, which can begin by checking impedance values. A low individual electrode impedance, e.g., <5 kΩ per electrode, suggests good electrode contact with the patient. If the impedance is higher, the electrode might be in poor contact, and repositioning is worth considering. Both sides should read <5 kΩ with an imbalance between electrodes of <1 kΩ. Please note that impedance typically only implies adequate electrode contact, not necessarily the correct positioning.

When preparing the monitor box initially, the stimulus can be set at 1.0 mA, which is usually sufficient, although 2.0 mA is also an option. Recall from the discussion above that these values are safely above the measured thresholds for nerve stimulation. Event triggers can be set at 100 μV or 200 μV to minimize false-positive readings. Awareness is required when monitoring the superior laryngeal nerve as thresholds may need to be less than 100 μV; recall that the superior laryngeal nerve has differing amplitude numbers compared to the recurrent laryngeal nerve, as discussed earlier in this chapter. Experience has shown that most equipment-related problems encountered during the setup phase are caused by malpositioned endotracheal tube recording electrodes.

Anesthesia

Maintaining an open dialogue with anesthesia during the procedure is critical, as it is in any case. Intubation in IONM procedures can be performed with or without a stylet. Since significant changes in tube positioning may occur after intubation as the patient is taken from a neutral intubating position to extended position, tube malpositioning is a common cause of a monitoring problem. If an endotracheal tube placement problem is suspected, vagal or nerve stimulation by the surgeon can be helpful feedback for an anesthesiologist who is readjusting the tube. The tube position can be assessed initially through its appearance at the lips as compared to its appearance at the beginning of the case and ultimately through direct visualization of the glottis via laryngoscopy. Endotracheal tube placement errors also include rotational errors, which can be detected by rechecking monitor settings for correct impedance values [8]. A right-handed anesthesiologist tends to rotate the tube clockwise, as much as 30°, which means that rotational error usually needs a counterclockwise correction [9]. A recent study showed that when initial tube placement is performed carefully, optimal tube placement was possible in 94% of cases. The tube readjustment rate was just 5.7%, half of which required advancement and half of which required withdrawal. In addition, it was shown that men had a very slightly greater depth of insertion than women. However, there was no significant association between the desired depth of insertion and height, age, weight, or body mass index [10]. Also, pooled saliva at the glottis may result in altered signal. Therefore, a perioperative drying agent and intraoperative suction can also be very helpful. For that reason, the use of lubrication gel on the tube also should be avoided [8].

Conclusions

Intraoperative nerve monitoring is an advanced technology which bolsters the surgeon's skill set when seeking to prevent perioperative nerve damage. To successfully implement this technique, an understanding of the electrophysiological wave forms, composed of its key elements – amplitude, latency, and duration – is warranted. Impediments to detecting the standard biphasic wave form, such as artifact and/or abnormal impendence values, require expertise, and endotracheal tube/electrode positioning can be optimized for intraoperative monitoring. Ensuring proper setup, endotracheal tube placement, patient positioning, and electrode contact require effective communication and vigilance from the healthcare team.

References

1. Kirsch DeVore E, Carroll TL, Rosner B, Shin JJ. Can voice disorders matter as much as life-threatening comorbidities to patients' general health? Laryngoscope. 2020;130(10):2405–11.
2. Ma EP, Yiu EM. Voice activity and participation profile: assessing the impact of voice disorders on daily activities. J Speech Lang Hear Res. 2001;44(3):511–24.
3. Isette D, Eadie T. The Americans with Disabilities Act and voice disorders: practical guidelines for voice clinicians. J Voice. 2016;30(3):293–300.
4. Roswandowitz C, Kappes C, Obrig H, von Kriegstein K. Obligatory and facultative brain regions for voice-identity recognition. Brain. 2018;141(1):234–47.
5. Rosen CA, Lee AS, Osborne J, Zullo T, Murray T. Development and validation of the voice handicap index-10. Laryngoscope. 2004;114(9):1549–56.
6. Deniwar A, Kandil E, Randolph G. Electrophysiological neural monitoring of the laryngeal nerves in thyroid surgery: review of the current literature. Gland Surg. 2015;4(5):368–75. https://doi.org/10.3978/j.issn.2227-684X.2015.04.04. PMID: 26425449; PMCID: PMC4561657.
7. Darr EA, Tufano RP, Ozdemir S, Kamani D, Hurwitz S, Randolph G. Superior laryngeal nerve quantitative intraoperative monitoring is possible in all thyroid surgeries. Laryngoscope. 2014;124:1035–41.
8. Randolph GW, Dralle H, Abdullah H, et al. Electrophysiologic recurrent laryngeal nerve monitoring during thyroid and parathyroid surgery: international standards guideline statement. Laryngoscope. 2011;121(suppl 1):S1–S16.
9. Iowa Head and Neck Protocols [Internet]. [Updated 2020 Nov 29]. Available from: https://medicine.uiowa.edu/iowaprotocols/thyroidectomy-and-thyroid-lobectomy.
10. Lu IC, Chu KS, Tsai CJ, et al. Optimal depth of NIM EMG endotracheal tube for intraoperative neuromonitoring of the recurrent laryngeal nerve during thyroidectomy. World J Surg. 2008;32:1935–9. https://doi.org/10.1007/s00268-008-9549-1.
11. Randolph GW. Surgery of the thyroid and parathyroid glands. 2nd ed. Philadelphia: Saunders; 2013.

Anesthetic Considerations and Setup for Cranial Nerve Monitoring

3

Anisha Rhea Noble and Juliana Bonilla-Velez

Introduction

Intraoperative nerve monitoring (IONM) may provide additional protection against injury to the cranial nerves during head and neck surgery and can be particularly advantageous to surgeons during revisions or other technically challenging procedures [1]. While visual identification remains the gold standard, occult and clinically significant damage can occur despite the appearance of an intact nerve [2]. In thyroid surgery, for example, it has been estimated that injury to the nerve occurs in 2–5% of cases in high-volume centers and typically occurs as a result of traction [3, 4]. IONM assists in nerve identification, neural mapping, surgical dissection, avoidance of transient nerve injuries, prognostication of nerve function, and lesion site identification [5, 6]. Efforts to ensure nerve preservation in complex head and neck cases – including parotid, thyroid, neck, and neuro-otologic surgery – influence and direct surgical approaches. Given the diversity of surgical techniques and anatomic complexities inherent to each of these procedures, an established standardized intraoperative nerve monitoring paradigm could serve as a high-fidelity adjunct in head and neck surgery.

This chapter will cover foundational knowledge for any surgeon using IONM in their practice. A clear understanding of anesthetic considerations and equipment setup is necessary to perform cranial nerve monitoring that is of high quality and useful intraoperatively. Application of standardized methods for IONM is essential to perform monitoring that is accurate and reliable. This knowledge can minimize surgeon frustration with IONM systems which may be a barrier to widespread use of the technology. Arguably, IONM is most useful in difficult cases; however, surgical complexity is not always identified preoperatively. Therefore, routine application of IONM is suggested in order to facilitate increased experience with setup, interpretation, use, and troubleshooting malfunction [6]. The goal of this chapter is to provide an in-depth review of IONM for major nerves in the head and neck in order to promote high-fidelity application of this technology. The information provided in this chapter describes a review of published lit-

A. R. Noble
Department of Otolaryngology–Head and Neck Surgery, University of Washington School of Medicine, Seattle, WA, USA
e-mail: noble1@uw.edu

J. Bonilla-Velez (✉)
Department of Otolaryngology–Head and Neck Surgery, University of Washington School of Medicine, Seattle, WA, USA

Division of Pediatric Otolaryngology, Seattle Children's Hospital, Seattle, WA, USA

Center for Clinical and Translational Research, Seattle Children's Research Institute, Seattle, WA, USA
e-mail: Juliana.bonilla-velez@seattlechildrens.org

© The Author(s), under exclusive license to Springer Nature Switzerland AG 2022
J. Scharpf, G. W. Randolph (eds.), *Intraoperative Cranial Nerve Monitoring in Otolaryngology-Head and Neck Surgery*, https://doi.org/10.1007/978-3-030-84916-0_3

erature and reflects recommendations from the International Neural Monitoring Study Group (INMSG).

Anesthetic Considerations

Critical to the successful employment of IONM is the partnership between the anesthesia and surgical teams. Coordination with the anesthesia team includes choice of agent and – in the event of vagus nerve/recurrent laryngeal nerve monitoring – endotracheal tube selection, placement, and positioning. Preoperative planning is required to ensure that the anesthetic plan is tailored to the individual patient and their comorbidities while being mindful to avoid agents that could impede adequate neural monitoring.

Anesthetic agents affect IONM modalities in a multitude of mechanisms: Agents affect synaptic function, and therefore effects can be predicted by examining their impact on neural pathways [7]. Changes in signals arising from anesthetic technique may affect neural monitoring globally, whereas iatrogenic changes can be mapped to the focal area at risk [8]. Recovery of signal from anesthetic technique may require time during which it may not be possible to detect the presence of a concomitant surgical injury [8]. When monitoring complex neural pathways involving the peripheral and central nervous systems, anesthetic agents can impact electrophysiologic monitoring through several proposed mechanisms, briefly described here. Anesthetic agents can influence synaptic functioning of the monitored neural pathways, which in turn can affect other pathways that can enhance or depress the signal on the pathway of interest. Anesthesia may have global effects that alter cortical and spinal cord neural processing, affecting upper motor neurons in the efferent pathway. Neuromuscular blockade (NMB) agents take effect at the level of the lower motor neurons, altering function at the neuromuscular junction therefore dampening the final limb of a motor pathway. Also, important to consider is the effect that general anesthesia may have on neural functioning through physiologic effects such as changes in blood pressure or hypothermia [7]. For these reasons, the choice of anesthetic agents should be guided by the modality of neurophysiologic monitoring employed. Auditory evoked brainstem response can be measured during anesthesia with inhalational agents or NMB. Somatosensory evoked potentials (SSEP) may be used to monitor the integrity of the dorsal columns during spine surgery and brachial plexus during transaxillary thyroid surgery and are sensitive to inhalational agents [9]. Transcranial motor evoked potentials (tcMEP) – described in more detail below – can be used to monitor the integrity of the motor system and are sensitive to inhalational agents, high-doses of propofol or benzodiazepines, and NMB [6–8, 10]. Perhaps most relevant to head and neck surgery is the use of electromyography (EMG) to monitor muscle activity from peripheral cranial nerve stimulation; EMG is primarily sensitive to the use of NMB and will be described in more detail below.

Neuromuscular Blockade and IONM

Agents used for NMB cause a synaptic block at the neuromuscular junction that impedes transmission of the neural signal from the lower motor neuron to the muscle (effector). The efferent signal may originate from the central nervous system (e.g., during volitional movement), in response to transcranial stimulation, or from peripherally evoked motor responses such as mechanical or electric stimulation of cranial nerves in the surgical field [11]. Because NMB agents act at the neuromuscular junction, their use is relevant in peripheral nerve monitoring: Use of NMB agents block physiologic neuromuscular transmission and therefore results in ineffective IONM.

A discussion on NMB requires a basic understanding of neuromuscular physiology. Depolarization of a peripheral nerve results in release of acetylcholine contained in presynaptic vesicles. Acetylcholine diffuses across the synaptic cleft to bind to postsynaptic acetylcholine receptors; this results in depolarization of the muscle and contraction. Acetylcholine is degraded by acetylcholinesterase in the synaptic cleft; NMB agents act by interfering with this pathway [11]. NMB agents can be classified into three groups based on chemical structure and depolarizing effects (specifically depolarizing or non-depolarizing agents). The only depolarizing agent routinely used is succinylcholine. Succinylcholine is analogous to two acetylcholine molecules fused together and acts by diffusing and binding to the postsynaptic nicotinic receptor causing depolarization. It has a rapid onset of action and results in sustained depolarization, fasciculations, and flaccid paralysis with recovery of function within 7–12 minutes [12]. Succinylcholine is degraded by plasma cholinesterase. Inherited abnormalities of this enzyme can prolong the effects of succinylcholine to up to 4–6 hours [11]. Non-depolarizing agents function by serving as reversible binders to postsynaptic nicotinic receptors. These agents reach the synaptic cleft through diffusion and compete with acetylcholine for receptor binding leading to flaccid paralysis. Action of non-depolarizing agents is terminated by diffusion away from the cleft, metabolism, and elimination. Such medications are classified as "intermediate duration of action" given that the onset and duration of the effect is longer than that of succinylcholine. The third group of NMB agents includes cisatracurium which has a chemical composition that allows for spontaneous decomposition without requiring renal or hepatic function and is therefore preferentially used when these organs are impaired [11, 12]. An understanding of the pharmacokinetics of NMB agents has been applied to develop medications that can reverse their effects in the neuromuscular junction. Anticholinesterases such as neostigmine have been used to block the degradation of acetylcholine thereby increasing its concentration in the synaptic cleft, creating more competition with residual NMB agent [13]. This may also disrupt the metabolism of succinylcholine therefore prolonging its effect. Despite their theoretic pharmacokinetic benefits, anticholinesterases are somewhat limited in clinical practice given their side effect profile [13, 14]. Sugammadex is a cyclodextrin molecule that binds rocuronium and vecuronium removing them from the synaptic cleft and is used to reverse NMB [14, 15]. Sugammadex has been used with good results during intraoperative monitoring of the recurrent laryngeal and facial nerves [14–20]. Muscular groups have different sensitivities to NMB in terms of onset time, maximum degree, and duration of neuromuscular blockade. Centrally located muscles such as the laryngeal muscles and diaphragm have a faster onset of NMB but are less sensitive, while facial, abdominal, and limb musculature are most sensitive [13, 21–23]. Studies have shown that the impact of partial NMB on responses to facial nerve stimulation is lower than for responses to stimulation of the ulnar nerve [24, 25]. Laryngeal muscles have a shorter response time and recover more quickly from neuromuscular blockade than systemic musculature [26–29]. Marusch et al. (2005) found that with NMB, there was a measurable EMG from the vocalis muscle, but at systemic muscular relaxation degrees of >90%, vocalis muscle EMG amplitude became reduced; this supported the feasibility of laryngeal monitoring during NMB [26]. Differences in the sensitivity of muscle groups to NMB agents are thought to arise from variability in acetylcholine receptor density, blood flow with increased perfusion and earlier peak concentrations at respiratory muscles [29], muscle temperature, acetylcholine release with stimulation, and acetylcholinesterase activity [30].

Some authors have suggested that IONM may be possible with use of partial NMB [11, 26]. Sloan (2013) performed a thoughtful review of available evidence on NMB during IONM and noted that partial NMB is possible with EMG monitoring of muscle responses when the single twitch response (T1) is 10–20% or the train of four (TOF) response is two out of four twitches, the patient has no underlying neuromuscular disease, there is tight control of the drug effect by the anesthesiologist, and assessment of TOF is performed directly on the muscles being monitored [11]. It should be noted that cranial nerve monitoring may require a higher stimulation current and therefore less NMB to adequately monitor myogenic responses. Proposed benefits of NMB include facilitated surgical exposure, reduced unexpected movement, and reduction of excessive EMG noise which in turn could improve the signal to noise ratio [11]. Despite this finding, INMSG recommends strongly *against* the use of any NMB during a case where IONM is being employed [5, 6, 31]. Cranial nerve monitoring is designed to be sensitive to mechanical stimulation of the nerves; it is therefore preferable that after induction NMB is allowed to wear off and no further NMB used for the rest of the case [6]. The administration of any paralytic agent intraoperatively has the potential to attenuate EMG responses. Reduced EMG amplitude could lead to decreased sensitivity in detecting impending neural injury and may also reduce the amplitude of evoked responses [32]. Changes in EMG data could make postoperative prognostic schemes less accurate. It is also important to consider that the depth of anesthesia needed to avoid spontaneous activity of the vocal cords may be deeper than usually employed when using inhaled anesthetics and intravenous narcotics in the absence of NMB [6]. These agents do not affect EMG readings, but if the patient is in a lighter plane of anesthesia, spontaneous activity could be difficult to differentiate from a stimulated response [6]. Furthermore, a myriad of factors can result in variability in the desired NMB effect which could result in a more profound neuromuscular blockade than anticipated [11]. The INMSG recommends avoiding the risk of inaccurate IONM and, therefore, avoiding NMB beyond the need for intubation [6].

The anesthesia team must therefore balance this need for temporary NMB while allowing return of full muscular activity within a few minutes after induction and intubation to facilitate IONM. Lu et al. (2020) propose four regimens for IONM during thyroid surgery that could theoretically achieve these goals:

(a) Relaxant-free regimen: This suggests avoidance of NMB for the entire perioperative period [16]. This option is not suitable for routine clinical use due to concern for upper airway injury during intubation as well as limitation of the ability to ensure the exact position the nerve monitoring endotracheal tube needed for recurrent laryngeal nerve monitoring [33–35].
(b) Use of a depolarizing NMB succinylcholine: This option suggests that a single dose of succinylcholine (2–2.5 mg/kg) for endotracheal intubation provides adequate relaxation for endotracheal intubation as well as restoring neuromuscular function within 5 minutes. The disadvantage of using succinylcholine and therefore a limitation to this option lie in potential adverse events including myalgia, hyperkalemia, increased intracranial or intraocular pressure, cardiac dysrhythmia, or malignant hyperthermia [36, 37]. Additionally, as noted before, patients with abnormal function of plasma cholinesterase may endure prolonged blockade [11].
(c) This option proposes titration of non-depolarizing NMB: A single dose of intermediate-duration NMB (rocuronium or atracurium) could serve as an alternative that provides relaxation while avoiding adverse effects of succinylcholine. [27] The limitation lies in the unpredictable duration of NMB between individuals. Residual paralysis has been reported in 10% of patients 2 hours after a single dose of an intermediate-duration NMB agent [38]. Because of this there is a risk of inaccurate EMG neural monitoring. Alternatively, one effective dose of rocuronium (0.3 mg/kg) may be used in this setting. Pharmacokinetic advantages of rocuronium include faster onset and shorter duration of action supporting this as an alternative to achieve appropriate relaxation for intubation while allowing for adequate EMG functioning [39].
(d) Finally, there is the option of rocuronium combined with sugammadex: Sugammadex is a selective relaxant binding agent that encapsulates rocuronium and prevents its action on the acetylcholine receptor, rapidly reversing NMB [14]. Although sugammadex has been used to reverse NMB for IONM, the timing of administration, dosing, and use

remain topics of debate in the anesthesia literature [16, 40–44]. Additionally, its high cost may limit universal use.

Pediatric Anesthetic Considerations for IONM

The pharmacology and electrophysiology of NMB and IONM follow the same principles in adults and children. However, a couple of notable anesthetic considerations are important in the pediatric population that may influence the anesthetic plan as it relates to avoidance of NMB agents intraoperatively, and are therefore relevant knowledge for pediatric surgeons. First, ketamine is more commonly used in pediatric anesthesia than in adults as it provides good analgesia and hypnosis while having less hallucinatory effects in children. It can therefore serve as a good adjunct to the anesthetic plan [7]. Second, use of propofol can lead to the propofol-related infusion syndrome (PRIS) more commonly in children, which consists of a reversible lactic acidosis with acute refractory bradycardia that can lead to asystole, cardiac failure, rhabdomyolysis, renal failure, and death [45, 46]. Risk factors include prolonged high-dose infusions, airway infection, head injury, and increased levels of glucocorticoids or catecholamines. However, PRIS can also occur with short-term infusions of high-dose propofol [47]. In a survey of 40 pediatric centers who perform anesthesia in cases using IONM, none specifically avoided using propofol, but some centers expressed concern with propofol use due to the risk of PRIS. These concerns were addressed by avoiding propofol use in specific cases, such as patients with mitochondrial myopathy, and use of other agents to decrease overall dosage of propofol used [7].

Intraoperative Nerve Monitoring Equipment Setup

Intraoperative nerve monitoring (IONM) equipment and setup can vary by institution and surgical procedure. Equipment setup should be standardized in order to optimize accuracy and quality of nerve monitoring [6]. The use of non-standard monitoring techniques has resulted in inaccuracies presented in the literature [48–50]. Adoption of a standardized approach to IONM improves the fidelity of the system and may contribute to improved clinical outcomes. Regarding IONM in head and neck surgeries, electrode positioning varies depending on the procedure and the nerve(s) of interest. Reviewed below are an overview of the equipment and setup for monitoring the facial nerve (CN VII), glossopharyngeal nerve (IX), recurrent laryngeal nerve (RLN), accessory nerve (CN XI), hypoglossal nerve (CN XII), brachial plexus and spine monitoring.

Brief Overview of Nerve Monitoring Equipment and Systems

Historically, a myriad of methods has been used to assess neural function, as detailed in Chap. 1. The most commonly employed methods in clinical practice include systems that are composed of a monitoring system that integrates information from recording and stimulation electrodes. Monitoring systems are broadly categorized into audio-only or audio and visual systems that present a display of the evoked EMG waveform. Inherent limitations of the audio-only system curtail its regular use in clinical practice and have been described well in the literature [6]. Advantages of the visual and audio system include the ability to assess the evoked EMG waveform to monitor changes in amplitude, threshold, and latency. This can help determine response quantification, precision in determining loss of signal, and difference on a real signal from artifact, which are key pieces of information that can inform intraoperative decision-making [6].

The recording electrodes most frequently used are needle or surface electrodes (Fig. 3.1). Needle electrodes generally record higher amplitude than surface electrodes, but this difference has not been clinically significant [6]. Traumatic consequences from traversing the skin or mucosa

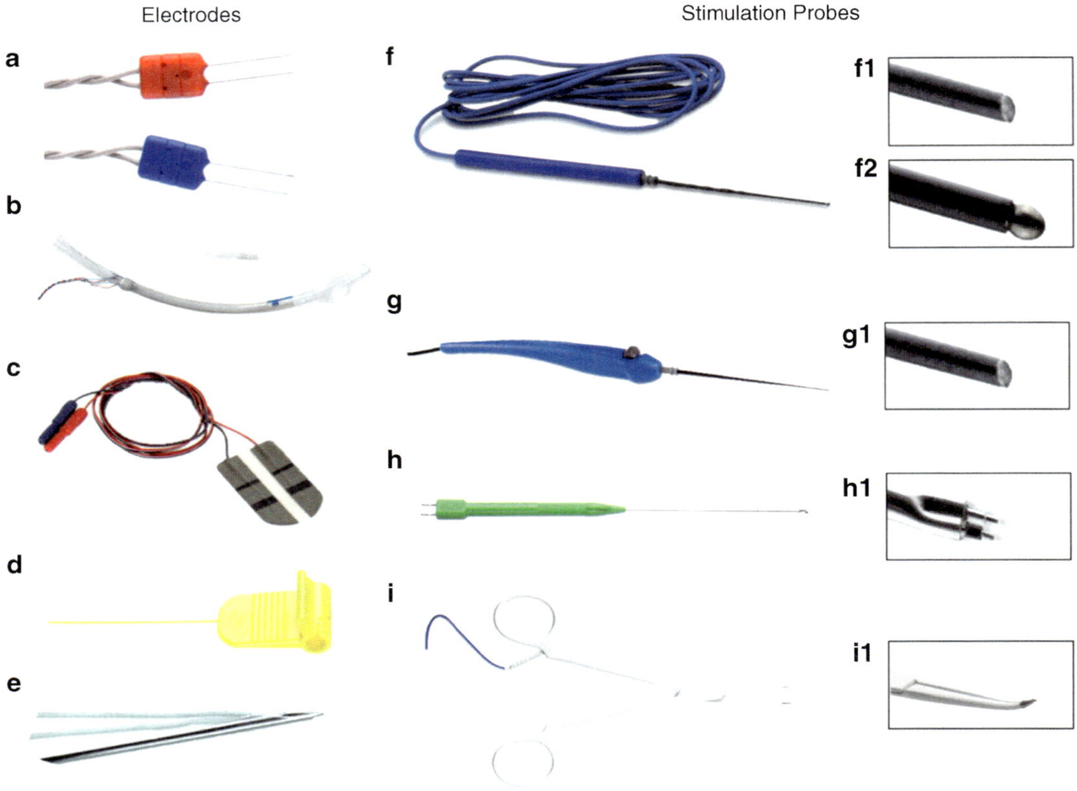

Fig. 3.1 Common intraoperative nerve monitoring electrodes and stimulation probes. Example of paired subdermal needle electrodes (**a**), endotracheal tube-based electrodes (**b**), adhesive surface electrodes for placement on endotracheal tubes (**c**), automatic periodic stimulation electrode (**d**), and endolaryngeal hookwire electrode (**e**). Monopolar (**f**) with a prass standard tip (F1) or a ball-tip (F2), monopolar incrementing (**g**), bipolar (**h**) and dissector-based (**i**) stimulation probes

could arise and include bleeding, hematoma, infection, laceration, and the potential risk of needlestick injury to healthcare professionals managing the equipment.

Special consideration is warranted when considering nerve monitoring in the larynx; options available include needle electrodes, endotracheal tube-based surface electrodes, and post-cricoid electrode surface arrays. Additional details regarding vagal IONM are described in the section entitled "Monitoring Side Setup: Nerve-Specific IONM Electrode Placement."

Stimulation probes can be broadly categorized into monopolar or bipolar neural stimulators and can be configured as isolated stimulation units or incorporated into dissecting instruments (Fig. 3.1). Monopolar stimulators are most commonly used and can be standard or ball tipped. This probe allows diffuse current spread over a larger anatomic area and may therefore be the most sensitive for nerve identification and mapping in the surgical field [51]. Bipolar stimulators provide stimulation current precisely between instrument prongs. Appropriate orientation of the positive and negative stimulating electrodes on the nerve is critical for nerve stimulation [6]. Stimulating dissecting instruments are similar to monopolar electrodes with slightly less sensitivity but perhaps more specificity in neural stimulation. Bipolar and dissecting instruments need to be placed directly on the nerve to generate evoked EMG potentials; these instruments may have added utility in minimizing false-positive stimulation and are most useful during subtle dissection (e.g., dissection around the ligament of Berry). The need for proximity to the nerve, however, limits use in initial nerve identification and mapping. In a comparative study of stimulator probes, the prass standard tip probe was recommended as the best overall stimulating electrode option because of its low threshold and high amplitude [51]. Bipolar stimulators are the most sensitive and may optimally be used as a confirmatory final stimulation in the neck, for example in thyroid surgery using it prior to proceeding to the contralateral side. Dissecting instruments have been recommended as an alternative for use during critical portions of the case when the nerve is at highest risk because they provide real-time feedback on EMG response, allowing the surgeon to have early detection of EMG changes and, in response, decrease traction on the nerve [52].

An alternative set up is to work with a team of neurophysiologists during the case to perform intraoperative nerve mapping – for example, in neurosurgical cases, in posterior fossa dissection, and during resection of complex cervicofacial vascular anomalies. With this modality nerves are percutaneously delineated by a neurophysiologist who is continuously interpreting neural activity and communicates directly with the surgical team throughout the case [53–55]. This highlights the value of teamwork and real-time feedback, greater ease for intraoperative nerve interrogation that can be modified accordingly based on proximity to the nerve, for example using high-amplitude stimulation to rule out presence of nerve versus low-amplitude confirmatory stimulation and allows the surgeon to focus solely on the operative field.

Recording Side Setup

Preoperative setup of nerve monitoring systems requires attention to both the recording side (i.e., monitoring system tower) and the monitoring side (i.e., the patient and electrodes). To ensure accurate, reproducible results, setup should be performed prior to prepping the anesthetized patient. The operating room must be arranged such that the recording side of the monitoring system is viewable and audible to the surgical team while far enough away to maintain sterility and provide unfettered access to the patient. Various monitoring systems are used across institutions; commonly, there is an IONM tower which supports a monitor screen for visual display of EMG evoked potentials, an attached patient interface box with electrode receiver ports, and drawers containing the electrodes and/or other equipment. The monitoring tower is optimally located about 6–10 feet away from the patient; electrode wires are long enough to accommodate this distance.

Depending on the system utilized, the monitor screen will present options for procedure type and recommended electrode and ground electrode placement. Once selected, the user can customize monitoring measures including stimulator intensity current (typically 0.5 mA, 1.0 mA, 1.5 mA, 2.0 mA, or 2.5 mA) as well as stimulation threshold (μV). An attached patient interface box with electrode receiver ports should be connected to the monitoring tower; the patient interface box often has an extension cable allowing for close placement near patient, ideal for troubleshooting during the case if necessary.

Monitoring Side Setup: Nerve-Specific IONM Electrode Placement

Electrode placement for various nerves commonly monitored in head and neck surgeries (i.e., CN VII, CN IX, CN X, CN XI, CN XII) will be described here. A brief review of nerve monitoring for brachial plexus and spinal monitoring will follow. Recommended locations for electrode placement to monitor cranial nerves are presented (Fig. 3.2). For intramuscular electrode placement, there are monitoring electrodes as well as ground and stimulator electrodes. Typically, the ground electrode is green in color, whereas the stimulator anode is white; this may be remembered using the mnemonic "ground is green" [56]. Prior to the use of any electrode monitoring, confirmation that the patient is appropriately grounded to the monopolar electrocautery unit is

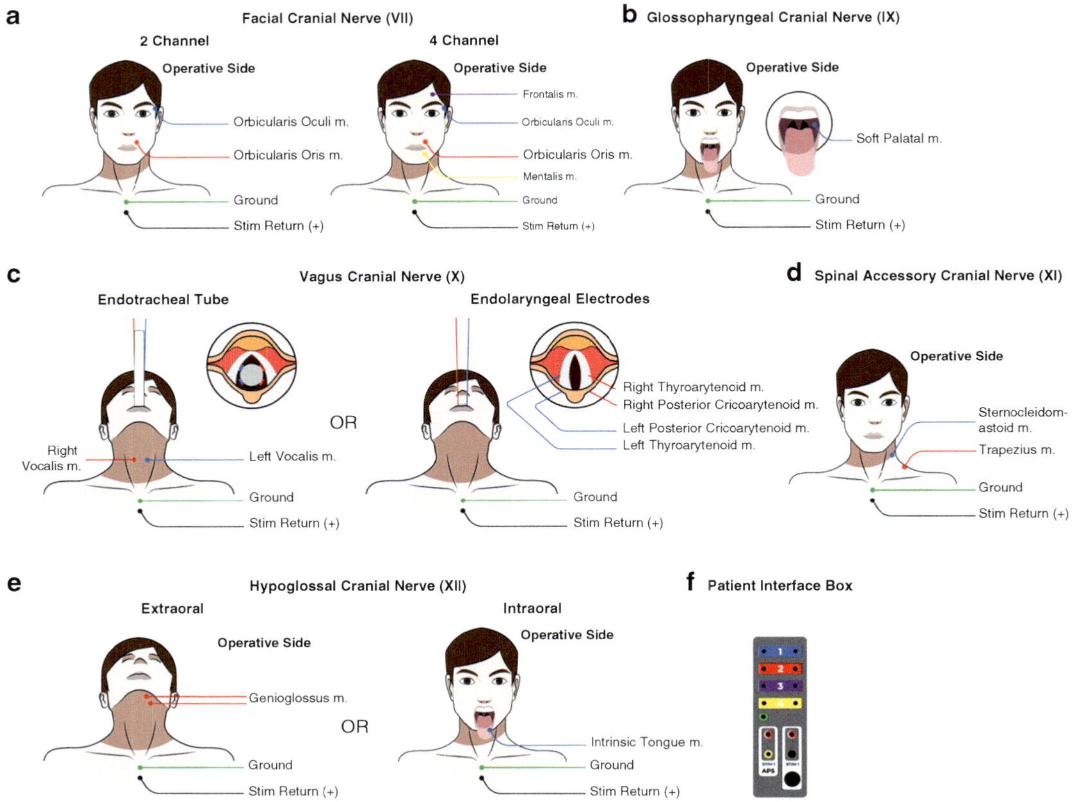

Fig. 3.2 Nerve-specific IONM electrode placement. Recommended placement of electrodes for cranial nerve monitoring of the facial nerve (**a**, using 2 and 4 channels), glossopharyngeal nerve (**b**), vagus nerve (**c**, for the recurrent and superior laryngeal nerves using an endotracheal tube with surface electrodes in contact with the vocal folds or endolaryngeal hookwire electrodes), spinal accessory nerve (**d**) and hypoglossal nerve (**e**, intraoral and extraoral options). The electrodes are connected to the patient interface box (**f**) at the color-coded electrode receiver ports (1, blue; 2, red; 3, purple; and 4, yellow for electrodes placed on target musculature; green for the ground electrode, and white for the cathode (−) of the stimulus output jack (on STIM1 and STIM2 stimulator ports). Note that stimulator probes should be connected on its corresponding anode (+) port. The patient interface box is placed in close proximity to the operative field. Abbreviations: m muscle. (Adapted from *Medtronic NIM 2.0 systems: Protocol and Troubleshooting guide*, 2007, http://electroneurodiagnostics.org/page2/styled-16/files/nim-2.0-system-and-et-tube-placement.pdf, copyright 2007, Medtronic, Inc. Adapted with permission)

necessary to avoid current transfer through the nerve monitoring electrodes causing burns [57].

Facial Nerve (CN VII) Monitoring

The facial nerve (CN VII) and parasympathetic (CN VII) provides motor innervation to mimetic muscles, sensation and taste to the anterior two-thirds of the tongue and parasympathetic innervation to the lacrimal, submandibular and sublingual glands. Motor facial nerve monitoring is commonly employed during middle ear surgery, excision of cerebellopontine angle tumors, parotidectomy, and resection of other cervicofacial masses. Prior to any procedure, a comprehensive and well-documented facial nerve examination is tantamount; one might consider the use of House-Brackmann and/or Sunnybrook facial grading systems to maximize objectivity and promote examination consistency [58, 59]. Sequelae of facial nerve injury range from mild weakness to disfiguring asymmetry and may have a significant impact on quality of life [60].

While several techniques for facial nerve monitoring have been described in the literature, subdermal needle electrode monitoring will be described here given its popularity and feasibility. Advantages to this approach include ease of use, low impedance, and redundancy given monitoring of multiple muscles [61]. Facial nerve monitoring may be achieved using either a two- or four-channel subdermal needle electrode system (Fig. 3.2). In the two-channel system, a pair of blue electrodes monitors the orbicularis oculi muscle with electrodes in the lateral orbital rim and upper eyelid separated by 1.5 cm; a pair of red electrodes is used to monitor the orbicularis oris, placed approximately 5 mm lateral to the oral commissure and along the lower lip separated by 2 cm [62]. Electrode placement is important and may impact the magnitude of recorded EMG signals [62]. The locations of colored electrodes may be remembered using the mnemonic "red lips, blue eyes." Care is taken to avoid placement of needle electrodes in close proximity to the orbit therefore potentially causing damage to the globe and/or postoperative bruising. The ground electrode ("ground is green") may be placed in the forehead and/or alongside the white cathode to the stimulator probe in the deltoid to avoid interference with access to the surgical site [57]. Surgeons may prefer having this prepped into the field to allow for manipulation and troubleshooting during surgery if necessary; in this case, the electrodes may be positioned in the ipsilateral trapezius muscle. For four-channel electrode mapping of the facial nerve, additional electrodes are placed in the frontalis and mentalis muscles to provide comprehensive monitoring of the mimetic musculature (Fig. 3.2). Electrodes may be secured to the skin with clear adhesive therefore allowing identification of electrode displacement if encountered during the case. Confirmation of system integrity can be performed with a firm tap of the overlying skin perpendicular to the electrode eliciting a tonal and/or visual response on the EMG [56]. Of note, this "tap test" assesses the integrity of connection from the electrodes to the monitoring system tower – this is *not* a true assessment of the nerve as it will present with a tonal/visual response even in the event of temporary muscle paralysis (e.g., during muscle relaxation). Stimulation on or around the facial nerve with a sufficient stimulation current (ranging between 0.05 and 0.5 mA for exposed nerve [61]) is necessary to ensure that the neural circuitry is intact and is recommended prior to more extensive dissection around the nerve [56, 57]. Higher stimulation currents may be required if the nerve is surrounded by bone, fascia, or granulation tissue [57, 61, 63].

Systematic use of CN VII monitoring has yet to be uniformly employed; therefore, there are no current guidelines for perioperative facial nerve examinations. Nevertheless, brief postoperative evaluation immediately following patient recovery followed by a more comprehensive and well-documented graded exam at the first postoperative visit is advised.

Glossopharyngeal Nerve (CN IX) Monitoring

The glossopharyngeal nerve (CN IX) is a mixed nerve that provides general, special sensory, parasympathetic, and motor innervation primarily along the posterior tongue and soft palatal region. It exclusively provides motor fibers to the stylopharyngeus muscle, known to assist in swallowing by elevating the larynx and expanding the pharynx [64]. Injury to the glossopharyngeal nerve can contribute to dysphagia. Because of its location proximal to pharyngeal musculature (otherwise supplied by branches of the vagus nerve), it is recommended that both nerves be monitored simultaneously to assist in the selective activation of the glossopharyngeal nerve. Intraoperative nerve monitoring for CN IX may be pursued in skull base surgeries involving the lower brain stem, cerebellopontine angle, jugular foramen, and petroclival region.

Accurate CN IX monitoring entails placement of electrodes along the lateral aspect of the soft palate which can be somewhat challenging given the narrow access to this area and the highly vascular mucosa. Several techniques have been proposed to isolate monitoring of this nerve: Manually curved subdermal electrodes or specially designed hook wire electrodes may be placed into the soft palate following intubation (Fig. 3.2) [65]. Alternatively, use of adhesive electrodes attached to either side of a laryngeal mask airway (LMA) therefore abutting pharyngeal musculature may be used; this can be done in conjunction with electrode-embedded endotracheal tube intubation to simultaneously monitor CN X [66]. Because of the inherent challenges of accurate and safe electrode placement in the posterior pharyngeal wall (risk of hematoma, bleeding, dislodgment with subsequent edema), alternate techniques using a modified endotracheal tube with adherent electrodes have been trialed to better characterize pharyngeal muscle evoked potentials (PhMEP) – which may be useful in predicting early postoperative swallowing outcomes [67]. Pitfalls of CN IX stimulation include bradycardia and hypotension secondary to the afferent input CN IX provides to the carotid body baroreceptors. It is therefore recommended that low stimulus rate and intensity are employed when stimulating CN IX [65].

Vagus Nerve (CN X) Monitoring

The vagus nerve (CN X) is a mixed nerve that carries motor, parasympathetic, and sensory neurons to the head, neck, and thorax. Although branches of the vagus nerve may be at risk in a multitude of head and neck procedures, IONM has been most robustly described in thyroid and parathyroid surgery and will therefore be the context provided here. Two important branches of CN X are the recurrent laryngeal nerve (RLN) which innervates the majority of intrinsic laryngeal musculature and provides sensation to the larynx distal to the glottis and the external branch of the superior laryngeal nerve (EBSLN) which innervates the cricothyroid muscle and provides sensation to the larynx proximal to the glottis.

Guidelines from various associations vary somewhat regarding the role of preoperative laryngoscopy in thyroid surgery. For example, the 2015 American Thyroid Association (ATA) and 2013 American Academy of Otolaryngology-Head and Neck Surgery (AAO-HNS) recommend preoperative laryngoscopy for high-risk patients only [5, 68]. Conversely, the 2011 British Association of Endocrine and Thyroid Surgery and 2016 American Head and Neck Society (AHNS) guidelines recommend preoperative laryngeal examination for all patients undergoing thyroidectomy [69]. Per the INMSG, preoperative flexible laryngoscopy is recommended for a baseline examination prior to undergoing surgery that could potentially affect laryngeal function. The rationale for this recommendation is multifaceted: First, vocal cord paralysis may be asymptomatic, thus use of voice as a predictor for normal vocal fold function is insufficient. Second, identification of vocal cord paralysis in standard preoperative laryngoscopy may denote neural invasion – a finding that can influence surgical planning, shed light upon the extent of disease prior to surgery, and direct patient counseling. Of note, computed tomography yields poor sensitivity for identification of vocal cord paralysis (25%) and for detection of airway invasion by thyroid malignancy (23%) [70] thereby strengthening the recommendation for preoperative laryngoscopy. Also important is the potential for identification of idiopathic vocal cord paralysis. Although this incidence is relatively low, postoperative identification without preoperative baseline documentation could be incorrectly attributed to the surgeon [70]. Finally, and perhaps most importantly, standardization of preoperative laryngoscopy provides a baseline for comparison of postoperative laryngoscopy.

Vagal injury – depending on how proximal along its course it occurs – can be very clinically impactful with sequelae including severe dysphagia, aspiration pneumonia, transient or permanent dysphonia, and breathing difficulties requiring tracheostomy [71]. The INMSG recommends use of endotracheal tube-based systems with audio and visual monitoring of the RLN during surgery [72]. This approach is generally preferred over the use of laryngeal needle electrodes given the risk of vocal cord/laryngeal hematoma, vocal cord laceration, cuff deflation requiring reintubation, retained fractured needle segments, and accidental needle aspiration. Hook electrodes have been used for pediatric laryngeal monitoring when endotracheal-based approaches are not available (Fig. 3.2). Endotracheal tube surface electrodes record EMG data from the thyroarytenoid or vocalis muscle (Fig. 3.2). Monitoring of the posterior cricoarytenoid muscle has been performed using post-cricoid electrode surface arrays. This method has been shown to obtain robust and reliable posterior cricoarytenoid muscle EMG waveforms. This has the potential to directly convey laryngeal abductor functional analysis as well as functional branch assessment in the presence of extra-laryngeal vagal branching [73]. This may be particularly useful in thyroid surgery requiring bilateral neck dissections – during which the risk of bilateral abductor dysfunction must be considered given the risk of acute or chronic central airway obstruction [73, 74]. However additional equipment is required, and its role in clinical practice has yet to be defined.

Additional considerations are required for RLN monitoring in pediatric patients. Use of standard endotracheal tube-based systems is limited in children due to the restricted availability of endotracheal tube sizes (inner diameter ≥5-0, outer diameter ≥6.5, no half-sizes). Endolaryngeal hook wire electrodes have been described as options for pediatric oncologic and/or endocrine resections, or in RLN reinnervation; however, this is not without aforementioned risks of needle-based electrodes in the airway [75–77]. Continuous monitoring with automatic periodic stimulation has also been explored in pediatric patients as a promising option that may be more accurate than intermittent monitoring but requires dissection of the vagus nerve in the carotid sheath [78]. A comprehensive study of adhesive endotracheal surface electrodes in tubes as small as 4.0 mm inner diameter (5.6 mm outer diameter) demonstrated the feasibility of this method in the pediatric population [76].

Because endotracheal tube-dependent monitoring relies on precise positioning of electrodes at the level of the true vocal cords, it requires close partnership with the anesthesia team. Optimal depth of ETT varies by gender: Electrodes are presumably in appropriate position in males when the ETT is 20.6 cm ± 0.97 cm deep and in females at an ETT depth of 19.6 cm ± 1 cm [79]. However these distances can vary considerably between individuals. It is recommended that the anesthesiologist and/or surgeon perform direct laryngoscopy following intubation after the patient is appropriately positioned to ensure accurate ETT location. An alternative is to perform intubation via videolaryngoscopy, such that the surgeon and anesthesia teams can use a high-quality image to visualize and confirm correct placement of the ETT, with electrodes abutting the vocal cords. In addition to glottic inspection, electrode placement may be confirmed by using respiratory variation. Respiratory variation refers to a pattern of small waveforms that range from 30 to 70 μV seen in both monitoring channels if there is appropriate effacement of the electrodes along the vocal cords and the patient is in an appropriately light plane of anesthesia [80]. Following intubation, the patient is lightened from anesthesia enough to confirm respiratory variation, and then anesthesia is deepened in anticipation of surgery. Once confirmed to be in the correct position, the ETT can be directed cephalad and secured, to avoid undue manipulation while operating in the neck (Fig. 3.3). Optimization of the ETT positioning begins with maintaining the tube in the midline position to avoid rotation and therefore disorientation of the red and blue electrode wires at the right and left of the patient, respectively. Conventionally, the red wire denotes the electrodes monitoring the right vocal fold, and the blue wire denotes the left vocal cord; this can be remembered by the mnemonic "red is right." A sponge and/or towels can be used to support the ETT and protect the patient's skin as the tube courses cephalad along the forehead. Ensure that the ETT is securely connected to the circuit – use of a straight connector may facilitate this. Surgeons may consider use of a one- or two-towel head wrap to further stabilize the endotracheal tube (Fig. 3.3). Care

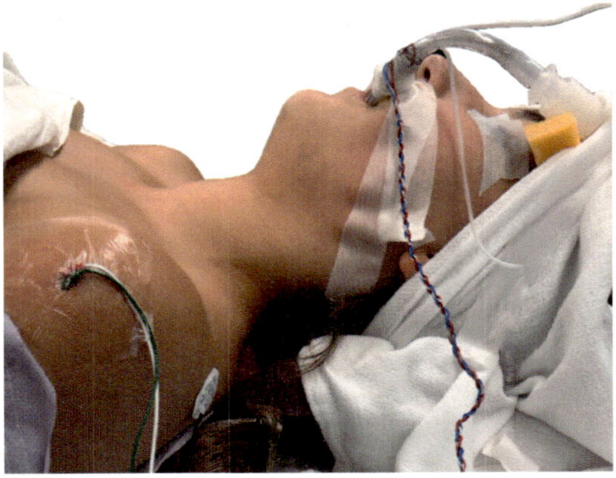

Fig. 3.3 Suggestion for optimization of endotracheal tube positioning

should be taken to avoid undue pressure on the nasal tip nor excessive bend on the endotracheal tube that could limit ventilation prior to proceeding with surgery.

Monitoring of the EBSLN is important to avoid injury which can result in cricothyroid dysfunction – affecting the fundamental frequency of the voice, production of high-frequency phonation, and vocal projection – and loss of sensation to laryngeal mucosa proximal to the glottis [72, 81]. EBSLN dysfunction is challenging to confirm on endoscopic and/or clinical examination alone; IONM provides an objective means of identifying and documenting EBSLN integrity. The INMSG recommends a two-pronged approach to intraoperative EBSLN monitoring: cricothyroid muscle twitch and EMG-glottic waveform confirmation [72]. Because identification of EBSLN during dissection may be challenging, stimulation (with current at 1 mA) of tissues 1–2 mm parallel to the oblique laryngeal attachment of the sternothyroid muscle is recommended. Blind stimulation in this area has been found to reliably stimulate the EBSN and therefore result in cricothyroid muscle twitch [72]. This stimulation may be accompanied by EMG-glottic waveform in 70–80% of patients; this is due to a small branch of EBSLN that extends into the larynx to innervate the anterior one-third of the ipsilateral vocal cord [82–84]. The depolarization measured on the glottic surface endotracheal tube electrodes is of small amplitude and short latency and sensitive to positioning of the endotracheal tube, possibly contributing to the inconsistent stimulation [72]. If cricothyroid muscle twitch is observed (with or without EMG-glottic waveform) at the time of presumed EBSLN stimulation around 1 mA, this is thought to be a true positive. Similarly, a true-negative response is defined as absence of cricothyroid muscle twitch with stimulation of non-EBLSN tissue. Use of currents greater than 1 mA may result in a false-positive stimulation (positive cricothyroid muscle twitch in absence of true EBSLN stimulation); therefore, use of a stimulation current between 0.8 and 1 mA is recommended [72].

Prior to initiation of dissection, it is recommended that suprathreshold vagal stimulation is performed to ensure that the nerve is appropriately being monitored and to validate negative stimulations during the dissection when a candidate nerve is being interrogated [6]. Doing so demonstrates intact neural circuitry and confirms nerve integrity prior to onset of dissection. This can be done without extensive vagal dissection by placement of the stimulator probe (current ranging 1–2 mA) between the carotid artery and internal jugular vein [85]. For accurate prognostication of postoperative glottic function, suprathreshold stimulation of the vagal pathway should also be performed at the end of the case [6, 86]. This does not replace the value of postoperative flexible laryngoscopy which remains important. Similar to preoperative laryngoscopy, guidelines vary somewhat regarding the need for symptoms to justify routine laryngoscopic assessment following surgery [87]. It is the recommendation of the authors that postoperative laryngoscopy be performed because it remains the only sufficient RLN outcome measure that denotes significant clinical implications and informs on the risk of contralateral surgery in the future [85]. Although the ideal timing of laryngoscopic evaluation remains somewhat elusive, postoperative day 2 has been suggested [88].

Finally, continuous vagal nerve monitoring (c-IONM) merits brief discussion. Continuous IONM permits ongoing monitoring of the RLN and vagal circuitry during surgery and provides real-time feedback by way of an implantable vagal electrode [89]. Electrodes vary in composition and size but are designed to provide a safe, augmentable nerve monitoring system that may be more effective than intermittent IONM in preventing vocal cord dysfunction [90]. Continuous IONM requires baseline amplitudes greater than 500 μV; this is in comparison to suggested monitor event thresholds of 100 μV with use of intermittent IONM. Ideally, c-IONM may serve as a warning system during dissection around the nerve, alerting the surgeon to impending injury before it happens via continuous EMG [91]. Continuous IONM has also been used successfully in the pediatric population [78]. Use of c-IONM is inherently limited by the need for identification and dissection of the vagus nerve prior to implantable electrode positioning – which can present its own challenges. However, with ongoing studies and modifications of this more recently described method of IONM, surgeons are likely to see continuous monitoring employed more frequently as an adjunct to open, endoscopic, and robotic surgery moving forward [92, 93]. For additional details, refer to Chaps. 7, 8, and 9.

Spinal Accessory Nerve (CN XI)

The spinal accessory nerve is unique in that it receives motor efferent fibers from the C6 and C7 cervical roots to innervate the trapezius and sternocleidomastoid muscles. Its trajectory through the neck puts it at risk of traction injuries during oncologic dissections with functional sequelae including shoulder droop, weakness of contralateral head rotation, and limited abduction of the upper extremity and scapula flaring despite CN XI preservation [94, 95]. A correlation between IONM of CN XI and postoperative shoulder function has been described – specifically, significant EMG changes during dissection portending poorer short-term functional outcomes [96]. However, more robust, randomized studies are warranted to understand the role of IONM in greater detail.

For IONM of CN XI, subdermal electrodes can be placed into the trapezius muscle at the level of C7, approximately 5 cm from midline (Fig. 3.2). Ground and stimulating electrodes can be placed in deltoid musculature, as previously described. Preoperatively, shoulder and head range of motion and strength testing should be performed as part of the extended cranial nerve examination. Postoperatively a similar examination should occur. Because shoulder dysfunction is relatively common in patients undergoing surgery for head and neck cancers, several rehabilitative measures have been investigated including intraoperative brief electrical stimulation (BES) of the nerve to promote neural regrowth in the event of injury [97].

Hypoglossal Nerve (CN XII)

The hypoglossal nerve provides motor innervation to the intrinsic tongue muscles (styloglossus, genioglossus, and hyoglossus). Hypoglossal weakness is characterized by tongue deviation toward the side of the lesion and can result in dysarthria and oral phase dysphagia. Surgeries of the posterior fossa and suprahyoid neck dissection can result in injury to the proximal and distal extent of the hypoglossal nerve, respectively. Use of IONM, although less commonly employed for lower cranial nerves, may minimize this risk [98, 99].

For intraoperative monitoring of CN XII, needle electrodes should be placed along the midline of the tongue and secured to the perioral skin with adhesive tape to prevent displacement (Fig. 3.2). Consider use of a bite block to prevent clenching and resultant dislodgment of electrodes. Alternatively, extra-oral monitoring may be achieved by isolating the genioglossus muscle, which extends from the genial/mental spine of the mandible to the hyoid bone and dorsum of the tongue. Paired monopolar EMG electrodes can be inserted 1 cm lateral to the submandibular midline and 1 cm dorsal to the chin with forceful protrusion of the tongue assisting in genioglossus identification (Fig. 3.2) [100].

Review of Brachial Plexus and Spinal Monitoring

Minimally invasive approaches to the thyroid and parathyroid glands require vagal IONM as well as monitoring of the brachial plexus given the risk of position-related traction and compression injuries during transaxillary approaches [101]. Transaxillary robotic thyroid surgery requires nearly a 180° flexion of the shoulder with internal rotation and a 90° flexion at the elbow; it is not surprising that transient brachial plexopathies may occur as a result of this positioning [102]. SSEP has been applied to robotic thyroidectomies and has been found to be a safe method for identification and prevention of injuries from brachial plexus traction [9]. SSEP utilizes intraoperative neurophysiologic monitoring and uses amplitude and latency patterns to predict neural injury. When applied to robotic thyroid and parathyroid surgery, SSEP monitors three brachial plexus branches (median, radial, and ulnar nerves) ipsilateral to the site of transaxillary approach with the contralateral median nerve serving as a control. Huang et al. (2019) reviewed use of SSEP in a large cohort of transaxillary robotic thyroid cases and highlighted its ability to intraoperatively identify a modifiable decline in brachial plexus SSEP – consistent with impending injury – that improved with patient repositioning [9].

Similar principles are employed with use of intraoperative nerve monitoring in spine surgery – in which neurologic injury is one of the most feared outcomes [103, 104]. The most commonly used form of IONM in spinal surgery is SSEP with evidence of improved neurologic outcomes and a reported clinically relevant neurologic event detection rate of 90% [105–107]. However, there are limitations with use of SSEP in spinal monitoring – in particular, concern for errors associated with false-positive and false-negative events [108, 109]. To address this, multimodal IONM has been proposed: Use of continuous intraoperative evoked EMG – highly sensitive to nerve root manipulation but nonspecific in predicting persistent neurologic defects – may be used in conjunction with SSEP, which has low sensitivity but high specificity in detecting neurologic events [108]. Further details regarding brachial plexus and spinal monitoring can be found in Chap. 19.

Conclusion

This chapter has provided a review of anesthetic considerations and nerve monitoring setup with the goal of creating a feasible and accessible approach to IONM during head and neck surgery. Additional details on the rationale for IONM, indications for monitoring, and risks of injury to the major nerves of the head and neck are elucidated in more detail throughout this book.

References

1. Chung TK, Rosenthal EL, Porterfield JR, Carroll WR, Richman J, Hawn MT. Examining national outcomes after thyroidectomy with nerve monitoring. J Am Coll Surg. 2014;219(4):765–70.
2. Chiang FY, Lu IC, Kuo WR, Lee KW, Chang NC, Wu CW. The mechanism of recurrent laryngeal nerve injury during thyroid surgery--the application of intraoperative neuromonitoring. Surgery. 2008;143(6):743–9.
3. Snyder SK, Sigmond BR, Lairmore TC, Govednik-Horny CM, Janicek AK, Jupiter DC. The long-term impact of routine intraoperative nerve monitoring during thyroid and parathyroid surgery. Surgery. 2013;154(4):704–11; discussion 711–703.
4. Chan WF, Lang BH, Lo CY. The role of intraoperative neuromonitoring of recurrent laryngeal nerve during thyroidectomy: a comparative study on 1000 nerves at risk. Surgery. 2006;140(6):866–72; discussion 872–863.
5. Chandrasekhar SS, Randolph GW, Seidman MD, et al. Clinical practice guideline: improving voice outcomes after thyroid surgery. Otolaryngol Head Neck Surg. 2013;148(6 Suppl):S1–37.
6. Randolph GW, Dralle H, Group wtIIMS, et al. Electrophysiologic recurrent laryngeal nerve monitoring during thyroid and parathyroid surgery: international standards guideline statement. Laryngoscope. 2011;121(S1):S1–S16.
7. Sloan T. Anesthesia and intraoperative neurophysiological monitoring in children. Childs Nerv Syst. 2010;26(2):227–35.
8. Deiner S. Highlights of anesthetic considerations for intraoperative neuromonitoring. Semin Cardiothorac Vasc Anesth. 2010;14(1):51–3.
9. Huang S, Garstka ME, Murcy MA, et al. Somatosensory evoked potential: preventing brachial plexus injury in transaxillary robotic surgery. Laryngoscope. 2019;129(11):2663–8.
10. Deletis V, Sala F. Intraoperative neurophysiological monitoring of the spinal cord during spinal cord and spine surgery: a review focus on the corticospinal tracts. Clin Neurophysiol. 2008;119(2):248–64.
11. Sloan TB. Muscle relaxant use during intraoperative neurophysiologic monitoring. J Clin Monit Comput. 2013;27(1):35–46.
12. Ortega R, Brull SJ, Prielipp R, Gutierrez A, De La Cruz R, Conley CM. Monitoring neuromuscular function. N Engl J Med. 2018;378(4):e6.

13. Bevan DR, Donati F, Kopman AF. Reversal of neuromuscular blockade. Anesthesiology. 1992;77(4):785–805.
14. Suy K, Morias K, Cammu G, et al. Effective reversal of moderate rocuronium- or vecuronium-induced neuromuscular block with sugammadex, a selective relaxant binding agent. Anesthesiology. 2007;106(2):283–8.
15. Carron M, Zarantonello F, Tellaroli P, Ori C. Efficacy and safety of sugammadex compared to neostigmine for reversal of neuromuscular blockade: a meta-analysis of randomized controlled trials. J Clin Anesth. 2016;35:1–12.
16. Lu IC, Wu SH, Wu CW. Neuromuscular blockade management for intraoperative neural monitoring. Kaohsiung J Med Sci. 2020;36(4):230–5.
17. Gunes ME, Dural AC, Akarsu C, et al. Effect of intraoperative neuromonitoring on efficacy and safety using sugammadex in thyroid surgery: randomized clinical trial. Ann Surg Treat Res. 2019;97(6):282–90.
18. Pavoni V, Gianesello L, Martinelli C, et al. Recovery of laryngeal nerve function with sugammadex after rocuronium-induced profound neuromuscular block. J Clin Anesth. 2016;33:14–9.
19. Lu IC, Chang PY, Su MP, et al. The feasibility of sugammadex for general anesthesia and facial nerve monitoring in patients undergoing parotid surgery. Kaohsiung J Med Sci. 2017;33(8):400–4.
20. Fabregat López J, Porta Vila G, Martin-Flores M. Reversal of moderate and intense neuromuscular block induced by rocuronium with low doses of sugammadex for intraoperative facial nerve monitoring. Rev Esp Anestesiol Reanim. 2013;60(8):465–8.
21. Donati F, Meistelman C, Plaud B. Vecuronium neuromuscular blockade at the diaphragm, the orbicularis oculi, and adductor pollicis muscles. Anesthesiology. 1990;73(5):870–5.
22. Donati F, Meistelman C, Plaud B. Vecuronium neuromuscular blockade at the adductor muscles of the larynx and adductor pollicis. Anesthesiology. 1991;74(5):833–7.
23. Plaud B, Debaene B, Donati F. The corrugator supercilii, not the orbicularis oculi, reflects rocuronium neuromuscular blockade at the laryngeal adductor muscles. Anesthesiology. 2001;95(1):96–101.
24. Cai YR, Xu J, Chen LH, Chi FL. Electromyographic monitoring of facial nerve under different levels of neuromuscular blockade during middle ear microsurgery. Chin Med J. 2009;122(3):311–4.
25. Kizilay A, Aladag I, Cokkeser Y, Miman MC, Ozturan O, Gulhas N. Effects of partial neuromuscular blockade on facial nerve monitorization in otologic surgery. Acta Otolaryngol. 2003;123(2):321–4.
26. Marusch F, Hussock J, Haring G, Hachenberg T, Gastinger I. Influence of muscle relaxation on neuromonitoring of the recurrent laryngeal nerve during thyroid surgery. Br J Anaesth. 2005;94(5):596–600.
27. Chu KS, Wu SH, Lu IC, et al. Feasibility of intraoperative neuromonitoring during thyroid surgery after administration of nondepolarizing neuromuscular blocking agents. World J Surg. 2009;33(7):1408–13.
28. Meistelman C. Effects on laryngeal muscles and intubating conditions with new generation muscle relaxants. Acta Anaesthesiol Belg. 1997;48(1):11–4.
29. Bragg P, Fisher DM, Shi J, et al. Comparison of twitch depression of the adductor pollicis and the respiratory muscles. Pharmacodynamic modeling without plasma concentrations. Anesthesiology. 1994;80(2):310–9.
30. Wright PM, Caldwell JE, Miller RD. Onset and duration of rocuronium and succinylcholine at the adductor pollicis and laryngeal adductor muscles in anesthetized humans. Anesthesiology. 1994;81(5):1110–5.
31. Macdonald DB, Skinner S, Shils J, Yingling C, American Society of Neurophysiological Monitoring. Intraoperative motor evoked potential monitoring – a position statement by the American Society of Neurophysiological Monitoring. Clin Neurophysiol. 2013;124(12):2291–316.
32. Sloan TB, Erian R. Effect of atracurium-induced neuromuscular block on cortical motor-evoked potentials. Anesth Analg. 1993;76(5):979–84.
33. Hanci V, Erdoğan G, Okyay RD, et al. Effects of fentanyl-lidocaine-propofol and dexmedetomidine-lidocaine-propofol on tracheal intubation without use of muscle relaxants. Kaohsiung J Med Sci. 2010;26(5):244–50.
34. Mencke T, Echternach M, Kleinschmidt S, et al. Laryngeal morbidity and quality of tracheal intubation: a randomized controlled trial. Anesthesiology. 2003;98(5):1049–56.
35. Mencke T, Knoll H, Schreiber JU, et al. Rocuronium is not associated with more vocal cord injuries than succinylcholine after rapid-sequence induction: a randomized, prospective, controlled trial. Anesth Analg. 2006;102(3):943–9.
36. Orebaugh SL. Succinylcholine: adverse effects and alternatives in emergency medicine. Am J Emerg Med. 1999;17(7):715–21.
37. Miller R. Will succinylcholine ever disappear? Anesth Analg. 2004;98(6):1674–5.
38. Debaene B, Plaud B, Dilly MP, Donati F. Residual paralysis in the PACU after a single intubating dose of nondepolarizing muscle relaxant with an intermediate duration of action. Anesthesiology. 2003;98(5):1042–8.
39. Lu IC, Tsai CJ, Wu CW, et al. A comparative study between 1 and 2 effective doses of rocuronium for intraoperative neuromonitoring during thyroid surgery. Surgery. 2011;149(4):543–8.
40. Brunaud L, Fuchs-Buder T. In reference to reversal of rocuronium-induced neuromuscular blockade by sugammadex allows for optimization of neural monitoring of the recurrent laryngeal nerve. Laryngoscope. 2017;127(1):E50.
41. Lu IC, Wu CW, Chang PY, et al. In response to reversal of rocuronium-induced neuromuscular blockade by sugammadex allows for optimization of

neural monitoring of the recurrent laryngeal nerve. Laryngoscope. 2017;127(1):E51–e52.
42. Empis de Vendin O, Schmartz D, Brunaud L, Fuchs-Buder T. Recurrent laryngeal nerve monitoring and rocuronium: a selective sugammadex reversal protocol. World J Surg. 2017;41(9):2298–303.
43. Errando CL, Blanco T, Díaz-Cambronero Ó. Repeated sugammadex reversal of muscle relaxation during lumbar spine surgery with intraoperative neurophysiological multimodal monitoring. Rev Esp Anestesiol Reanim. 2016;63(9):533–8.
44. Trifa M, Krishna S, Mello A, Hakim M, Tobias J. Sugammadex to reverse neuromuscular blockade and provide optimal conditions for motor-evoked potential monitoring. Saudi J Anaesth. 2017;11(2):219–21.
45. Fudickar A, Bein B, Tonner PH. Propofol infusion syndrome in anaesthesia and intensive care medicine. Curr Opin Anaesthesiol. 2006;19(4):404–10.
46. Kam PC, Cardone D. Propofol infusion syndrome. Anaesthesia. 2007;62(7):690–701.
47. Liolios A, Guérit JM, Scholtes JL, Raftopoulos C, Hantson P. Propofol infusion syndrome associated with short-term large-dose infusion during surgical anesthesia in an adult. Anesth Analg. 2005;100(6):1804–6.
48. Echeverri A, Flexon PB. Electrophysiologic nerve stimulation for identifying the recurrent laryngeal nerve in thyroid surgery: review of 70 consecutive thyroid surgeries. Am Surg. 1998;64(4):328–33.
49. Hamelmann WH, Meyer T, Timm S, Timmermann W. A critical estimation of intraoperative neuromonitoring (IONM) in thyroid surgery. Zentralbl Chir. 2002;127(5):409–13.
50. Thomusch O, Sekulla C, Machens A, Neumann HJ, Timmermann W, Dralle H. Validity of intra-operative neuromonitoring signals in thyroid surgery. Langenbeck's Arch Surg. 2004;389(6):499–503.
51. Abt NB, Puram SV, Kamani D, Modi R, Randolph GW. Neuromonitored thyroid surgery: optimal stimulation based on intraoperative EMG response features. Laryngoscope. 2020;130(12):E970–e975.
52. Chiang FY, Lu IC, Chang PY, et al. Stimulating dissecting instruments during neuromonitoring of RLN in thyroid surgery. Laryngoscope. 2015;125(12):2832–7.
53. Bly RA, Holdefer RN, Slimp J, et al. Preoperative facial nerve mapping to plan and guide pediatric facial vascular anomaly resection. JAMA Otolaryngol Head Neck Surg. 2018;144(5):418–26.
54. Chiara J, Kinney G, Slimp J, Lee GS, Oliaei S, Perkins JA. Facial nerve mapping and monitoring in lymphatic malformation surgery. Int J Pediatr Otorhinolaryngol. 2009;73(10):1348–52.
55. Sala F, Krzan MJ, Deletis V. Intraoperative neurophysiological monitoring in pediatric neurosurgery: why, when, how? Childs Nerv Syst. 2002;18(6–7):264–87.
56. Kartush J, Benscoter B. Intraoperative Facial Nerve Monitoring. In: Guntinas-Lichius O, Schaitkin BM. Facial Nerve Disorders and Diseases: Diagnosis and Management. 1st ed. Thieme; 2016:200–12.
57. Eshraghi AA, Connell SS, Chang RC, Telischi FF. Chapter 64 – Intraoperative neurophysiologic monitoring. In: Brackmann DE, Shelton C, Arriaga MA, editors. Otologic surgery. 3rd ed. Philadelphia: W.B. Saunders; 2010. p. 773–84.
58. Neely JG, Cherian NG, Dickerson CB, Nedzelski JM. Sunnybrook facial grading system: reliability and criteria for grading. Laryngoscope. 2010;120(5):1038–45.
59. House JW, Brackmann DE. Facial nerve grading system. Otolaryngol Head Neck Surg. 1985;93(2):146–7.
60. Ryzenman JM, Pensak ML, Tew JM Jr. Facial paralysis and surgical rehabilitation: a quality of life analysis in a cohort of 1,595 patients after acoustic neuroma surgery. Otol Neurotol. 2005;26(3):516–21; discussion 521.
61. Prass RL. Iatrogenic facial nerve injury: the role of facial nerve monitoring. Otolaryngol Clin N Am. 1996;29(2):265–75.
62. Guo L, Jasiukaitis P, Pitts LH, Cheung SW. Optimal placement of recording electrodes for quantifying facial nerve compound muscle action potential. Otol Neurotol. 2008;29(5):710–3.
63. Choung YH, Park K, Cho MJ, Choung PH, Shin YR, Kahng H. Systematic facial nerve monitoring in middle ear and mastoid surgeries: "surgical dehiscence" and "electrical dehiscence". Otolaryngol Head Neck Surg. 2006;135(6):872–6.
64. Erman AB, Kejner AE, Hogikyan ND, Feldman EL. Disorders of cranial nerves IX and X. Semin Neurol. 2009;29(1):85–92.
65. Singh R, Husain AM. Neurophysiologic intraoperative monitoring of the glossopharyngeal and vagus nerves. J Clin Neurophysiol. 2011;28(6):582–6.
66. Husain AM, Wright DR, Stolp BW, Friedman AH, Keifer JC. Neurophysiological intraoperative monitoring of the glossopharyngeal nerve: technical case report. Neurosurgery. 2008;63(4 Suppl 2):277–8; discussion 278.
67. Fukuda M, Oishi M, Hiraishi T, Saito A, Fujii Y. Pharyngeal motor evoked potentials elicited by transcranial electrical stimulation for intraoperative monitoring during skull base surgery. J Neurosurg. 2012;116(3):605–10.
68. Haugen BR, Alexander EK, Bible KC, et al. 2015 American Thyroid Association management guidelines for adult patients with thyroid nodules and differentiated thyroid Cancer: the American Thyroid Association guidelines task force on thyroid nodules and differentiated thyroid cancer. Thyroid. 2016;26(1):1–133.
69. Sinclair CF, Bumpous JM, Haugen BR, et al. Laryngeal examination in thyroid and parathyroid surgery: an American Head and Neck Society Consensus Statement: AHNS Consensus Statement. Head Neck. 2016;38(6):811–9.
70. Randolph GW, Kamani D. The importance of preoperative laryngoscopy in patients undergoing thyroidectomy: voice, vocal cord function, and the preoperative detection of invasive thyroid malignancy. Surgery. 2006;139(3):357–62.

71. Nouraei SAR, Allen J, Kaddour H, et al. Vocal palsy increases the risk of lower respiratory tract infection in low-risk, low-morbidity patients undergoing thyroidectomy for benign disease: a big data analysis. Clin Otolaryngol. 2017;42(6):1259–66.
72. Barczyński M, Randolph GW, Cernea CR, et al. External branch of the superior laryngeal nerve monitoring during thyroid and parathyroid surgery: International Neural Monitoring Study Group standards guideline statement. Laryngoscope. 2013;123(S4):S1–S14.
73. Liddy W, Barber SR, Lin BM, et al. Monitoring of the posterior cricoarytenoid muscle represents another option for neural monitoring during thyroid surgery: normative vagal and recurrent laryngeal nerve posterior cricoarytenoid muscle electromyographic data. Laryngoscope. 2018;128(1):283–9.
74. Eckel HE, Thumfart M, Wassermann K, Vössing M, Thumfart WF. Cordectomy versus arytenoidectomy in the management of bilateral vocal cord paralysis. Ann Otol Rhinol Laryngol. 1994;103(11): 852–7.
75. Caloway CL, Diercks GR, Randolph G, Hartnick CJ. Vagal stimulation and laryngeal electromyography for recurrent laryngeal reinnervation in children. Laryngoscope. 2020;130(3):747–51.
76. Propst EJ, Gorodensky J, Wasserman JD, Glazman EF, Tilis LA, Wolter NE. Recurrent laryngeal nerve monitoring with surface electrodes in pediatric thyroid surgery. Laryngoscope. 2020;130(6):1583–9.
77. Ritter A, Hod R, Reuven Y, et al. Role of intraoperative recurrent laryngeal nerve monitoring for pediatric thyroid surgery: comparative analysis. Head Neck. 2020;43:849–57.
78. Schneider R, Machens A, Sekulla C, Lorenz K, Weber F, Dralle H. Twenty-year experience of paediatric thyroid surgery using intraoperative nerve monitoring. Br J Surg. 2018;105(8):996–1005.
79. Lu IC, Chu KS, Tsai CJ, et al. Optimal depth of NIM EMG endotracheal tube for intraoperative neuromonitoring of the recurrent laryngeal nerve during thyroidectomy. World J Surg. 2008;32(9):1935–9.
80. Chambers KJ, Pearse A, Coveney J, et al. Respiratory variation predicts optimal endotracheal tube placement for intra-operative nerve monitoring in thyroid and parathyroid surgery. World J Surg. 2015;39(2):393–9.
81. Barczyński M, Konturek A, Stopa M, Honowska A, Nowak W. Randomized controlled trial of visualization versus neuromonitoring of the external branch of the superior laryngeal nerve during thyroidectomy. World J Surg. 2012;36(6):1340–7.
82. Maranillo E, León X, Quer M, Orús C, Sañudo JR. Is the external laryngeal nerve an exclusively motor nerve? The cricothyroid connection branch. Laryngoscope. 2003;113(3):525–9.
83. Morton RP, Whitfield P, Al-Ali S. Anatomical and surgical considerations of the external branch of the superior laryngeal nerve: a systematic review. Clin Otolaryngol. 2006;31(5):368–74.
84. Kochilas X, Bibas A, Xenellis J, Anagnostopoulou S. Surgical anatomy of the external branch of the superior laryngeal nerve and its clinical significance in head and neck surgery. Clin Anat. 2008;21(2):99–105.
85. Randolph GW, Kamani D, Wu C-W, Schneider R. Chapter 36 – Surgical anatomy and monitoring of the recurrent laryngeal nerve. In: Randolph GW, editor. Surgery of the thyroid and parathyroid glands. 3rd ed. Philadelphia: Elsevier; 2021. p. 326–359.e310.
86. Dralle H, Sekulla C, Haerting J, et al. Risk factors of paralysis and functional outcome after recurrent laryngeal nerve monitoring in thyroid surgery. Surgery. 2004;136(6):1310–22.
87. Shonka DC Jr, Terris DJ. The American Thyroid Association guidelines on voice assessment-have we done enough? JAMA Otolaryngol Head Neck Surg. 2016;142(2):115–6.
88. Dionigi G, Boni L, Rovera F, Rausei S, Castelnuovo P, Dionigi R. Postoperative laryngoscopy in thyroid surgery: proper timing to detect recurrent laryngeal nerve injury. Langenbeck's Arch Surg. 2010;395(4):327–31.
89. Lamadé W, Meyding-Lamadé U, Buchhold C, et al. First continuous nerve monitoring in thyroid gland surgery. Chirurg. 2000;71(5):551–7.
90. Schneider R, Sekulla C, Machens A, Lorenz K, Nguyen Thanh P, Dralle H. Postoperative vocal fold palsy in patients undergoing thyroid surgery with continuous or intermittent nerve monitoring. Br J Surg. 2015;102(11):1380–7.
91. Schneider R, Przybyl J, Hermann M, Hauss J, Jonas S, Leinung S. A new anchor electrode design for continuous neuromonitoring of the recurrent laryngeal nerve by vagal nerve stimulations. Langenbeck's Arch Surg. 2009;394(5):903–10.
92. Dionigi G, Kim HY, Wu CW, et al. Neuromonitoring in endoscopic and robotic thyroidectomy. Updat Surg. 2017;69(2):171–9.
93. Lörincz BB, Möckelmann N, Busch CJ, Hezel M, Knecht R. Automatic periodic stimulation of the vagus nerve during single-incision transaxillary robotic thyroidectomy: feasibility, safety, and first cases. Head Neck. 2016;38(3):482–5.
94. Cappiello J, Piazza C, Giudice M, De Maria G, Nicolai P. Shoulder disability after different selective neck dissections (levels II–IV versus levels II–V): a comparative study. Laryngoscope. 2005;115(2):259–63.
95. Leipzig B, Suen JY, English JL, Barnes J, Hooper M. Functional evaluation of the spinal accessory nerve after neck dissection. Am J Surg. 1983;146(4):526–30.
96. Birinci Y, Genc A, Ecevit MC, et al. Spinal accessory nerve monitoring and clinical outcome results of nerve-sparing neck dissections. Otolaryngol Head Neck Surg. 2014;151(2):253–9.
97. Barber B, Seikaly H, Ming Chan K, et al. Intraoperative Brief Electrical Stimulation of the

Spinal Accessory Nerve (BEST SPIN) for prevention of shoulder dysfunction after oncologic neck dissection: a double-blinded, randomized controlled trial. J Otolaryngol Head Neck Surg. 2018; 47(1):7.

98. Topsakal C, Al-Mefty O, Bulsara KR, Williford VS. Intraoperative monitoring of lower cranial nerves in skull base surgery: technical report and review of 123 monitored cases. Neurosurg Rev. 2008;31(1):45–53.
99. Ishikawa M, Kusaka G, Takashima K, Kamochi H, Shinoda S. Intraoperative monitoring during surgery for hypoglossal schwannoma. J Clin Neurosci. 2010;17(8):1053–6.
100. Skinner SA. Neurophysiologic monitoring of the spinal accessory nerve, hypoglossal nerve, and the spinomedullary region. J Clin Neurophysiol. 2011;28(6):587–98.
101. Kandil E, Abdelghani S, Noureldine SI, et al. Transaxillary gasless robotic thyroidectomy: a single surgeon's experience in North America. Arch Otolaryngol Head Neck Surg. 2012;138(2):113–7.
102. Landry CS, Grubbs EG, Morris GS, et al. Robot assisted transaxillary surgery (RATS) for the removal of thyroid and parathyroid glands. Surgery. 2011;149(4):549–55.
103. Ahn H, Fehlings MG. Prevention, identification, and treatment of perioperative spinal cord injury. Neurosurg Focus. 2008;25(5):E15.
104. Fehlings MG, Brodke DS, Norvell DC, Dettori JR. The evidence for intraoperative neurophysiological monitoring in spine surgery: does it make a difference? Spine (Phila Pa 1976). 2010;35(9 Suppl):S37–46.
105. Nuwer MR, Dawson EG, Carlson LG, Kanim LE, Sherman JE. Somatosensory evoked potential spinal cord monitoring reduces neurologic deficits after scoliosis surgery: results of a large multicenter survey. Electroencephalogr Clin Neurophysiol. 1995;96(1):6–11.
106. Dawson EG, Sherman JE, Kanim LE, Nuwer MR. Spinal cord monitoring. Results of the Scoliosis Research Society and the European Spinal Deformity Society survey. Spine (Phila Pa 1976). 1991;16(8 Suppl):S361–4.
107. Herdmann J, Deletis V, Edmonds HL Jr, Morota N. Spinal cord and nerve root monitoring in spine surgery and related procedures. Spine (Phila Pa 1976). 1996;21(7):879–85.
108. Gunnarsson T, Krassioukov AV, Sarjeant R, Fehlings MG. Real-time continuous intraoperative electromyographic and somatosensory evoked potential recordings in spinal surgery: correlation of clinical and electrophysiologic findings in a prospective, consecutive series of 213 cases. Spine (Phila Pa 1976). 2004;29(6):677–84.
109. Lesser RP, Raudzens P, Lüders H, et al. Postoperative neurological deficits may occur despite unchanged intraoperative somatosensory evoked potentials. Ann Neurol. 1986;19(1):22–5.

Neural Injury Mechanisms

4

Kevin J. Contrera, Tomislav Novosel,
and Joseph Scharpf

Injuries to cranial nerves range from 3% to 12% after thyroidectomy [1–4] and 6% to 46% after other head and neck surgeries [5–8]. Depending on the cranial nerve involved, it is estimated that only one-tenth of injuries are recognized intraoperatively [9, 10]. An even lower number of these will have a known source of injury. Nevertheless, understanding the different types and mechanisms of nerve injury will aid in surgeons' ability to not only manage but also reduce the risk of harm.

Basic Anatomy and Physiology of Peripheral Nerves

Familiarity with the most basic anatomic elements of a peripheral nerve is necessary for comprehension of the distinct locations of neural injury. Axons, sometimes referred to as nerve fibers, are the basic conduction units of the neuron. These are encased in a connective tissue layer called the endoneurium. Multiple of these units are bunched into a fascicle, which is in turn wrapped in another layer of connective tissue, known as the perineurium. Numerous fascicles are encased in a third layer and final layer along with vessels by the epineurium. The peripheral nerves of greatest interest to the head and neck surgeon (e.g., vagus, facial, glossopharyngeal, and hypoglossal) are predominantly motor but also include sensory, sympathetic, and parasympathetic fibers.

When the axon is injured (Fig. 4.1), subsequent loss of signal occurs distal to the site of injury due to degradation of the myelin sheath and infiltration of macrophages. This is known as Wallerian degeneration, which begins within 24–36 hours of the insult and is completed in 3–4 days. Importantly, this means that a nerve can be stimulated intraoperatively distal, but not proximal, to the site of injury, allowing for localization of the site of damage. This is sometimes referred to as Type I injury, particularly within literature specific to the recurrent laryngeal nerve (RLN) [11–13]. It is contrast to Type II injury, where the nerve is globally damaged, inhibiting stimulation at any segment of the nerve, usually with no localized appearance of injury.

Classification of Injury

Seddon Classification

The first modern organization of peripheral nerve injuries was defined by Dr. Herbert Seddon in

K. J. Contrera (✉) · J. Scharpf
Head and Neck Institute, Cleveland Clinic, Cleveland, OH, USA
e-mail: contrek@ccf.org; scharpj@ccf.org

T. Novosel
Thyroid and Parathyroid Center, Klinikum Bad Salzungen GmbH, Bad Salzungen, Germany

© The Author(s), under exclusive license to Springer Nature Switzerland AG 2022

J. Scharpf, G. W. Randolph (eds.), *Intraoperative Cranial Nerve Monitoring in Otolaryngology-Head and Neck Surgery*, https://doi.org/10.1007/978-3-030-84916-0_4

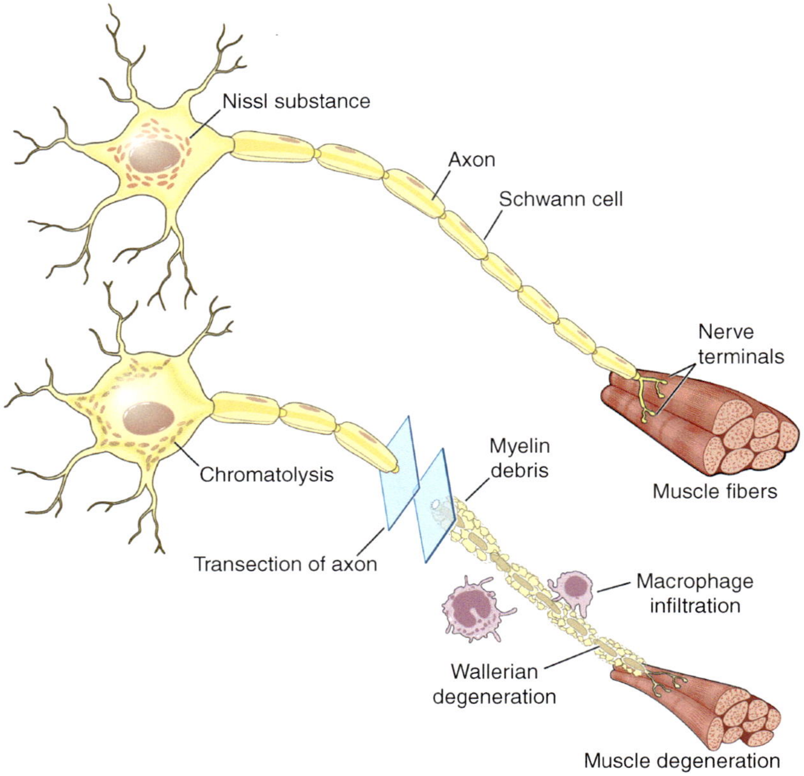

Fig. 4.1 Peripheral nerve injury induced by transection. (Illustration by David Schumick, BS, CMI. Reprinted with the permission of the Cleveland Clinic Center for Medical Art & Photography ©2020/2021. All Rights Reserved)

1943 [14]. He standardized nomenclature surrounding three types of neural insults based on the severity of tissue damage and potential for recovery: neuropraxia, axonotmesis, and neurotmesis.

Neuropraxia ("praxis" is "to perform") refers to the inability of the nerve to conduct an impulse. There is no violation of the axon or perineurium. It is the mildest form of injury with degeneration limited to the myelin sheath. Expected recovery is complete and relatively rapid, typically ranging from days to weeks [15].

Axonotmesis ("tmesis" is "to cut") is defined as a disruption of axonal continuity, including the myelin sheath, but with preservation of the surrounding supportive structures—namely, the endoneurium, perineurium, and epineurium. Although Wallerian degradation occurs, the signal begins to return in several weeks, demonstrated by fibrillation potential and sharp waves on EMG. Recovery is usually gradual, lasting weeks to months [15].

Neurotmesis is injury to the entire nerve and support structure. Although the term derives from "cut nerve," neurotmesis does not necessitate that the nerve is transected, only that injury extends beyond the axon. It is the most severe type and spontaneous recovery is limited.

Sunderland Classification

The work of Seddon was expanded by Dr. Sunderland, who introduced a five-tiered classification in 1951 [16]. While this system is also based on the severity of the injury, it allowed greater anatomic specificity with grading. A comparison of the two classifications is found on Fig. 4.2.

First-degree injury is synonymous with neuropraxia and is likewise defined as a block in electrical conduction without axonal injury. The disruption is restricted to the immediately affected area with no Wallerian degeneration or

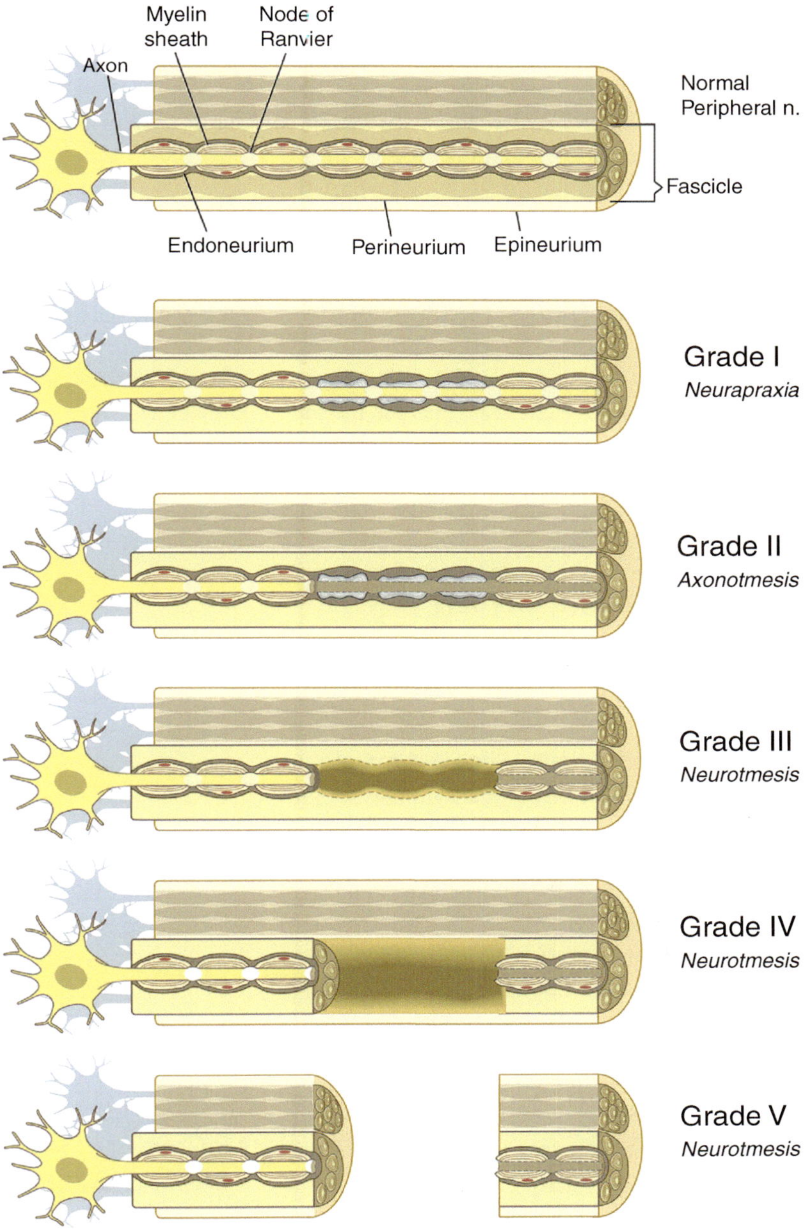

Fig. 4.2 Classification of peripheral nerve injury based on Seddon (italics) and Sunderland (grade). (Illustration by David Schumick, BS, CMI. Reprinted with the permission of the Cleveland Clinic Center for Medical Art & Photography ©2020/2021. All Rights Reserved)

distal decay of function. Second-degree injury mirrors axonotmesis. Thus, it consists of injury to the axon without damage to the axon sheath.

Third-degree injury includes not only the axon but also the endoneurium. This results in incomplete regeneration due to the disorganization of fibers, which can lead to synkinesis. However, the endoneurium and perineurium are spared for third-degree injury. Damage to these structures constitutes fourth-degree injury. Although the nerve remains in continuity, severely disorganized regeneration and fibrosis can result in traumatic neuromas and aberrant function. Fifth-degree injury is defined as a complete transection, or axonotomy, including all nerve layers through the epineurium. Dr. Susan Mackinnon subsequently proposed a sixth-degree of injury, which is a combination of at least two of the above types [17].

Mechanisms of Neural Injury

There are considered to be six mechanisms to nerve injury: compression, ischemia, ligation, thermal, traction, and transection [18–21]. These etiologies are not entirely disparate—it is likely some combinations of the different types of nerve injury are involved with each event. Nevertheless, prevention of damage to the nerve necessitates familiarity with each of the potential means of harm.

Compression

Nerve compression, or "crush injury," has been attributed to a host of neurologic symptoms, ranging from trigeminal neuralgia to facial palsies [22, 23]. Compression, which has been estimated to make up 6–40% of RLN injuries, can occur from primarily two methods [2, 12, 20]. First is when the nerve is opposed between two ends of an instrument. This most often occurs when a nerve is being mobilized or "followed," maneuvers that are particularly relied upon in head and neck surgery. There is inadvertent closure of an instrument (e.g., Schnidt tonsil forceps or McCabe facial nerve dissector) on a nerve. It is for this reason that meticulous surgical technique necessitates closure of the nerve dissector only when the instrument has been withdrawn from the tissue. Other possible causes include mistakenly grasping a nerve due to failure to recognize it as such [20].

The second means by which compression can occur is when the nerve is opposed between firm or immobile tissue and a second object, such as an instrument or even adjacent tissue. For example, the RLN can be compressed when medially displaced against the trachea during tracheal retraction. Similarly, in narrow anatomic regions, such as the stylomastoid foramen or laryngeal entry point of the RLN, nerves can be compressed due to mobilization of surrounding vasculature. The risk of such injuries is reduced through optimized visualization when working near the cranial nerves [24].

Ischemia/Idiopathic

When a cranial nerve injury occurs without a known mechanism, it is theorized that it is due to vascular compromise [18]. Blood flow can be obstructed when at least 30 mmHg are applied to a vessel [25]. Ischemic injury is impossible to demonstrate in an intraoperative setting, and the frequency of such an insult is not known. Nevertheless, it remains a reasonable concern that nerves at greatest risk of vascular compromise are those that are circumferentially dissected or "skeletonized." This is consistent with rates of injury being greater with extended surgeries, such as those involving neck dissections [26, 27]. However, it is important to note that there is no clear correlation between nerves that are "followed" and nerve injury, which may be secondary to the robust vasa nervorum preventing frequent ischemic insults.

Ligation

Ligation of a nerve can occur due to misidentification and poor visualization. This can account for 0–16% of RLN injuries and can be secondary to suture or surgical clips [11, 12, 20]. Nerves that are tortuous, branching, or anatomically variant are at greater risk, so it is important to circumferentially expose each vessel before ligation. Attention to hemostasis, particularly in tight surgical fields, will help reduce this risk.

If ligation is suspected due to loss of signal, removal of the suture or clip is imperative to minimize the potential for long-term injury. Return of function is estimated to occur in 2–3 months if the inciting source is corrected [20].

Thermal

Thermal injury is reported to account for approximately one-tenth of RLN injuries [2, 11]. Two millimeters of separation is often referenced as the necessary distance between the heat source and nerve to avoid harm [28]. However, the severity of the injury is directly related to both the distance of the instrument to the nerve and the temperature. Electrical spread (e.g., bipolar vs. monopolar) should also be considered. Expanded use of energy-based devices, such as the Harmonic Focus® and Medtronic LigaSure™, has likely increased this incidence of thermal injury [29]. The distance of heat spread with these instruments is approximately 2 millimeters so the 4 millimeters of distance from the nerve may be the safest. Thermal injuries may be less likely to have complete recovery than the other types. Standardization of equipment and multidisciplinary familiarity with instrumentation can help reduce the risk of harm [30].

Traction

Traction is frequently cited as the most common mechanism of cranial nerve injury [2, 11, 20]. Within thyroid and parathyroid surgery, traction injuries appear to be most common with the anterior motor branch of a bifurcated RLN near the ligament of Berry [2, 20]. This can be demarcated with intraoperative nerve monitoring by a gradual decrease in amplitude and increase in latency [31]. For this reason, frequent stimulation during high-risk maneuvers can help surgeons quickly recognize when traction insults are occurring.

When it does take place, intraoperative return of function can occur if the traumatic force is discontinued [20]. For this reason, continuous intraoperative nerve monitoring may help reduce the risk of damage from traction [18]. Periodically releasing traction and alternating the vector of force may help reduce the incidence of harm. If sustained traction forces result in the absence of nerve function in the operating room, complete recovery can still be expected in 2–3 months [20].

Transection

When intraoperative loss of signal is identified, transection appears to account for a decreasing percentage of cases with time, ranging from 1% to 10% [1, 2, 12, 20]. These are defined as a Sunderland fifth-degree injury. It is primarily attributed to misidentification due to variant anatomy, such as a non-recurrent RLN, history of radiation, or atherosclerotic artery which mirrors the whitish appearance of a nerve [18].

Transection can be avoided by stimulation of tissues prior to division. When transection occurs, intraoperative primarily neurorrhaphy is recommended when the nerve can be re-approximated without tension. After an injury, patients can expect 2–3 weeks of fibrillation potentials, which are a sign of denervation [32]. Patients should also be counseling regarding the risk of synkinesis or aberrant innervation, such as with Frey syndrome after injury to the auriculotemporal nerve.

Risk of Nerve Injury

Not all patients are at the same risk of nerve injury. Recognizing preoperative factors associated with postoperative palsies will aid in the appropriate escalation of caution and counseling. Table 4.1 depicts the demographics, comorbidities, and medications associated with nerve injury. Age, particularly >70 years, has been associated with nerve injury; however, other demographic factors such as sex and race have not [33, 34]. Medical conditions that predispose to neuropathies, such as diabetes, put patients at greatest risk [7]. Surgeon volume has also been shown to play a role in the frequency of nerve injury, with lower incidences of RLN injury for surgeons performing more than 50 thyroid or parathyroid surgeries a year [35]. The likelihood of injury increases with surgical difficulty, including larger lesions, revision procedures, and extended resections [7, 26, 33, 34, 36].

Few interventions have demonstrated a reduced risk of nerve injury. Shorter operative time may be related to improved outcomes, but it

Table 4.1 Factors associated with risk of nerve injury

Characteristics	Comorbidities	Medications
Age	Diabetes mellitus	Amiodarone
Size of lesion	Hypoglycemia	Cisplatin
Revision surgery	Hypothyroidism	Dapsone
Extended resections	Dyscrasias	Disulfiram
Operative time	Chronic lung disease	Hydralazine
	Liver disease	Isoniazid
	Amyloidosis	Metronidazole
	Acromegaly	Phenytoin
	Acromegaly	Pyridoxine (B6)
		Vincristine

is likely that this association has more to do with surgical difficulty [33, 34, 37]. Having patients hold risk-associated medications could help lower the incidence of nerve injury, but this has not been empirically demonstrated, and it is unclear what duration is required to obtain this benefit [18]. Intraoperative nerve monitoring (discussed separately in this book) has frequently been associated with lower risk of injury [4, 8, 21]. In particular, nerve monitoring may bring the quality of inexperienced surgeons up to that of more experienced surgeons [38]. Although nerve monitoring is not universally mandated, it should be strongly considered for higher-risk patients based on the aforementioned factors [39].

References

1. Chiang FY, Wang LF, Huang YF, Lee KW, Kuo WR. Recurrent laryngeal nerve palsy after thyroidectomy with routine identification of the recurrent laryngeal nerve. Surgery. 2005;137(3):342–7. https://doi.org/10.1016/j.surg.2004.09.008.
2. Liu N, Chen B, Li L, Zeng Q, Sheng L, Zhang B, et al. Mechanisms of recurrent laryngeal nerve injury near the nerve entry point during thyroid surgery: a retrospective cohort study. Int J Surg. 2020;83:125–30. https://doi.org/10.1016/j.ijsu.2020.08.058.
3. Moreira A, Forrest E, Lee JC, Paul E, Yeung M, Grodski S, et al. Investigation of recurrent laryngeal palsy rates for potential associations during thyroidectomy. ANZ J Surg. 2020;90(9):1733–7. https://doi.org/10.1111/ans.16166.
4. Chan WF, Lang BH, Lo CY. The role of intraoperative neuromonitoring of recurrent laryngeal nerve during thyroidectomy: a comparative study on 1000 nerves at risk. Surgery. 2006;140(6):866–72; discussion 72–3. https://doi.org/10.1016/j.surg.2006.07.017.
5. Liu J, Li Y, Yang L, Cai H. Surgical resection of carotid body tumors with versus without preoperative embolization: retrospective case-control study. Head Neck. 2018;40(12):2590–5. https://doi.org/10.1002/hed.25387.
6. Kligerman MP, Song Y, Schoppy D, Divi V, Megwalu UC, Haughey BH, et al. Retrograde Parotidectomy and facial nerve outcomes: a case series of 44 patients. Am J Otolaryngol. 2017;38(5):533–6. https://doi.org/10.1016/j.amjoto.2017.05.003.
7. Yuan X, Gao Z, Jiang H, Yang H, Lv W, Wang Z, et al. Predictors of facial palsy after surgery for benign parotid disease: multivariate analysis of 626 operations. Head Neck. 2009;31(12):1588–92. https://doi.org/10.1002/hed.21134.
8. Savvas E, Hillmann S, Weiss D, Koopmann M, Rudack C, Alberty J. Association between facial nerve monitoring with postoperative facial paralysis in parotidectomy. JAMA Otolaryngol Head Neck Surg. 2016;142(9):828–33. https://doi.org/10.1001/jamaoto.2016.1192.
9. Bergenfelz A, Jansson S, Kristoffersson A, Martensson H, Reihner E, Wallin G, et al. Complications to thyroid surgery: results as reported in a database from a multicenter audit comprising 3,660 patients. Langenbeck's Arch Surg. 2008;393(5):667–73. https://doi.org/10.1007/s00423-008-0366-7.
10. Lo CY, Kwok KF, Yuen PW. A prospective evaluation of recurrent laryngeal nerve paralysis during thyroidectomy. Arch Surg. 2000;135(2):204–7. https://doi.org/10.1001/archsurg.135.2.204.
11. Dionigi G, Wu CW, Kim HY, Rausei S, Boni L, Chiang FY. Severity of recurrent laryngeal nerve injuries in thyroid surgery. World J Surg. 2016;40(6):1373–81. https://doi.org/10.1007/s00268-016-3415-3.
12. Chiang FY, Lu IC, Kuo WR, Lee KW, Chang NC, Wu CW. The mechanism of recurrent laryngeal nerve injury during thyroid surgery--the application of intraoperative neuromonitoring. Surgery. 2008;143(6):743–9. https://doi.org/10.1016/j.surg.2008.02.006.
13. Chiang FY, Lee KW, Chen HC, Chen HY, Lu IC, Kuo WR, et al. Standardization of intraoperative neuromonitoring of recurrent laryngeal nerve in thyroid operation. World J Surg. 2010;34(2):223–9. https://doi.org/10.1007/s00268-009-0316-8.
14. Seddon HJ. Three types of nerve injury. Brain. 1943;66(4):237–88.
15. Robinson LR. Trauma rehabilitation. Diagnosis and rehabilitation of peripheral nerve injuries. Philadelphia: Lippincott Williams & Wilkins; 2006.
16. Sunderland S. A classification of peripheral nerve injuries producing loss of function. Brain. 1951;74(4):491–516. https://doi.org/10.1093/brain/74.4.491.
17. Mackinnon SE, Dellon AL. Surgery of the peripheral nerve. New York: Thieme Medical Publishers; 1988.

18. Randolph G. The recurrent and superior laryngeal nerves. Cham: Springer; 2016.
19. Myssiorek D. Recurrent laryngeal nerve paralysis: anatomy and etiology. Otolaryngol Clin N Am. 2004;37(1):25–44, v. https://doi.org/10.1016/S0030-6665(03)00172-5.
20. Snyder SK, Lairmore TC, Hendricks JC, Roberts JW. Elucidating mechanisms of recurrent laryngeal nerve injury during thyroidectomy and parathyroidectomy. J Am Coll Surg. 2008;206(1):123–30. https://doi.org/10.1016/j.jamcollsurg.2007.07.017.
21. Chiesa-Estomba CM, Larruscain-Sarasola E, Lechien JR, Mouawad F, Calvo-Henriquez C, Diom ES, et al. Facial nerve monitoring during parotid gland surgery: a systematic review and meta-analysis. Eur Arch Otorhinolaryngol. 2020; https://doi.org/10.1007/s00405-020-06188-0.
22. Celik O, Ulkumen B, Eskiizmir G, Can F, Pabuscu Y, Kamiloglu U, et al. The ratio of facial nerve to facial canal as an indicator of entrapment in Bell's palsy: a study by CT and MRI. Clin Neurol Neurosurg. 2020;198:106109. https://doi.org/10.1016/j.clineuro.2020.106109.
23. Jannetta PJ. Neurovascular compression in cranial nerve and systemic disease. Ann Surg. 1980;192(4):518–25. https://doi.org/10.1097/00000658-198010000-00010.
24. Jatzko GR, Lisborg PH, Muller MG, Wette VM. Recurrent nerve palsy after thyroid operations--principal nerve identification and a literature review. Surgery. 1994;115(2):139–44.
25. Rydevik B, Lundborg G, Bagge U. Effects of graded compression on intraneural blood blow. An in vivo study on rabbit tibial nerve. J Hand Surg Am. 1981;6(1):3–12. https://doi.org/10.1016/s0363-5023(81)80003-2.
26. ErbilY, Barbaros U, Issever H, Borucu I, Salmaslioglu A, Mete O, et al. Predictive factors for recurrent laryngeal nerve palsy and hypoparathyroidism after thyroid surgery. Clin Otolaryngol. 2007;32(1):32–7. https://doi.org/10.1111/j.1365-2273.2007.01383.x.
27. Thomusch O, Sekulla C, Walls G, Machens A, Dralle H. Intraoperative neuromonitoring of surgery for benign goiter. Am J Surg. 2002;183(6):673–8. https://doi.org/10.1016/s0002-9610(02)00856-5.
28. Jiang H, Shen H, Jiang D, Zheng X, Zhang W, Lu L, et al. Evaluating the safety of the harmonic scalpel around the recurrent laryngeal nerve. ANZ J Surg. 2010;80(11):822–6. https://doi.org/10.1111/j.1445-2197.2010.05436.x.
29. Dionigi G. Energy based devices and recurrent laryngeal nerve injury: the need for safer instruments. Langenbeck's Arch Surg. 2009;394(3):579–80; author reply 81–6. https://doi.org/10.1007/s00423-008-0454-8.
30. Wu CW, Chai YJ, Dionigi G, Chiang FY, Liu X, Sun H, et al. Recurrent laryngeal nerve safety parameters of the harmonic focus during thyroid surgery: porcine model using continuous monitoring. Laryngoscope. 2015;125(12):2838–45. https://doi.org/10.1002/lary.25412.
31. Genther DJ, Kandil EH, Noureldine SI, Tufano RP. Correlation of final evoked potential amplitudes on intraoperative electromyography of the recurrent laryngeal nerve with immediate postoperative vocal fold function after thyroid and parathyroid surgery. JAMA Otolaryngol Head Neck Surg. 2014;140(2):124–8. https://doi.org/10.1001/jamaoto.2013.6139.
32. Volk GF, Hagen R, Pototschnig C, Friedrich G, Nawka T, Arens C, et al. Laryngeal electromyography: a proposal for guidelines of the European Laryngological Society. Eur Arch Otorhinolaryngol. 2012;269(10):2227–45. https://doi.org/10.1007/s00405-012-2036-1.
33. Guntinas-Lichius O, Gabriel B, Klussmann JP. Risk of facial palsy and severe Frey's syndrome after conservative parotidectomy for benign disease: analysis of 610 operations. Acta Otolaryngol. 2006;126(10):1104–9. https://doi.org/10.1080/00016480600672618.
34. Dulguerov P, Marchal F, Lehmann W. Postparotidectomy facial nerve paralysis: possible etiologic factors and results with routine facial nerve monitoring. Laryngoscope. 1999;109(5):754–62. https://doi.org/10.1097/00005537-199905000-00014.
35. Stavrakis AI, Ituarte PH, Ko CY, Yeh MW. Surgeon volume as a predictor of outcomes in inpatient and outpatient endocrine surgery. Surgery. 2007;142(6):887–99; discussion –99. https://doi.org/10.1016/j.surg.2007.09.003.
36. Dralle H, Sekulla C, Haerting J, Timmermann W, Neumann HJ, Kruse E, et al. Risk factors of paralysis and functional outcome after recurrent laryngeal nerve monitoring in thyroid surgery. Surgery. 2004;136(6):1310–22. https://doi.org/10.1016/j.surg.2004.07.018.
37. Terrell JE, Kileny PR, Yian C, Esclamado RM, Bradford CR, Pillsbury MS, et al. Clinical outcome of continuous facial nerve monitoring during primary parotidectomy. Arch Otolaryngol Head Neck Surg. 1997;123(10):1081–7. https://doi.org/10.1001/archotol.1997.01900100055008.
38. Alesina PF, Hinrichs J, Meier B, Cho EY, Bolli M, Walz MK. Intraoperative neuromonitoring for surgical training in thyroid surgery: its routine use allows a safe operation instead of lack of experienced mentoring. World J Surg. 2014;38(3):592–8. https://doi.org/10.1007/s00268-013-2372-3.
39. Randolph GW, Dralle H, International Intraoperative Monitoring Study Group, Abdullah H, Barczynski M, Bellantone R, et al. Electrophysiologic recurrent laryngeal nerve monitoring during thyroid and parathyroid surgery: international standards guideline statement. Laryngoscope. 2011;121(Suppl 1):S1–16. https://doi.org/10.1002/lary.21119.

Neuromonitoring Usage Patterns and Education

5

Michael C. Singer

The last two decades have seen intraoperative neuromonitoring (IONM) become a widely adopted surgical adjunct in a range of otolaryngology operations. A number of IONM methods are employed by surgeons, relying on different observable, palpable, or measurable responses, to assess nerve integrity and function. Regardless of particular technique, these approaches are all intended to aid in reduction of injury to cranial nerves at risk during surgery. While the precise value of IONM continues to be debated, its use has become particularly widespread in certain fields of otolaryngology. This likely reflects the direct exposure that residents and fellows receive to IONM during their training.

Usage Patterns

While IONM for a range of procedures is available, it is most commonly utilized in thyroid gland, otologic, neurotologic, and parotid gland surgeries.

The use of IONM in thyroid surgery has been most robustly examined. A series of studies have demonstrated that adoption of IONM in thyroid surgery has consistently increased over time [1–6]. This is true among both general surgeons and otolaryngologists [3, 5, 6]. A recent international survey of surgeons, belonging to the American Association of Otolaryngology–Head and Neck Surgery (AAO-HNS), American Head and Neck Society (AHNS), or International Association of Endocrine Surgeons, found that 83% of respondents reported using IONM in at least some of their thyroid procedures [5].

Interestingly, high-volume surgeons are among those most likely to utilize IONM on a routine basis [3, 4, 6]. This large-scale usage of IONM likely reflects its multidimensional functionality in thyroid surgery, as it can facilitate nerve identification, potentially reduce risk of neuropraxia and transection injuries, and aid in prognostication of postoperative function. This routine use of IONM also suggests that experienced surgeons recognize that trying to select prior to surgery which thyroidectomy cases might most benefit from use of IONM is difficult. Another group that reports a high rate of IONM utilization is younger surgeons [3, 6]. This appears to reflect a correlation with exposure to IONM during their training.

Utilization of IONM in other head and neck surgeries has been less well documented. In parotid surgery, a single study from 2005 found that approximately 60% of surgeons were using facial nerve monitoring [7]. In this study, use during training and higher procedural volume were

M. C. Singer (✉)
Department of Otolaryngology–Head and Neck Surgery, Henry Ford Hospital, Detroit, MI, USA
e-mail: MSINGER1@hfhs.org

© The Author(s), under exclusive license to Springer Nature Switzerland AG 2022
J. Scharpf, G. W. Randolph (eds.), *Intraoperative Cranial Nerve Monitoring in Otolaryngology-Head and Neck Surgery*, https://doi.org/10.1007/978-3-030-84916-0_5

associated with a greater likelihood of IONM utilization.

The incorporation of facial nerve monitoring in otologic and neurotologic surgery mirrors the trends that have occurred with recurrent laryngeal nerve monitoring [8–10]. Surveys done several years apart of different surgical cohorts have shown an increasing trend of IONM employment. The most recent study from 2018 demonstrated that the vast majority of chronic ear disease and neurotologic surgeries in the United States are performed with IONM.

Education

Given that the use and benefit of IONM in otolaryngology surgeries remain controversial, the adoption rates might be viewed as unexpectedly high. To a large degree, this is likely the result of residents and fellows training with attending surgeons who incorporate IONM techniques in their practices. Several studies have shown a strong correlation between IONM exposure during training and continued use when training is completed [2, 6, 7, 9, 10]. However, while IONM instruction is prescribed by a number of surgical organizations, the details of what knowledge is necessary to be considered competent with IONM are not defined.

For residents and fellows in otolaryngology, there is a clear call for training in IONM by several key educational groups. For residents, the American Board of Otolaryngology (ABOTO) curriculum prescribes training in the use of IONM for otologic surgery [11]. This curriculum serves as the basis for the written and oral certification examinations for board certification. In the otology section, the stated objective is that the resident "understands the indications, techniques, and pitfalls of intraoperative cranial nerve monitoring." This includes the technique for monitoring cranial nerves VII, IX, X, XI, and XII. Specifically, residents are supposed to be able to interpret the results of IONM and troubleshoot common causes of inaccurate monitoring.

A more recent guide, named OTOSource, developed by the Comprehensive Curriculum Task Force and Work Group of Otolaryngology of the AAO-HNS provides a compilation of topics and learning objectives appropriate for both residents and practicing otolaryngologists [12]. Similar to the ABOTO's curriculum, in the otology section of OTOSource, there is a requirement for knowledge of IONM of the cranial nerves. This section refers to cranial nerves III–VI and IX–XII. In OTOSource, a need for awareness of facial nerve monitoring is also described in the head and neck surgery section discussing parotid gland disease.

Understanding and performing recurrent laryngeal nerve IONM is mandatory in those fellowships under the auspices of both the AHNS and the American Association of Endocrine Surgeons [13, 14]. These organizations both require fellows to obtain knowledge of IONM as well as experience using it surgically.

Studies suggest that this training with IONM is indeed occurring in residency programs [4, 10]. However, what is unclear is the extent that this exposure is consistent across departments. In a survey performed in 2018, residency program directors reported universal exposure of residents to IONM (in otologic/neurotologic procedures), but only 61% of programs described providing formal IONM training.

Conclusion

Use of IONM techniques is already widespread in a number of sub-specialties of otolaryngology. As IONM education is an established goal of residency and fellowship programs, trainees are acquiring experience with IONM. Given the association between exposure to IONM and adoption in practice, the utilization of these techniques is likely only to increase in the future.

References

1. Horne SK, Gal TJ, Brennan JA. Prevalence and patterns of intraoperative nerve monitoring for thyroidectomy. Otolaryngol Head Neck Surg. 2007;136(6):952–6.
2. Sturgeon C, Sturgeon T, Angelos P. Neuromonitoring in thyroid surgery: attitudes, usage patterns, and pre-

dictors of use among endocrine surgeons. World J Surg. 2009;33(3):417–25.
3. Singer MC, Rosenfeld RM, Sundaram K. Laryngeal nerve monitoring: current utilization among head and neck surgeons. Otolaryngol Head Neck Surg. 2012;146:895–9.
4. Ho Y, Carr MM, Goldenberg D. Trends in intraoperative neural monitoring for thyroid and parathyroid surgery amongst otolaryngologists and general surgeons. Eur Arch Otorhinolaryngol. 2013;270:2525–30.
5. Feng AL, Puram SV, Singer MC, Modi R, Kamani D, Randolph GW. Increased prevalence of neural monitoring during thyroidectomy: global surgical survey. Laryngoscope. 2020;130(4):1097–104.
6. Marti JL, Holm T, Randolph GW. Universal use of intraoperative nerve monitoring by recently fellowship-trained thyroid surgeons is common, associated with higher surgical volume, and impacts intraoperative decision-making. World J Surg. 2016;40(2):337–43.
7. Lowry TR, Gal TJ, Brennan JA. Patterns of use of facial nerve monitoring during parotid gland surgery. Otolaryngol Head Neck Surg. 2005;133(3):313–8.
8. Greenberg JS, Manolidis S, Stewart MG, Kahn JB. Facial nerve monitoring in chronic ear surgery: US practice patterns. Otolaryngol Head Neck Surg. 2002;126(2):108–14.
9. Hu J, Fleck TR, Xu J, Hsu JV, Xu HX. Contemporary changes with the use of facial nerve monitoring in chronic ear surgery. Otolaryngol Head Neck Surg. 2014;151(3):473–7.
10. Gidley PW, Maw J, Gantz B, Kaylie D, Lambert P, Malekzadeh S, Chandrasekhar SS. Contemporary opinions on intraoperative facial nerve monitoring. Oto Open. 2018;2(3):2473974X18791803.
11. The American Board of Otolaryngology – Head and Neck Surgery. www.ABOTO.org.
12. The American Academy of Otolaryngology – Head and Neck Surgery Foundation. www.OTOSOURCE.org.
13. The American Head & Neck Society. www.AHNS.info.
14. The American Association of Endocrine Surgeons. www.ENDOCRINESURGERY.org.

Part II

Vagus/Recurrent Laryngeal Nerve Monitoring

Greg Randolph

Rationale and Indications for Vagus/Recurrent Laryngeal Nerve Monitoring

6

Che-Wei Wu, Feng-Yu Chiang, Amanda Silver Karcioglu, Ayaka J. Iwata, Amr H. Abdelhamid Ahmed, and Gregory W. Randolph

Introduction

Recurrent laryngeal nerve (RLN) injury and vocal cord paralysis after thyroid surgery remain a significant source of morbidity and is a leading cause for medicolegal action [1]. Intraoperative neural monitoring (IONM) has gained widespread acceptance as a tool to assist in identifying and mapping the external branch of the superior laryngeal nerve (EBSLN), RLN, and vagus nerve (VN), detecting RLN anatomic variations, confirming and elucidating mechanisms of RLN injury, and predicting the outcome of vocal cord function [2–13]. By providing real-time functional information, IONM empowers surgeons beyond what is available to them through visual information alone. This chapter reviews the surgical anatomy of the VN, the carotid sheath, and the RLN as well as the surgical anatomy-based classifications and variations relevant to thyroid/parathyroid surgery, discusses the rationale and indications for VN and RLN monitoring, and also reviews basic laryngeal nerve monitoring equipment setup, standard procedures, and LOS definition and classification to facilitate accurate and efficient IONM. This chapter also summarizes the current standards and guidelines of VN and RLN monitoring.

C.-W. Wu
Department of Otorhinolaryngology-Head and Neck Surgery, Kaohsiung Municipal Siaogang Hospital, Faculty of Medicine, College of Medicine, Kaohsiung Medical University, Kaohsiung, Taiwan
e-mail: cwwu@kmu.edu.tw

F.-Y. Chiang
Department of Otolaryngology, E-Da Hospital, School of Medicine, College of Medicine, I-Shou University, Kaohsiung, Taiwan
e-mail: fychiang@kmu.edu.tw

A. S. Karcioglu
Division of Thyroid and Parathyroid Endocrine Surgery, Department of Otolaryngology-Head & Neck Surgery, Massachusetts Eye and Ear Infirmary, Harvard Medical School, Boston, MA, USA

A. J. Iwata
Department of Otolaryngology-Head and Neck Surgery, Kaiser Permanente, Santa Clara, CA, USA
e-mail: Ayaka.J.Iwata@kp.org

A. H. Abdelhamid Ahmed
Division of Thyroid and Parathyroid Endocrine Surgery, Department of Otolaryngology-Head & Neck Surgery, Massachusetts Eye and Ear Infirmary, Harvard Medical School, Boston, MA, USA
e-mail: Amr_ahmed@meei.harvard.edu

G. W. Randolph (✉)
Thyroid and Parathyroid Endocrine Surgery Division, Department of Otolaryngology, Massachusetts Eye and Ear Infirmary, Boston, MA, USA

Division of Surgical Oncology, Endocrine Surgery Service, Department of Surgery, Massachusetts General Hospital, Boston, MA, USA

Otolaryngology-Head and Neck Surgery, Claire and John Bertucci Endowed Chair in Thyroid Surgical Oncology, Harvard Medical School, Boston, MA, USA
e-mail: gregory_randolph@meei.harvard.edu

© The Author(s), under exclusive license to Springer Nature Switzerland AG 2022

J. Scharpf, G. W. Randolph (eds.), *Intraoperative Cranial Nerve Monitoring in Otolaryngology-Head and Neck Surgery*, https://doi.org/10.1007/978-3-030-84916-0_6

Anatomy

Vagal Nerve and Carotid Sheath Anatomy

A better understanding of the anatomy and variability in the position of the VN within the carotid sheath is necessary not only to minimize complications but also to ensure accurate, efficient, and safe use of IONM [14]. The carotid sheath refers to the fibrous connective tissue that surrounds the vascular compartment of the neck and is part of the deep cervical fascia. The medial location of the common carotid artery (CCA) and anterolateral or lateral location of the internal jugular vein (IJV) are the most common configurations in the carotid sheath. Rare cases of medial IJV positions have been observed [15, 16]. In the largest series to date, Dionigi et al. [16] proposed an anatomical classification of the VN based on its position relative to the great vessels and offered a reproducible methodology for identifying the VN and its course in the carotid sheath. The relative location of the VN has been classified into various configurations where **A** denotes a VN anterior to the CCA and IJV (4%), **P** denotes a VN posterior to the CCA and the IJV (73%), **Pj** denotes a VN posterior to the internal jugular vein (8%), and **Pc** denotes a VN posterior to the CCA (15%) (Fig. 6.1). Such classification is useful in the intraoperative setting to localize the VN for IONM. During intermittent IONM, VN identification may also be expedited without formally dissecting the carotid sheath by placing the stimulation probe on the carotid sheath and blindly stimulating at 2–3 mA [11], as shown in Fig. 6.1.

RLN Surgical Anatomic Trajectory in the Neck Base

The RLN is a branch of VN that normally loops around the aorta at the ligamentum arteriosum on the left side and around the subclavian artery on the right side before coursing to the larynx. In 2016, Randolph et al. [14] published the basic classification of the RLN surgical anatomic pathway in the neck as it relates to thyroid surgery. This classification incorporates normal anatomy as well as embryological and acquired variations in the trajectory of the right and left RLN. It is simple and surgically relevant, presenting a valuable framework for the surgeon. This classification broadly categorizes the RLNs as having a(n):

1. Normal trajectory
2. Abnormal trajectory – acquired
3. Abnormal trajectory – embryological

The details of the classification system and the estimated prevalence of each category are depicted in Fig. 6.2 and Table 6.1, respectively.

Normal Trajectory L1, R1

As the heart and great vessels descend during early embryologic life, the RLN is dragged down

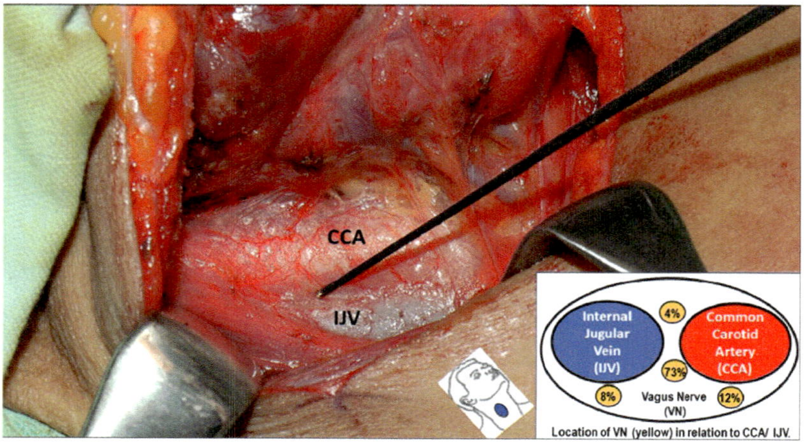

Fig. 6.1 Common locations of vagal nerve (VN) within the carotid sheath and procedure of VN stimulation by using the ball-tip stimulation probe mapping on the carotid sheath

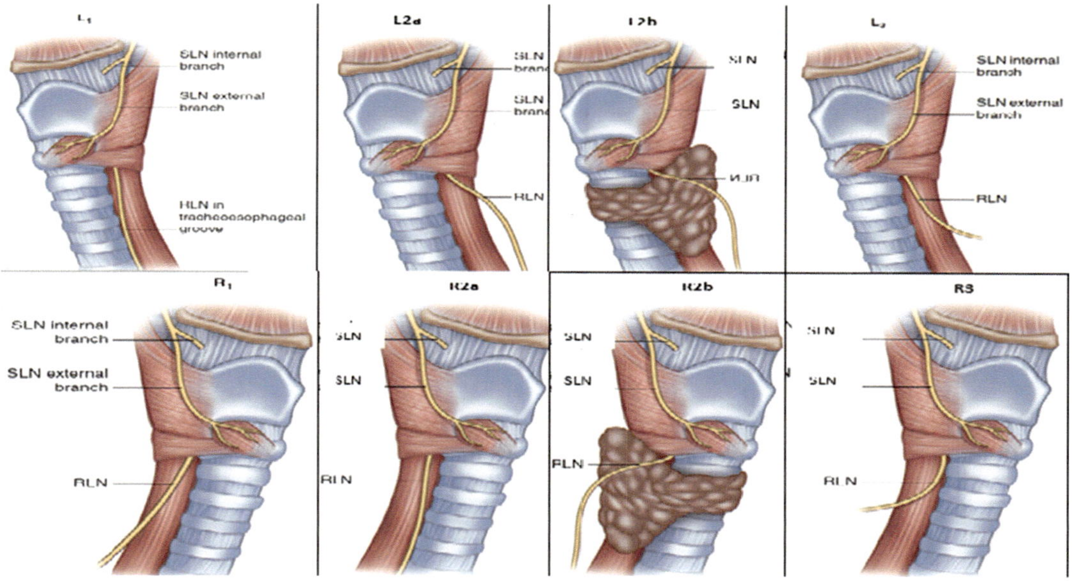

Fig. 6.2 Basic classification of RLN surgical anatomic path in the neck base as it relates to the thyroid surgical procedure [14]

Table 6.1 The international RLN anatomic classification and the estimated prevalence of each class [14]

Class	Description	Estimated prevalence
I/II. Left/right RLN basic surgical anatomic path		
L1/R1	Normal trajectory	95%/90%
L2a/R2a	Abnormal acquired – lateral/medial	5%/5–10%
L2b/R2b	Abnormal acquired – ventral	<1%/<1%
L3/R3	Abnormal embryologic – nonrecurrent	0.04%/0.5–1%
III. Clinically important neural features		
Anatomical		
F – Fixed/splayed/entrapped	Capsular association through fascial bands, vessels, or goitrous change	15% (with substernal goiter)
I – Invaded	Neural invasion	< 5% (with cancer)
L – Posterior ligament	Posterior ligament of Berry or associated vessel neural entrapment	10%
B – Branched	Extralaryngeal RLN branching	24.3–72%
T – Thin	Neural caliber <1 mm	<2.5%
Dynamic		
LOS – Loss of signal	Loss of EMG signal	
D – Extensive neural dissection	Extensive nerve dissection or 360° dissection	

by the persistent aortic arch. The right VN runs from the posterior aspect of the carotid sheath in the neck base and crosses anterior to the first segment of the subclavian artery. The RLN branches off, traversing posterior to the subclavian artery (the fourth branchial arch remnant) to course supero-medially behind the CCA as it ascends through the right thoracic inlet to cross obliquely from lateral to medial as it ascends the neck. The left VN courses from the posterior aspect of the left carotid sheath in the left neck base anterior to the aortic arch (sixth arch ligament and arteriosus). The left RLN then branches underneath the aortic arch just lateral to the obliterated ductus arteriosus and ascends into the paratracheal region in a direct cranial-caudal trajectory within the tracheoesophageal (TE) groove. This should be distinguished from the more oblique path of its right counterpart. In general, the normal trajectory of the left RLN (**L1**) travels in a path that is parallel to the TE groove at an angle less than 30° in at least 80% of cases, whereas the normal trajectory of the right RLN (**R1**) travels in a path between 15 and 45° relative to the TE groove in approximately 80% of cases.

Acquired Variations of L2a/R2a (Lateral/Medial)

L2a If a goiter on the left side extends significantly into the TE groove, a more lateral displacement (more than 30°) of the left RLN may occur.

R2a Goitrous changes of certain aspects of the right normal thyroid lobe, especially the more dorsal aspects of the mid-inferior pole region, may displace the normally oblique nerve more medially into a newly acquired medial position more parallel to the TE groove (less than 15°).

Acquired Variations of L2b/R2b (Ventral)

L2b/R2b When thyroid tissue extends deep to the trachea due to a dorsally oriented tubercle of Zuckerkandl and forms a retrotracheal cervical goiter or posterior mediastinal goiter, the RLN may be excavated posteriorly by this segment of dorsal tissue. This can potentially result in a significant displacement of the RLN ventrally.

Embryologic Variations of L3/R3 (Nonrecurrent)

L3 A nonrecurrent left RLN embryologically requires a simultaneous occurrence of other anomalies, namely, situs invertus, aberrant subclavian artery, and ductus arteriosus. This is extraordinarily rare.

R3 A nonrecurrent right RLN occurs when the right subclavian artery arises from the distal aortic arch and extends to the right side in a retroesophageal course. In this case, the right RLN runs in a more direct and medial course from the VN to its laryngeal entry point.

Clinically Important RLN Features

In addition to the L1–L3 and R1–R3 classes described above, other factors are also a crucial part of the surgical anatomic classification system. These can be denoted by additional lettering added to the L or R notations and can be classified as **anatomical** (*F*, fixed/splayed/entrapped; *I*, invaded; *L*, posterior ligament of Berry, entrapped; *B*, branched; *T*, thin caliber) or **dynamic** (*LOS*, loss of electrophysiologic signal; *D*, extensive nerve dissection) (Table 6.1).

Rationale of Vagus and Recurrent Laryngeal Nerve Monitoring

The RLN contains motor fibers that enable abduction and adduction of intrinsic vocal fold muscles and provides sensory fibers to the larynx. Intraoperative injury of the RLN or invasion of the nerve may result in RLN dysfunction, including vocal cord paralysis (VCP) with or without clinical symptoms [12, 14]. Unilateral RLN injury and VCP can cause significant dysphonia and dysphagia, while bilateral RLN injuries and VCP are potentially life-threatening due to airway compromise.

The use of VN and RLN IONM during thyroid and parathyroid surgery provides surgeons with a tool to better understand the possible mechanisms of RLN injury [6, 7, 17–19]. Previously, the surgeon was only aware of RLN injury if there were visible trauma to the identified nerve. Nerves that appear intact however are not always functionally intact. With IONM, the surgeon can confirm that nerve stimulation results in contraction of the laryngeal muscles, which can be palpated or recorded electrophysiologically. The amplitude of the vocal fold contraction can be measured in microvolts, and the latency of nerve conduction can be measured in microseconds [2, 20]. During intermittent IONM (IIONM), repeated stimulation of the VN or RLN during thyroidectomy can help the surgeon identify an impending RLN injury by identifying a decrease in the amplitude of the vocal fold contraction and increased latency of nerve conduction. A similar result may be obtained during continuous IONM (CIONM), which provides automated stimulation to the nerves. In the event of total loss or impending loss of nerve signal (LOS), the surgeon can evaluate the surgical maneuver that produced the impending or actual RLN injury and modify the maneuver [21–23]. Such real-time intraoperative feedback of RLN function also provides an opportunity to understand the mechanisms of RLN injury. Experience with IONM has demonstrated RLN injury occurs more frequently to a visually intact nerve than a visually damaged nerve [6, 7, 14, 17–19]. By enabling early detection of RLN injury and prediction of nerve outcome, IONM can help clinicians plan and modify intra- and postoperative treatments [2–5, 8, 14, 19].

Indications and Benefits of VN/RLN Monitoring

Appropriate use of VN/RLN monitoring during thyroid/parathyroid surgery should be considered for all cases. Certainly, cases that can be recognized preoperatively as likely having greater risk to the RLN should be monitored. However, many cases lacking these preoperative features may well present significant intraoperative difficulties and may benefit from monitoring. Routine application has been shown to shorten learning curves through greater experience in the interpretation of signal and troubleshooting system malfunction [24]. Although the impact of IONM on rates of RLN injury is generally accepted as lower, many studies have not shown statistical significance [25–27], possibly due to the power needed to detect a statistically significant difference (9 million patients per arm for benign goiter and 40 million per arm for malignant thyroid disease) [28].

In addition to thyroid/parathyroid surgery, RLN monitoring can be considered for open approaches to address Zenker's diverticulum, carotid endarterectomy, surgery for laryngotracheal stenosis, anterior cervical approaches to the cervical spine, and certain skull base, cardiac, and upper chest procedures [29].

Given the potential implications on intraoperative decision-making, especially in total thyroidectomy, the use of IONM should be included in informed consent. Most patients appreciate and wish to actively take part in shared decision making regarding the management of their disease [30]. Adequate informed consent and use of IONM documentation have been reported to favorably impact malpractice suits against surgeons [31, 32].

Basic VN/RLN Monitoring Equipment Setup
Various methods have been applied to intraoperative VN and RLN monitoring during thyroid and parathyroid surgery. These different nerve monitoring formats include laryngeal palpation, glottic observation, glottic pressure monitoring, endoscopically placed intramuscular vocal cord electrodes (hookwires), intramuscular electrodes placed through the cricothyroid membrane, postcricoid surface electrodes, and endotracheal tube (ET)-based surface electrodes [2]. Basic VN/RLN monitoring involves multifaceted electronic stimulation and recording equipment (Fig. 6.3) which can be divided into the following categories: (i) the recording side and (ii) the stimulation side.

The recording side involves the recording electrodes (Figs. 6.3 and 6.4a, b), the grounding electrode, and associated connections at the interface-connector box and monitor [2]. ET-based surface electrodes are the most popular and have several advantages including the ease of setup, their noninvasive nature, and the large EMG potentials recordable with such electrodes. Electrodes are incorporated into the wall of the ET or fixed to the side of the endotracheal wall with adhesives and are exposed at the level of the glottis for optimal bilateral vocal cord mucosal contact. This allows evoked surface electromyography (EMG) monitoring of the vocal muscles' contraction during stimulation of RLN and VN [2]. Several kinds of ET-based electrodes have been commercialized for recording during IONM, including adhesive, wire, and ink surface electrodes. A limitation of the clinical use of ET-based surface electrodes is the need to maintain constant contact between the electrodes and vocal cords

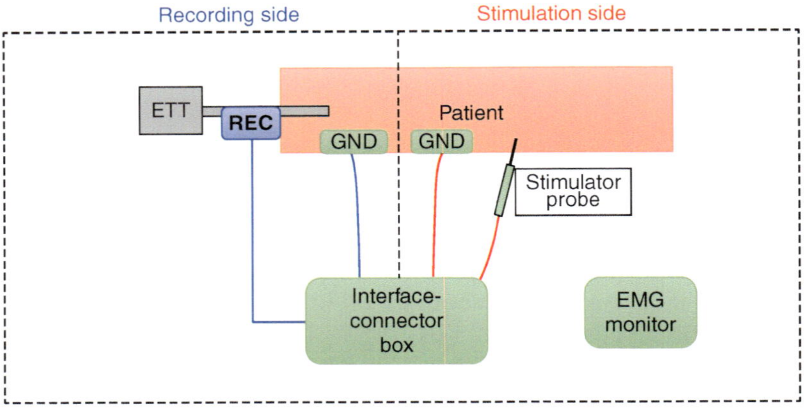

Fig. 6.3 Multifaceted electronic stimulation and recording equipment for laryngeal nerve monitoring. Abbreviations: ETT, endotracheal tube; EMG, electromyogram; GND, ground

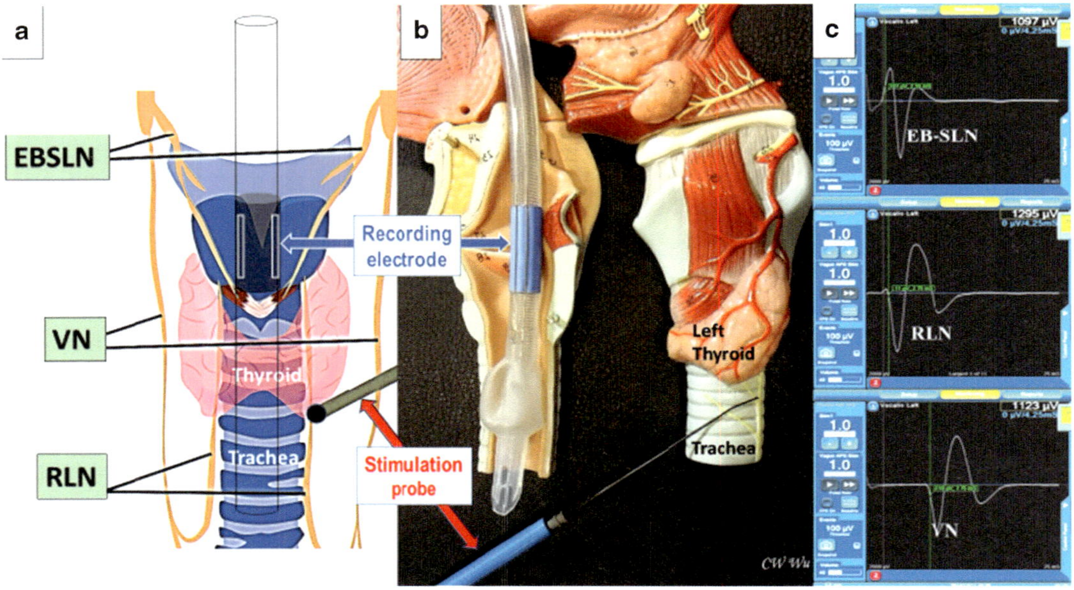

Fig. 6.4 The multifaceted electronic equipment and principle of the IONM system. (**a**) The basic equipment included the neural stimulating electrodes (stimulator) and the recording electrodes (connected to the ETT). (**b**) The stimulating electrodes can be used to determine the location and functional status of the EBSLN, RLN, and VN during IONM. (**c**) The evoked EMG response is displayed on an LCD screen

during surgery to obtain a high-quality recording [33, 34]. Alternative electrode systems that can circumvent the factors affecting ET-based neural monitoring accuracy have been sought, such as anterior laryngeal transcutaneous or trans-cartilaginous surface electrodes [20, 35, 36].

The stimulation side includes the neural stimulating electrodes (Figs. 6.3 and 6.4a, b), its grounding electrode, and associated connections to the interface box-connector and stimulation current pulse generator within the monitor. Recording ground and nerve stimulator anode surface electrodes are placed on the patient's shoulders and are interfaced with the monitor through a connector box. Stimulating electrodes may be monopolar or bipolar and may also be configured as dissecting instruments [37]. The selection of a stimulator can be based on the stimulation characteristics, the intended nerve monitoring application, and the surgeon's preference [38]. During thyroid and parathyroid surgery, the stimulating electrode can be used for mapping, localization, and identification of the EBSLN, RLN, and VN (Fig. 6.4a). The evoked laryngeal EMG waveform may be viewed on the EMG monitor screen (Fig. 6.4c) and the amplitude and latency changes monitored during surgery.

Continuous intraoperative nerve monitoring (CIONM) uses a newly configured electrode positioned on the VN to indirectly stimulate the RLN [39–41]. A laryngeal adductor reflex (LAR-C-IONM) EMG tube [42] has the advantage of assessing real-time nerve integrity and thus better indicates impending nerve injury compared to intermittent (IONM) stimulation techniques. A more complete description of alternative techniques and methods of IIONM and CIONM is presented in the following chapters.

Basic Standard VN and RLN Monitoring Procedures

According to current literature and international standards and guidelines [2], the standard procedure for performing IONM should include the following six steps: (i) preoperative laryngoscopy (L1); (ii) VN stimulation before surgical dissection (V1); (iii) RLN stimulation at initial identification (R1); (iv) RLN stimulation after completion of thyroid dissection and hemostasis (R2); (v) VN stimulation after completion of thyroidectomy and confirmation of hemostasis (V2); and (vi) postoperative laryngoscopy (L2) (Table 6.2).

Table 6.2 Basic standard VN/RLN monitoring procedures

Acronym	Description
L1	*Laryngoscopy* to check vocal cord movement before surgery
V1	*VN* stimulation before thyroid dissection
R1	*RLN* stimulation at initial identification
R2	*RLN* stimulation after complete thyroidectomy and hemostasis
V2	*VN* stimulation after complete thyroidectomy and hemostasis
L2	*Laryngoscopy* to check vocal cord movement after surgery

Abbreviations: *VN* vagus nerve, *RLN* recurrent laryngeal nerve

Preoperative laryngoscopy (L1) provides the baseline functional status of the vocal cords prior to surgery. Pre-RLN dissection vagal stimulation (V1) allows for the verification of system function and RLN mapping so that a negative stimulation can be interpreted as a true negative. Post-RLN dissection vagal stimulation (V2) is the most accurate prognostic test available for postoperative glottic function and has been shown to have higher sensitivity, slightly higher specificity, higher positive predictive value, and slightly higher negative predictive value compared to RLN stimulation [2, 8]. VN stimulation typically can be performed successfully without direct vagal dissection by placing the stimulator probe between the jugular vein and carotid artery at a level of stimulation between 1 and 2 mA (Fig. 6.1) [11]. On the right side a pattern of high vagal positive stimulation and lower vagal negative stimulation is the diagnostic for nonrecurrent right RLN [43]. Following the V1-R1-R2-V2 procedure during surgery, three evaluative events can be observed [6, 17]:

1. *Stable signal*: Improved or unchanged amplitude of R_2 and V_2 signals as compared with R_1 and V_1 signals confirms no RLN injury due to surgical dissection. It indicates normal intraoperative RLN function and postoperative vocal cord function.
2. *Weak or incomplete loss of signal (LOS)*: The RLN can be partially injured by certain surgical maneuvers including traction, compression, clamping, mechanical trauma, or cauterization. Despite a visually intact nerve, these maneuvers can lead to focally absent or weak points of nerve conduction, where the amplitude of proximal RLN stimulation is over 100 μV compared to a substantial amplitude reduction of the distal RLN stimulation [6, 7, 18]. The correlation between the percentage of EMG amplitude reduction and postoperative vocal cord function is highly variable, and vocal cord mobility can be normal, weak, or paralyzed. Recent studies recommend that if the final EMG amplitude reduction reaches 50–60% or more, surgeons should consider the possibility of postopera-

tive VCP [44, 45]. However, an incomplete LOS may occur if the recording electrodes are not contacting properly the vocal cords possibly due to surgical manipulation of the thyroid or trachea. This displacement can result in a substantial change of EMG amplitude. Thus, it is important to verify and when needed adjust the EMG tube and electrode position if a significant reduction in amplitude is noted [46].

3. *Loss of signal (LOS)*: LOS is defined in part as an amplitude of 100 μV or less (see Section VII). When R_2 and V_2 signals become lost after complete dissection of the RLN, it should be assumed that the RLN might have been injured during surgical manipulation. An effort should be made to identify the disrupted point of nerve conduction and elucidate the mechanism of injury. The disrupted point of nerve conduction may be located by testing the RLN from the distal portion near the entry point of the larynx. If a signal is obtained, the lower portion of the nerve should be tested until a response can no longer be elicited. In this manner, the disrupted point of nerve conduction may be located more precisely. If no disrupted point of nerve conduction is detected, contralateral VN stimulation should be used to exclude the possibility of false LOS, such as monitoring equipment dysfunction, EMG tube malposition, or misuse of neuromuscular blocking agents [2, 12, 14, 47].

Loss of Signal: Definition and Classifications

According to the 2011 International Neural Monitoring Study Group (INMSG) guidelines [2], the three basic criteria for LOS are (1) an EMG change from an initially satisfactory EMG, (2) absence of response or low response (i.e., 100 μV or less) to 1–2 mA stimulation on a dry field, and (3) absence of laryngeal and/or glottic twitch. According to a recent 2018 INMSG guideline for interpreting LOS [4], the optimal normative baseline at the beginning of surgery is an initial V1/R1 waveform with an amplitude of 500 μV or greater obtained under a stimulation current of 1–2 mA.

INMSG Impending Adverse EMG (IA-EMG) and Adverse EMG (A-EMG)

In the setting of continuous vagal IONM, the surgeon can use repeated pulsed stimulation to obtain the real-time EMG change during surgical dissection. The surgeon can set the threshold to a percentage (%) of amplitude reduction (fewer nerve fibers participating in the response) and latency increase (slower response) as an indicator of adverse EMG changes. The surgeon can then correct certain maneuvers immediately to prevent irreversible nerve injury. Animal studies using continuous IONM have demonstrated that amplitude and latency degradation under ongoing traction has potential for recovery if traction is released [23, 48–51]. Two clinical studies that have explored concordant amplitude decrease and latency increase indicate that these "combined events" are reliable early indicators of impending neurapraxia [21, 22]. Therefore, according to the recent INMSG LOS guideline [4], an amplitude decrease of >50% (with absolute amplitude >100 μV) and latency increase of >10% should be interpreted as an Impending Adverse EMG (IA-EMG) because they imply that the nerve is approaching a combined event status in which VCP risk is elevated. Immediate cessation of the surgical maneuver is recommended. The INMSG has also proposed that Adverse EMG (A-EMG) should be defined as 100 μV or less as this drop indicates a progression from the preceding IA-EMG and is known to have a strong association with subsequent VCP with limited recoverability of 17–23% [4].

Other Absolute and Relative Threshold Criteria

Different criteria for using LOS to predict VCP are reported in the literature, including absolute threshold values and relative threshold values. Absolute threshold value criteria include the occurrence of LOS (intraoperative LOS episodes [21, 52, 53] or persistent LOS at the end of surgery [2, 6, 17, 54–56]) and specific final V2 value (200 μV [57] or 280 μV [58]). Relative threshold value criteria involve comparing the signals from the most distal (R2d) and the most proximal (R2p) ends of the exposed RLN as a simple and useful method to evaluate type I LOS (or segmental RLN injury) after completion of thyroid lobectomy and for predicting RLN functional outcome [13, 59]. The positive predictive value of a R2p/R2d ratio >63% for postoperative VCP was 79.4% [59]. Therefore, when the relative threshold value R2p/R2d reduction exceeds 60%, the surgeon should consider the possibility of postoperative VCP, even if the EMG value exceeds 100 μV [13].

False LOS

Normal RLN function with no or very low EMG signal is called false LOS. False LOS is characterized by a lack of a point of injury on the exposed RLN and a lack of response to contralateral VN stimulation [2].

The most common three causes of false LOS are:

1. *Monitoring equipment malfunction.* The grounding, recording/stimulating electrodes and associated connections at the interface-connector box and monitor should be checked to ensure that they are not displaced, dislodged, or broken. The use of electrocauterization can also cause a broken fuse.
2. *ET malposition.* During ET-based recording, displacement of the EMG tube (up- or downward or due to rotation) during surgical manipulation may cause false LOS due to insufficient contact between EMG tube electrodes and vocal folds [46, 60, 61]. To correct a displaced ET EMG tube, the surgeon can perform vagal stimulation, while the anesthesiologist readjusts the tube [2]. If false LOS is suspected, fiber-optic laryngoscopy can be used to confirm the presence of laryngeal twitch and to adjust the electrode position [17].
3. *Repeated use of neuromuscular blocking agents (NMBAs).* Repeated intraoperative administration of NMBAs can cause a false LOS. Preoperative discussion with the anesthesiologist enables proper anesthetic planning. Intraoperatively, when LOS occurs, the surgeon should consult the anesthesiologist regarding any NMBA use. If an NMBA has been inadvertently administered intraoperatively, NMBA reversals (e.g., sugammadex) may be needed for rapid restoration of normal muscle twitch activity [62–65].

True LOS: Type I and Type II

True LOS is defined as an RLN injury resulting in an elicited EMG signal <100 μV. According to the troubleshooting algorithm described in the INSMSG guidelines [2, 4], a negative laryngeal/glottic twitch combined with a positive contralateral VN evoked EMG signal should be interpreted as an ipsilateral neural injury and the possibility of postoperative VCP.

Currently, true LOS and RLN injury are usually classified into two subtypes [2, 6, 17] according to the electrophysiology results observed during IONM. Type 1 LOS or RLN injury (i.e., segmental or localized RLN injury) is characterized by a nerve injury at a specific site, and it usually results from direct stress on the nerve. In type 1 LOS, distal RLN stimulation induces normal evoked activity, whereas proximal stimulation to the injured segment elicits a waveform no greater than 100 μV. In type 2 LOS, the exposed RLN shows no specific disruption site (i.e., diffuse or global RLN injury) and no visible change in appearance [2, 6, 17].

The reported proportion of type I and type II RLN LOS varies in the literature. Dionigi reported greater type I than type II LOS (I = 71% vs. II = 29%) [18] as did Snyder (I = 92% vs. II = 8%) [7]. In contrast, Schneider reported fewer type I LOS lesions (I = 44% vs. II = 56%) [45] as did Chiang (I = 33% vs. II = 67%) [6]. Differences in the reported prevalence may be due to differences in the extent of RLN exposure and whether the disrupted point of the RLN is checked routinely, surgical experience and technique or the use of certain surgical maneuvers, as well as variations in RLN anatomy (i.e., branching patterns, relationship to the ligament of Berry) among different study populations (e.g., different ethnicities) [66].

To establish true LOS with high certainty, the surgeon must use IONM LOS troubleshooting algorithms to exclude all possible causes of false LOS [2].

When a true LOS is confirmed, the following management principles should be applied: (1) Map lesion (type I or II) and elucidate the possible injury mechanism (2) Consider a staged contralateral procedure in cases of LOS with no or incomplete intraoperative recovery. Detailed information on the management of LOS and its troubleshooting algorithms will be introduced and discussed in the following chapters.

Clinically Significant Monitoring Applications

There is increasing adoption of nerve monitoring in endocrine and other head and neck surgery. In a recent survey of practice patterns in the United States, IONM is utilized in roughly 80% of thyroid surgeries performed by otolaryngology-head and neck surgeons and over 65% performed by general surgeons with the number rising significantly over the last 5 years [67, 68]. Over 95% of endocrine surgery fellows (general surgery and otolaryngology-head and neck surgery), exposed to nerve monitoring during their endocrine surgery fellowship, report utilizing IONM in some or all of their cases upon completion of fellowship [69]. Large survey studies suggest higher-volume surgeons more commonly utilize neural monitoring [70]. Strict adherence to IONM standards improves implementation [71].

The 2018 INMSG Guidelines [4] identified the following clinically significant IONM applications and benefits:

1. RLN mapping before its visual identification to facilitate subsequent visual identification and help avoid RLN injury [72]. Snyder et al. reported that electrical RLN neural identification preceded visual identification in nearly 35% of cases [73]. RLN identification speed is improved with IONM [74].
2. Identification of RLN anatomical variants with increased potential for iatrogenic injury.
3. Reducing the rate of tracheotomy in total thyroidectomy based on the prognostication of RLN function [75, 76].
4. Intraoperative alteration of surgical maneuver in case of impending neural injury [22, 77].
5. Identification and preservation of superior laryngeal nerve (SLN) [3, 78].
6. IONM may help younger or less experienced surgeons achieve outcomes similar to experienced surgeons [79].
7. IONM may assist in early and definitive intraoperative identification of nonrecurrent laryngeal nerve variations [80].

The 2018 INMSG Guidelines [4] further outlined the following conceptual domains for the use of IONM during thyroidectomy

1. Intraoperative nerve identification and nerve mapping
2. Differentiation between neural and non-neural structures
3. Identification of impeding nerve injury as well as the mechanism and site of injury
4. Reduction of tracheotomy risk based on the prognostication of nerve injury before proceeding with the contralateral side

Guidelines and Current Standards

In 2006, The International Neural Monitoring Study Group (INMSG) was founded as an international multidisciplinary collaboration to serve the emerging field of neurophysiologic monitoring of laryngeal nerves in head and neck endocrine surgery. Comprised of experts in the field of head and neck endocrine surgery, laryngology, electromyography, anesthesiology, and neurophysiology, the group has published several guidelines to promote uniform and standard IONM technique, to define standardized references of normative and pathological RLN neurophysiology parameters, to evaluate new technological developments, and to support standardized educational and research activities in the field of IONM for head and neck surgeries. It has published guidelines on basic RLN and EBSLN monitoring techniques and interpretations for monitored thyroid and parathyroid surgery [2, 3]. More recently, INMSG has published a two-part consensus guideline discussing nerve monitoring for thyroid and parathyroid surgery with a specific focus of its application on intraoperative strategy and disease management. Part I discusses the management of LOS including its relevance to the staging of thyroid surgery. Part II discusses optimal IONM in the setting of invasive thyroid cancer [4, 5].

These guidelines together with continued advances in monitoring equipment as well as the increasing body of literature supporting the application of IONM in head and neck surgery have led to increasing organizational support for IONM in thyroid and parathyroid surgeries. Both INMSG Guidelines and the German Association of Endocrine Surgery guidelines recommend neural monitoring in all cases of thyroid and parathyroid surgery [2–5, 81]. Updating the 2009 American Thyroid Association (ATA) Thyroid Nodules and Differentiated Thyroid Cancer guidelines, the 2015 Guidelines Task Force on Thyroid Nodules and Differentiated Thyroid Cancer included seven surgical recommendations pertaining to voice optimization laryngeal exam, neural management, and IONM [82]. In addition, the ATA Surgical Affairs Committee Consensus Statement on Outpatient Thyroid Surgery and the ATA Statement on Optimal Surgical Management of Goiter highlight the role of neural monitoring in confirming intact neural function at the end of surgery including its role in discharge planning particularly in cases of bilateral LOS [83, 84]. The American Academy of Otolaryngology Head and Neck Surgery (AAOHNS) Clinical Practice Guideline: Improving Voice Outcomes After Thyroid Surgery as well as the Evidence-Based American Head and Neck Society (AHNS) Consensus Statement on the Management of Locally Invasive Well-Differentiated Thyroid Cancer discuss the utility of neural monitoring in neural identification, reduction of transient nerve paralysis rates, prognostication of nerve function, and avoidance of bilateral VCP [76, 85]. The AAOHNS supports the use of IONM in cases of (i) total thyroidectomy, (ii) revision surgery for thyroid cancer, and (iii) thyroid surgery on an only functioning nerve.

Conclusion

There has been much progress in the application of VN/RLN monitoring during thyroid and parathyroid surgery. Standardization and organizational support has been instrumental in promoting the use of IONM. This chapter provides an overview of the rationale and indications of IONM. Detailed information on the monitoring of the EBSLN and CIONM, troubleshooting system integrity, managing LOS, incorporating IONM into the intraoperative management of invasive thyroid cancer, and nerve monitoring in remote access thyroid surgery and parathyroid surgery are described in other chapters.

References

1. Swonke ML, Shakibai N, Chaaban MR. Medical malpractice trends in thyroidectomies among general surgeons and otolaryngologists. OTO Open. 2020;4(2):2473974x20921141.
2. Randolph GW, Dralle H, Abdullah H, Barczynski M, Bellantone R, Brauckhoff M, Carnaille B, Cherenko S, Chiang FY, Dionigi G, et al. Electrophysiologic recurrent laryngeal nerve monitoring during thyroid and parathyroid surgery: international standards guideline statement. Laryngoscope. 2011;121(Suppl 1):S1–16.
3. Barczynski M, Randolph GW, Cernea CR, Dralle H, Dionigi G, Alesina PF, Mihai R, Finck C, Lombardi D, Hartl DM, et al. External branch of the superior laryngeal nerve monitoring during thyroid and parathyroid surgery: International Neural Monitoring Study Group standards guideline statement. Laryngoscope. 2013;123(Suppl 4):S1–14.
4. Schneider R, Randolph GW, Dionigi G, Wu CW, Barczynski M, Chiang FY, Al-Quaryshi Z, Angelos P, Brauckhoff K, Cernea CR, et al. International neural monitoring study group guideline 2018 part I: staging bilateral thyroid surgery with monitoring loss of signal. Laryngoscope. 2018;128(Suppl 3):S1–s17.
5. Wu CW, Dionigi G, Barczynski M, Chiang FY, Dralle H, Schneider R, Al-Quaryshi Z, Angelos P, Brauckhoff K, Brooks JA, et al. International neuromonitoring study group guidelines 2018: Part II: optimal recurrent laryngeal nerve management for invasive thyroid cancer-incorporation of surgi-

cal, laryngeal, and neural electrophysiologic data. Laryngoscope. 2018;128(Suppl 3):S18–s27.
6. Chiang FY, Lu IC, Kuo WR, Lee KW, Chang NC, Wu CW. The mechanism of recurrent laryngeal nerve injury during thyroid surgery–the application of intraoperative neuromonitoring. Surgery. 2008;143(6):743–9.
7. Snyder SK, Lairmore TC, Hendricks JC, Roberts JW. Elucidating mechanisms of recurrent laryngeal nerve injury during thyroidectomy and parathyroidectomy. J Am Coll Surg. 2008;206(1):123–30.
8. Dralle H, Sekulla C, Lorenz K, Brauckhoff M, Machens A. Intraoperative monitoring of the recurrent laryngeal nerve in thyroid surgery. World J Surg. 2008;32(7):1358–66.
9. Chiang FY, Lu IC, Tsai CJ, Hsiao PJ, Lee KW, Wu CW. Detecting and identifying nonrecurrent laryngeal nerve with the application of intraoperative neuromonitoring during thyroid and parathyroid operation. Am J Otolaryngol. 2012;33(1):1–5.
10. Chiang FY, Lu IC, Chen HC, Chen HY, Tsai CJ, Hsiao PJ, Lee KW, Wu CW. Anatomical variations of recurrent laryngeal nerve during thyroid surgery: how to identify and handle the variations with intraoperative neuromonitoring. Kaohsiung J Med Sci. 2010;26(11):575–83.
11. Wu CW, Dionigi G, Chen HC, Chen HY, Lee KW, Lu IC, Chang PY, Hsiao PJ, Ho KY, Chiang FY. Vagal nerve stimulation without dissecting the carotid sheath during intraoperative neuromonitoring of the recurrent laryngeal nerve in thyroid surgery. Head Neck. 2013;35(10):1443–7.
12. Wu CW, Wang MH, Chen CC, Chen HC, Chen HY, Yu JY, Chang PY, Lu IC, Lin YC, Chiang FY. Loss of signal in recurrent nerve neuromonitoring: causes and management. Gland Surg. 2015;4(1):19–26.
13. Wu CW, Hao M, Tian M, Dionigi G, Tufano RP, Kim HY, Jung KY, Liu X, Sun H, Lu IC, et al. Recurrent laryngeal nerve injury with incomplete loss of electromyography signal during monitored thyroidectomy-evaluation and outcome. Langenbecks Arch Surg. 2017;402(4):691–9.
14. Randolph GW, Wu CW, Dionigi G, Kamani D, Modi RR, Chiang FY, Henry JF. The international RLN anatomic classification system. In: Randolph GW, editor. The recurrent and superior laryngeal nerves. Cham: Springer International Publishing; 2016. p. 125–38.
15. Shoja MM, Ardalan MR, Tubbs RS, Loukas M, Vahedinia S, Jabbary R, Jalilvand M, Shakeri A. The relationship between the internal jugular vein and common carotid artery in the carotid sheath: the effects of age, gender and side. Ann Anat. 2008;190(4):339–43.
16. Dionigi G, Chiang FY, Rausei S, Wu CW, Boni L, Lee KW, Rovera F, Cantone G, Bacuzzi A. Surgical anatomy and neurophysiology of the vagus nerve (VN) for standardised intraoperative neuromonitoring (IONM) of the inferior laryngeal nerve (ILN) during thyroidectomy. Langenbecks Arch Surg. 2010;395(7):893–9.
17. Chiang FY, Lee KW, Chen HC, Chen HY, Lu IC, Kuo WR, Hsieh MC, Wu CW. Standardization of intraoperative neuromonitoring of recurrent laryngeal nerve in thyroid operation. World J Surg. 2010;34(2):223–9.
18. Dionigi G, Alesina PF, Barczynski M, Boni L, Chiang FY, Kim HY, Materazzi G, Randolph GW, Terris DJ, Wu CW. Recurrent laryngeal nerve injury in video-assisted thyroidectomy: lessons learned from neuromonitoring. Surg Endosc. 2012;26(9):2601–8.
19. Dionigi G, Wu CW, Kim HY, Rausei S, Boni L, Chiang FY. Severity of recurrent laryngeal nerve injuries in thyroid surgery. World J Surg. 2016;40(6):1373–81.
20. Chiang F-Y, Lu IC, Chang P-Y, Dionigi G, Randolph GW, Sun H, Lee K-D, Tae K, Ji YB, Kim SW, et al. Comparison of EMG signals recorded by surface electrodes on endotracheal tube and thyroid cartilage during monitored thyroidectomy. Kaohsiung J Med Sci. 2017;33(10):503–9.
21. Schneider R, Randolph GW, Sekulla C, Phelan E, Thanh PN, Bucher M, Machens A, Dralle H, Lorenz K. Continuous intraoperative vagus nerve stimulation for identification of imminent recurrent laryngeal nerve injury. Head Neck. 2013;35(11):1591–8.
22. Phelan E, Schneider R, Lorenz K, Dralle H, Kamani D, Potenza A, Sritharan N, Shin J. G WR: continuous vagal IONM prevents recurrent laryngeal nerve paralysis by revealing initial EMG changes of impending neuropraxic injury: a prospective, multicenter study. Laryngoscope. 2014;124(6):1498–505.
23. Wu CW, Dionigi G, Sun H, Liu X, Kim HY, Hsiao PJ, Tsai KB, Chen HC, Chen HY, Chang PY, et al. Intraoperative neuromonitoring for the early detection and prevention of RLN traction injury in thyroid surgery: a porcine model. Surgery. 2014;155(2):329–39.
24. Dionigi G, Bacuzzi A, Boni L, Rovera F, Dionigi R. What is the learning curve for intraoperative neuromonitoring in thyroid surgery? Int J Surg. 2008;6(Suppl 1):S7–12.
25. Cirocchi R, Arezzo A, D'Andrea V, et al. Intraoperative neuromonitoring versus visual nerve identification for prevention of recurrent laryngeal nerve injury in adults undergoing thyroid surgery. Cochrane Database Syst Rev. 2019;1(1):CD012483. https://doi.org/10.1002/14651858.CD012483.pub2.
26. Zheng S, Xu Z, Wei Y, Zeng M, He J. Effect of intraoperative neuromonitoring on recurrent laryngeal nerve palsy rates after thyroid surgery–a meta-analysis. J Formos Med Assoc. 2013;112(8):463–72. https://doi.org/10.1016/j.jfma.2012.03.003.
27. Higgins TS, Gupta R, Ketcham AS, Sataloff RT, Wadsworth JT, Sinacori JT. Recurrent laryngeal nerve monitoring versus identification alone on post-thyroidectomy true vocal fold palsy: a meta-analysis. Laryngoscope. 2011;121(5):1009–17. https://doi.org/10.1002/lary.21578.
28. Dralle H, Sekulla C, Haerting J, et al. Risk factors of paralysis and functional outcome after recurrent laryngeal nerve monitoring in thyroid surgery. Surgery. 2004;136(6):1310–22. https://doi.org/10.1016/j.surg.2004.07.018.
29. Roberts JR, Wadsworth J. Recurrent laryngeal nerve monitoring during mediastinoscopy: predictors of

injury. Ann Thorac Surg. 2007;83(2):388–91. discussion 391-382

30. Uldry E, Schafer M, Saadi A, Rousson V, Demartines N. Patients' preferences on information and involvement in decision making for gastrointestinal surgery. World J Surg. 2013;37(9):2162–71.
31. Horne SK, Gal TJ, Brennan JA. Prevalence and patterns of intraoperative nerve monitoring for thyroidectomy. Otolaryngol Head Neck Surg. 2007;136(6):952–6.
32. Dralle H, Lorenz K, Machens A. Verdicts on malpractice claims after thyroid surgery: emerging trends and future directions. Head Neck. 2012;34(11):1591–6.
33. Randolph GW, Shin JJ, Grillo HC, Mathisen D, Katlic MR, Kamani D, Zurakowski D. The surgical management of goiter: part II. Surgical treatment and results. Laryngoscope. 2011;121(1):68–76.
34. Kim HY, Tufano RP, Randolph G, Barczynski M, Wu CW, Chiang FY, Liu X, Masuoka H, Miyauchi A, Park SY, et al. Impact of positional changes in neural monitoring endotracheal tube on amplitude and latency of electromyographic response in monitored thyroid surgery: results from the Porcine Experiment. Head Neck. 2016;38(Suppl 1):E1004–8.
35. Liddy W, Lawson BR, Barber SR, Kamani D, Shama M, Soylu S, Wu CW, Chiang FY, Scharpf J, Barczynski M, et al. Anterior laryngeal electrodes for recurrent laryngeal nerve monitoring during thyroid and parathyroid surgery: new expanded options for neural monitoring. Laryngoscope. 2018;128(12):2910–5.
36. Lee HS, Oh J, Kim SW, Jeong YW, Wu CW, Chiang FY, Lee KD. Intraoperative neuromonitoring of recurrent laryngeal nerve during thyroidectomy with adhesive skin electrodes. World J Surg. 2020;44(1):148–54.
37. Chiang FY, Lu IC, Chang PY, Sun H, Wang P, Lu XB, Chen HC, Chen HY, Kim HY, Dionigi G, et al. Stimulating dissecting instruments during neuromonitoring of RLN in thyroid surgery. Laryngoscope. 2015;125(12):2832–7.
38. Wu CW, Liu X, Barczynski M, Kim HY, Dionigi G, Sun H, Chiang FY, Kamani D, Randolph GW. Optimal stimulation during monitored thyroid surgery: EMG response characteristics in a porcine model. Laryngoscope. 2017;127(4):998–1005.
39. Lamade W, Ulmer C, Seimer A, Molnar V, Meyding-Lamade U, Thon KP, Koch KP. A new system for continuous recurrent laryngeal nerve monitoring. Minim Invasive Ther Allied Technol. 2007;16(3):149–54.
40. Ulmer C, Koch KP, Seimer A, Molnar V, Meyding-Lamade U, Thon KP, Lamade W. Real-time monitoring of the recurrent laryngeal nerve: an observational clinical trial. Surgery. 2008;143(3):359–65.
41. Schneider R, Przybyl J, Pliquett U, Hermann M, Wehner M, Pietsch UC, Konig F, Hauss J, Jonas S, Leinung S. A new vagal anchor electrode for real-time monitoring of the recurrent laryngeal nerve. Am J Surg. 2010;199(4):507–14.
42. Sinclair CF, Téllez MJ, Ulkatan S. Noninvasive, tube-based, continuous vagal nerve monitoring using the laryngeal adductor reflex: feasibility study of 134 nerves at risk. Head Neck. 2018;40(11):2498–506.
43. Brauckhoff M, Walls G, Brauckhoff K, Thanh PN, Thomusch O, Dralle H. Identification of the non-recurrent inferior laryngeal nerve using intraoperative neurostimulation. Langenbecks Arch Surg. 2002;386(7):482–7.
44. Wu CW, Hao M, Tian M, Dionigi G, Tufano RP, Kim HY, Jung KY, Liu X, Sun H, Lu IC, et al. Recurrent laryngeal nerve injury with incomplete loss of electromyography signal during monitored thyroidectomy-evaluation and outcome. Langenbecks Arch Surg. 2016; https://doi.org/10.1007/s00423-00016-01381-00428.
45. Schneider R, Sekulla C, Machens A, Lorenz K, Thanh PN, Dralle H. Dynamics of loss and recovery of the nerve monitoring signal during thyroidectomy predict early postoperative vocal fold function. Head Neck. 2016;38(Suppl 1):E1144–51.
46. Lu IC, Chu KS, Tsai CJ, Wu CW, Kuo WR, Chen HY, Lee KW, Chiang FY. Optimal depth of NIM EMG endotracheal tube for intraoperative Neuromonitoring of the recurrent laryngeal nerve during thyroidectomy. World J Surg. 2008;32(9):1935–9.
47. Randolph GW. Surgery of the thyroid and parathyroid glands. Philadelphia: Saunders, Elsevier; 2013.
48. Puram SV, Chow H, Wu CW, Heaton JT, Kamani D, Gorti G, Chiang FY, Dionigi G, Barczynski M, Schneider R, et al. Posterior cricoarytenoid muscle electrophysiologic changes are predictive of vocal cord paralysis with recurrent laryngeal nerve compressive injury in a canine model. Laryngoscope. 2016;126(12):2744–51.
49. Puram SV, Chow H, Wu CW, Heaton JT, Kamani D, Gorti G, Chiang FY, Dionigi G, Barczynski M, Schneider R, et al. Vocal cord paralysis predicted by neural monitoring electrophysiologic changes with recurrent laryngeal nerve compressive neuropraxic injury in a canine model. Head Neck. 2016;38(Suppl 1):E1341–50.
50. Brauckhoff K, Svendsen OS, Stangeland L, Biermann M, Aas T, Husby PJA. Injury mechanisms and electromyographic changes after injury of the recurrent laryngeal nerve: experiments in a porcine model. Head Neck. 2018;40(2):274–82.
51. Wu C-W, Randolph GW, Lu I-C, Chang P-Y, Chen Y-T, Hun P-C, Lin Y-C, Dionigi G, Chiang F-Y. Intraoperative neural monitoring in thyroid surgery: lessons learned from animal studies. Gland Surg. 2016;5(5):473–80.
52. Jonas J. Continuous vagal nerve stimulation for recurrent laryngeal nerve protection in thyroid surgery. Eur Surg Res. 2010;44(3-4):185–91.
53. Sitges-Serra A, Fontane J, Duenas JP, Duque CS, Lorente L, Trillo L, Sancho JJ. Prospective study on loss of signal on the first side during neuromonitoring of the recurrent laryngeal nerve in total thyroidectomy. Br J Surg. 2013;100(5):662–6.
54. Cernea CR, Brandao LG, Hojaij FC, De Carlucci D, et al. Negative and positive predictive values of nerve monitoring in thyroidectomy. Head Neck. 2012;34(2):175–9.

55. Melin M, Schwarz K, Lammers BJ, Goretzki PE. IONM-guided goiter surgery leading to two-stage thyroidectomyDOUBLEHYPHENindication and results. Langenbecks Arch Surg. 2013;398(3):411–8.
56. Caragacianu D, Kamani D, Randolph GW. Intraoperative monitoring: normative range associated with normal postoperative glottic function. Laryngoscope. 2013;123(12):3026–31.
57. Genther DJ, Kandil EH, Noureldine SI, Tufano RP. Correlation of final evoked potential amplitudes on intraoperative electromyography of the recurrent laryngeal nerve with immediate postoperative vocal fold function after thyroid and parathyroid surgery. JAMA Otolaryngol Head Neck Surg. 2014;140(2):124–8.
58. Pavier Y, Saroul N, Pereira B, Tauveron I, Gilain L, Mom T. Acute prediction of laryngeal outcome during thyroid surgery by electromyographic laryngeal monitoring. Head Neck. 2015;37(6):835–9.
59. Yuan Q, Wu G, Hou J, Liao X, Liao Y, Chiang FY. Correlation between electrophysiological changes and outcomes of vocal cord function in 1764 recurrent laryngeal nerves with visual integrity during thyroidectomy. Thyroid. 2020;30(5):739–45.
60. Tsai CJ, Tseng KY, Wang FY, Lu IC, Wang HM, Wu CW, Chiang HC, Chiang FY. Electromyographic endotracheal tube placement during thyroid surgery in neuromonitoring of recurrent laryngeal nerve. Kaohsiung J Med Sci. 2011;27(3):96–101.
61. Chang PY, Hu PY, Lin YC, Chen HY, Chiang FY, Wu CW, Dionigi G, Lu IC. Trachway video intubating stylet allows for optimization of electromyographic endotracheal tube placement for monitored thyroidectomy. Gland Surg. 2017;6(5):464–8.
62. Lu IC, Wu CW, Chang PY, Chen HY, Tseng KY, Randolph GW, Cheng KI, Chiang FY. Reversal of rocuronium-induced neuromuscular blockade by sugammadex allows for optimization of neural monitoring of the recurrent laryngeal nerve. Laryngoscope. 2016;126(4):1014–9.
63. Lu IC, Lin IH, Wu CW, Chen HY, Lin YC, Chiang FY, Chang PY. Preoperative, intraoperative and postoperative anesthetic prospective for thyroid surgery: what's new. Gland Surg. 2017;6(5):469–75.
64. Lu IC, Wu SH, Wu CW. Neuromuscular blockade management for intraoperative neural monitoring. Kaohsiung J Med Sci. 2020;36(4):230–5.
65. Lu IC, Wu SH, Chang PY, Ho PY, Huang TY, Lin YC, Kamani D, Randolph GW, Dionigi G, Chiang FY, et al. Precision neuromuscular block management for neural monitoring during thyroid surgery. J Invest Surg. 2020:1–8. https://doi.org/10.1080/08941939.2020.1805055.
66. Wu CW, Lee KD, Tae K, Ji YB, Kim SU, Lee HS, Lee KW, Chiang FY. Recurrent laryngeal nerve (RLN) injury in thyroid surgery: lessons learned from the intraoperative neural monitoring (IONM). Int J Head Neck Sci. 2017;1(1):19–26.
67. Singer MC, Rosenfeld RM, Sundaram K. Laryngeal nerve monitoring: current utilization among head and neck surgeons. Otolaryngol Head Neck Surg. 2012;146(6):895–9.
68. Ho Y, Carr MM, Goldenberg D. Trends in intraoperative neural monitoring for thyroid and parathyroid surgery amongst otolaryngologists and general surgeons. Eur Arch Otorhinolaryngol. 2013;270(9):2525–30.
69. Marti JL, Holm T, Randolph G. Universal use of intraoperative nerve monitoring by recently fellowship-trained thyroid surgeons is common, associated with higher surgical volume, and impacts intraoperative decision-making. World J Surg. 2016;40(2):337–43.
70. Sturgeon C, Sturgeon T, Angelos P. Neuromonitoring in thyroid surgery: attitudes, usage patterns, and predictors of use among endocrine surgeons. World J Surg. 2009;33(3):417–25.
71. Schneider R, Randolph GW, Barczynski M, Dionigi G, Wu C-W, Chiang F-Y, Machens A, Kamani D, Dralle H. Continuous intraoperative neural monitoring of the recurrent nerves in thyroid surgery: a quantum leap in technology. Gland Surg. 2016;5(6):607–16.
72. Chiang FY, Lu IC, Chen HC, Chen HY, Tsai CJ, Hsiao PJ, Lee KW, Wu CW. Intraoperative neuromonitoring for early localization and identification of the recurrent laryngeal nerve during thyroid surgery. Kaohsiung J Med Sci. 2010;26(12):633–9.
73. Snyder SK, Sigmond BR, Lairmore TC, Govednik-Horny CM, Janicek AK, Jupiter DC. The long-term impact of routine intraoperative nerve monitoring during thyroid and parathyroid surgery. Surgery. 2013;154(4):704–11. discussion 711–703
74. Sari S, Erbil Y, Sumer A, Agcaoglu O, Bayraktar A, Issever H, Ozarmagan S. Evaluation of recurrent laryngeal nerve monitoring in thyroid surgery. Int J Surg. 2010;8(6):474–8.
75. Goretzki PE, Schwarz K, Brinkmann J, Wirowski D, Lammers BJ. The impact of intraoperative neuromonitoring (IONM) on surgical strategy in bilateral thyroid diseases: is it worth the effort? World J Surg. 2010;34(6):1274–84.
76. Chandrasekhar SS, Randolph GW, Seidman MD, Rosenfeld RM, Angelos P, Barkmeier-Kraemer J, Benninger MS, Blumin JH, Dennis G, Hanks J, et al. Clinical practice guideline: improving voice outcomes after thyroid surgery. Otolaryngol Head Neck Surg. 2013;148(6 Suppl):S1–37.
77. Schneider R, Lamade W, Hermann M, Goretzki P, Timmermann W, Hauss J. Continuous intraoperative neuromonitoring of the recurrent laryngeal nerve in thyroid surgery (CIONM) – Where are we now? An update to the European Symposium of Continuous Neuromonitoring in Thyroid Surgery. Zentralbl Chir. 2012;137(1):88–90.
78. Cernea CR, Ferraz AR, Furlani J, Monteiro S, Nishio S, Hojaij FC, Dutra Junior A, Marques LA, Pontes PA, Bevilacqua RG. Identification of the external branch of the superior laryngeal nerve during thyroidectomy. Am J Surg. 1992;164(6):634–9.
79. Alesina PF, Hinrichs J, Meier B, Cho EY, Bolli M, Walz MK. Intraoperative neuromonitoring for surgical training in thyroid surgery: its routine use allows a

safe operation instead of lack of experienced mentoring. World J Surg. 2014;38(3):592–8.
80. Kamani D, Potenza AS, Cernea CR, Kamani YV, Randolph GW. The nonrecurrent laryngeal nerve: anatomic and electrophysiologic algorithm for reliable identification. Laryngoscope. 2015;125(2):503–8.
81. Musholt TJ, Clerici T, Dralle H, Frilling A, Goretzki PE, Hermann MM, Kussmann J, Lorenz K, Nies C, Schabram J, et al. German Association of Endocrine Surgeons practice guidelines for the surgical treatment of benign thyroid disease. Langenbecks Arch Surg. 2011;396(5):639–49.
82. Haugen BR, Alexander EK, Bible KC, Doherty GM, Mandel SJ, Nikiforov YE, Pacini F, Randolph GW, Sawka AM, Schlumberger M, et al. 2015 American thyroid association management guidelines for adult patients with thyroid nodules and differentiated thyroid cancer: the american thyroid association guidelines task force on thyroid nodules and differentiated thyroid cancer. Thyroid. 2016;26(1):1–133.
83. Chen AY, Bernet VJ, Carty SE, Davies TF, Ganly I, Inabnet WB III, Shaha AR. American thyroid association statement on optimal surgical management of goiter. Thyroid. 2014;24(2):181–9.
84. Terris DJ, Snyder S, Carneiro-Pla D, Inabnet WB, Kandil E, Orloff LA, Shindo M, Tufano RP, Tuttle RMM, Urken ML, et al. American thyroid association statement on outpatient thyroidectomy. Thyroid. 2013;23(10):1193–202.
85. Shindo ML, Caruana S, Kandil E, McCaffrey JC, Orloff L, Porterfield JR, Randolph G, Shaha A, Shin J, Terris D. Management of invasive well-differentiated thyroid cancer an American Head and Neck society consensus statement. Head Neck. 2014;36(10):1379–90.

Methods of Recurrent Laryngeal Nerve Monitoring

7

Betty Y. Chen and Brendan C. Stack

Injury of the recurrent laryngeal nerve (RLN) is one of the well-known risks of surgical procedures involving the thyroid, parathyroid, and central neck compartment. Unilateral injury results in variable degrees of impairments to the patient's voice, breathing, and swallowing, which can be associated with decreased quality of life [1]. Bilateral RLN injury is much more severe, leading to acute respiratory compromise often necessitating an emergent surgical airway in up to 50% of cases [1]. The incidence of temporary vocal cord injury has been reported to range from 2% to 13%, and permanent injury ranges from 0.4% to 5.2% after thyroidectomy [2]. However, these statistics are questionable from some series when universal postoperative laryngoscopy is not performed. Additional factors such as revision surgery, previous ipsilateral injury, patient anatomy, extent of oncologic resection, and a previous irradiated surgical field can increase the risk of nerve injury.

Meticulous dissection and visualization of the recurrent laryngeal nerve and its branches is largely accepted as the optimal method to avoid nerve injury. However, intact anatomy does not always correlate with intact function. Apart from transection, the intact nerve is susceptible to additional traumatic forces such as traction, thermal spread from cautery, compression, clamping, ligature, and suction injury [3, 4]. In fact, traction injury accounts for more than 75% of nerve injuries, with Berry's ligament implicated as the most frequent site of injury because it is a fixation point for the nerve [3–5]. This injury results from medial retraction and delivery of the partially dissected thyroid gland. Thus, the demand was born for reliable methods of recurrent laryngeal nerve monitoring to minimize the largely avoidable and potentially catastrophic risk of RLN injury.

History of Nerve Monitoring

Over time, the approaches for evaluation and prevention of recurrent laryngeal nerve injury have changed. Kocher, largely considered the father of thyroid surgery, routinely performed partial thyroidectomies under local anesthesia, where he would use the quality of the patient's voice as a measure of nerve injury [6]. This method was not accurate as there was no standardized assessment of postoperative nerve function. In addition, the timing between nerve injury and its functional sequelae can be variable and is often not detected immediately at the time of injury. In their 1939 paper, Lahey and Hoover presented a case series of 3000 thyroidectomies with a reported RLN injury rate of 0.3% [6]. They advocated for dis-

B. Y. Chen · B. C. Stack (✉)
Department of Otolaryngology-Head and Neck Surgery, Southern Illinois University School of Medicine, Springfield, IL, USA
e-mail: bchen63@siumed.edu; bcstackjr@gmail.com

© The Author(s), under exclusive license to Springer Nature Switzerland AG 2022

J. Scharpf, G. W. Randolph (eds.), *Intraoperative Cranial Nerve Monitoring in Otolaryngology-Head and Neck Surgery*, https://doi.org/10.1007/978-3-030-84916-0_7

Table 7.1 List of key personnel in the development of RLN and vagal nerve monitoring with their respective contributions, arranged in chronological order

Author (year)	Contribution to intraoperative nerve monitoring
Lahey and Hoover (1938)	Established direct RLN visualization as the gold standard for prevention of nerve injury
Durham and Shedd (1965)	Balloon pressure transducer as a surrogate tool to assess vocal fold function
Hedegaard et al.	Sound oscillator
Kratz (1973)	Rigid bronchoscope to visualize vocal fold motion
Premachandra et al. (1990)	Flexible endoscope suspended above the glottic airway to visualize vocal fold motion
Tanigawa et al. (1991)	LMA with bronchoscope, better view of vocal folds
Hillerman et al. (2003)	Double intubation with small ETT and LMA
Flisberg and Lindholm (1969)	First use of intraoperative EMG in thyroidectomy
Rea et al. (1998)	Postcricoid surface recording electrodes
Lamadé et al. (2000)	First surgical application of continuous intraoperative nerve monitoring
INSMG (2011)	Standardized guidelines for setup, equipment, interpretation of EMG-based intraoperative nerve monitoring

section and direct visualization of the recurrent laryngeal nerve intraoperatively as the gold standard of prevention of nerve injury [6] (Table 7.1). This has been codified in the current American Thyroid Association (ATA) thyroid nodule and cancer guidelines under recommendation 42, requiring visual identification of RLN during dissection in all cases [7].

Early Nerve Monitoring Technology

In 1965, Durham and Shedd developed a method for recording physiologic responses of the recurrent laryngeal nerve using a canine model [8]. They used a balloon pressure transducer attached to the endotracheal tube and positioned the apparatus at the level of the glottic opening to monitor vocal fold activity [8]. Stimulation of the intact and functional nerve corresponded with changes in the pressure transducer, which was measured and recorded by an external device [8, 9]. This was one of the first ways of indirectly identifying and monitoring the recurrent laryngeal nerve via electrical stimulation that was sensitive and specific.

Hvidegaard and colleagues also devised a method of nerve monitoring using an acoustic impedance monitoring system [10]. This involved placement of a sound oscillator into the trachea, which transmits pure tone frequency signals to a microphone sitting above the vocal cords. With RLN stimulation, the vocal cord motion changes air impedance inside the trachea, translating to measurable signals picked up by the microphone. Despite early promising results, this method has not been adopted into clinical settings.

Unlike facial nerve monitoring systems, where the functional integrity of the nerve is easily determined by visualization of facial movements upon direct stimulation, assessing RLN function requires visualization of the vocal cords. Multiple methods have been developed to provide direct view of the glottic airway intraoperatively. One involves a self-retaining rigid endoscope that is placed, draped, and suspended above the vocal folds [11]. Other setups have involved an intraoperative flexible laryngoscope positioned above the vocal cords beside the ETT for the duration of surgery [12]. Both methods offer the surgeon continuous visual feedback of vocal cord motion during dissection. However, these techniques provided a limited view of the vocal folds due to partial obstruction by the endotracheal tube. Using an LMA removed the obstructed view, but the airway was left relatively unsecured.

To optimize view of the visual cords during thyroidectomy, Tanigawa and colleagues have described the use of a laryngeal mask airway (LMA), which is positioned above the vocal folds in place of the traditional endotracheal tube [9, 13]. After proper placement, a rigid endoscope is passed through the lumen of the LMA and offers the surgical team an unobstructed view and easier assessment of vocal fold motion [13]. The major drawback to this technique is the risk of airway loss from factors such as extrinsic laryngeal compression during surgery, LMA displacement, laryngospasm, and intraoperative aspiration. The rate of conversion to endotracheal intubation during thyroidectomy using this technique has been reported up to 10% [9]. To mitigate the risk of intraoperative airway loss, Hillerman and colleagues introduced a double-intubation technique, where a small lumen microlaryngeal endotracheal tube is used to secure the airway [14]. Following intubation, a traditional LMA was placed, through which an endoscope was passed to visualize the vocal cord [14]. The LMA technique without double intubation has also been proven to be a feasible alternative to the ETT in intraoperative RLN monitoring by other authors [15].

Intermittent Electromyographic-Based Intraoperative Nerve Monitoring

Since intact nerve anatomy does not always correlate with function, intraoperative nerve monitoring was developed to enable assessment of RLN functional status. This information is particularly useful in intraoperative decision-making for bilateral surgeries in the setting of ipsilateral nerve injury. IONM involves stimulation of a nerve of interest to produce muscle response that is audibly and visually detectable as an electromyographic (EMG) waveform. Flisberg and Lindholm were one of the first to introduce EMG-based IONM to the operating room [16]. They placed intramuscular recording electrodes through the cricothyroid membrane into the vocalis muscle and recorded muscle action potentials induced by RLN stimulation. The main limitation of this method lies in the positioning of the recording electrodes, which are located in the operative field and prone to displacement during dissection.

Subsequently, various types of electrode equipment have been developed that enable endolaryngeal placement. For instance, Rea and colleagues developed postcricoid surface electrodes to monitor the activity of the posterior cricoarytenoid muscle during phonation and respiration [17]. However, visualization of the postcricoid larynx for electrode placement can be difficult depending on patient anatomical features such as limited cervical mobility and mouth opening [17]. These factors, combined with the presence of frequent motion artifacts, have limited widespread use of this technique [17, 18].

Currently, the most commonly employed apparatus for intraoperative nerve monitoring is an endotracheal tube-based recording system [19]. The ETT-based system is popular due to its ease of placement, safety from an established airway, and proven ability to generate a reliable electrophysiologic signals. The basic components of an EMG-based IONM system include recording electrodes, ground electrodes, stimulator probe, a monitor to display EMG data, and an interface-connector box (Fig. 7.1). In 2011, the International Neural Monitoring Study Group (INMSG) published a set of guidelines to standardize the equipment, reporting, and analysis of IONM in thyroid and parathyroid surgery [18]. Fundamental elements of a reliable IONM system include preoperative and postoperative suprathreshold vagal or RLN stimulation to verify integrity of the nerve monitoring system, along with preoperative and postoperative laryngoscopy to correlate EMG data with glottic function.

Historically, there has been variability in the application of recording and stimulation electrodes. As previously mentioned, recording electrodes used in the past have included needle electrodes placed into muscles innervated by RLN and surface electrodes placed to the postcricoid area or pre-fashioned surface electrodes attached to the ETT. Compared to surface electrodes, needle electrodes provide similar measurements but do confer additional risks related with placement, including laryngeal laceration and hematoma [18, 20]. Stimulation electrodes can be monopolar or bipolar. Monopolar instrumentation offers the advantage of diffuse spread of stimulating current, which enables neural mapping of a greater distance of the nerve of interest [18]. On the other hand, bipolar probes stimulate a focal area along the nerve. The INMSG recommends the use of an endotracheal tube-based recording electrode system with both

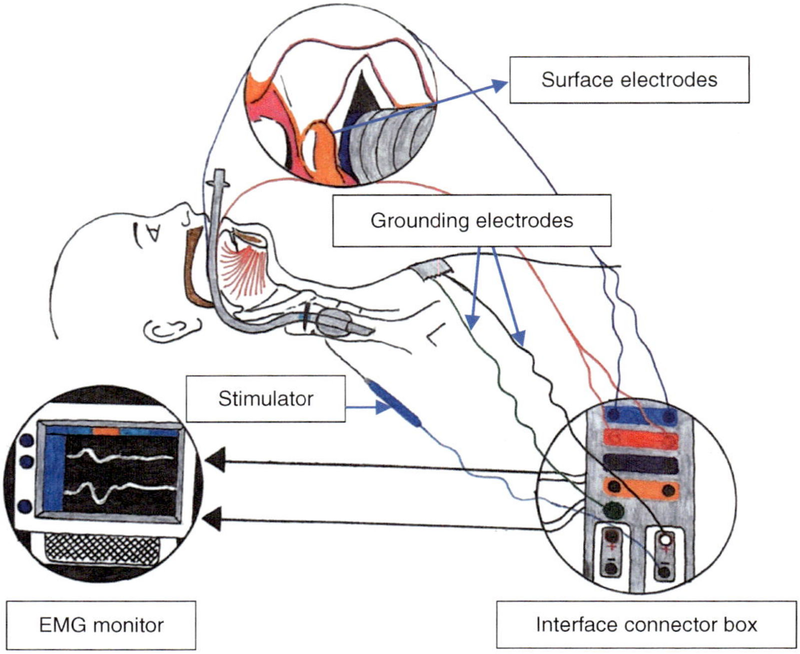

Fig. 7.1 Schematic of the setup and components of a typical ETT-based intraoperative nerve monitoring system. (Illustrated by B. Chen, MD)

audio feedback and waveforms for optimal neural monitoring [18].

Anesthesia and Intubation

The ideal anesthetic in IONM minimizes alterations in the neuromuscular signal while keeping the patient adequately sedated for surgery. Neuromuscular blockers have been shown to decrease the amplitude of the EMG waveform and would interfere with intraoperative interpretation of the neural signal [21]. Therefore, neuromuscular blockers are reserved only for short-term use during intubation, and long-acting paralytics should be avoided. Additional information on administration of anesthesia in nerve monitoring is provided in Chap. 3.

The integrity of the laryngeal EMG signal depends on proper positioning of the recording electrodes, which can be assessed by visualization of the endotracheal tube during intubation. Using GlideScope® (Verathon, Bothell, WA) visualization, the patient is intubated such that the surface electrodes attached to the endotracheal tube are at the level to contact the vocalis and thyroarytenoid muscles. This is achieved by placing the endotracheal tube mark at the level of the vocal cords. After optimal positioning of the patient on the operating bed, including shoulder extension and tucking of the upper extremities as needed, the position of the endotracheal tube can be re-examined using the GlideScope® (Verathon, Bothell, WA) and direct visualization, noting any displacements necessitating tube adjustments, and the tube is secured. Alternatively, the patient's shoulder roll can be placed prior to GlideScope® (Verathon, Bothell, WA) intubation after which the tube is secured in place. Verification testing is recommended when there is doubt based on EMG tracings following intubation. These maneuvers may include repeat laryngoscopy or assessing for presence of polyphasic waveforms, which is indicative of proper ETT placement [18] (Fig. 7.2).

EMG Waveform Parameters

For accurate interpretation of the EMG waveform, one needs to have knowledge of a standardized set of electrophysiologic properties, including amplitude, latency, and threshold.

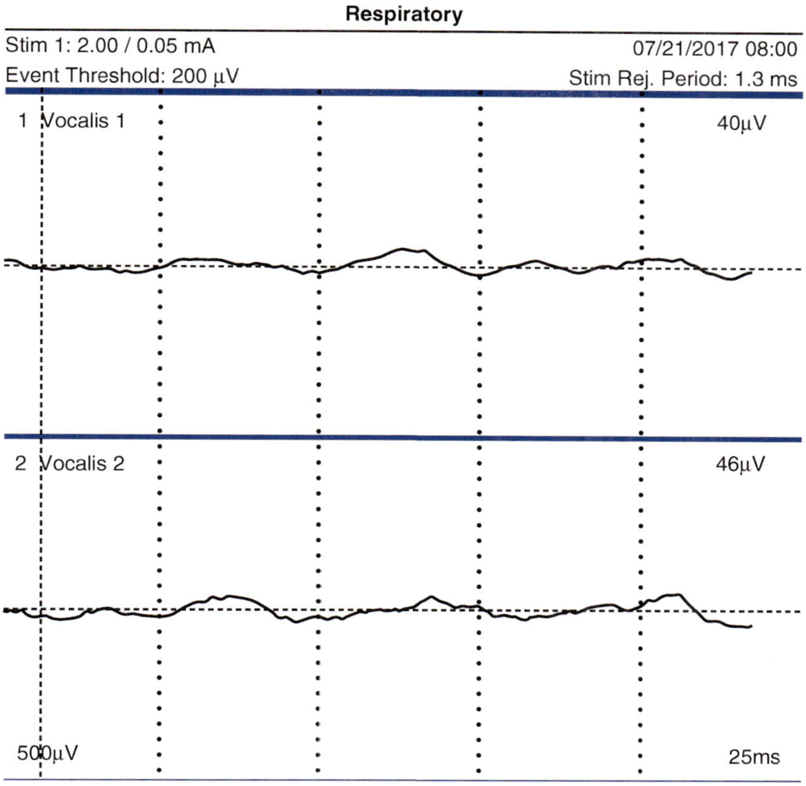

Fig. 7.2 Polyphasic waveform associated with respiratory variation

I. Amplitude

Amplitude is the maximum deflection from baseline EMG wave measurement, measured in millivolts (mV) [22] (Fig. 7.3). This value correlates with the number of muscle fibers recruited during stimulation. Based on previous studies in healthy volunteers during normal phonation, the mean amplitude of laryngeal EMG was measured as 350 µV in the thyroarytenoid muscle and 280 µV in the cricothyroid, with ranges from 100 µV to 800 µV [23].

II. Latency

Latency is defined as the time between stimulation artifact and onset of EMG signal, measured in milliseconds [22]. The value increases with increasing anatomic distance between the stimulation point and the vocal cord. This is evident in the significantly longer latency value of the left vagus nerve, given its longer anatomic course of the left vagus nerve with respect to the right [18]. Conversely, it is shorter for the superior laryngeal nerve (SLN). Variabilities in the latency values can be used to differentiate signals from the superior laryngeal, recurrent laryngeal, and vagal nerves.

III. Threshold

Threshold is the stimulation current applied to the RLN or vagal nerve that triggers minimal laryngeal EMG activity and is typically 0.3–0.4 mA in humans [18]. The maximal stimulation current is 0.8 mA, at which point all innervated muscle fibers are depolarized. The initial stimulus current is typically set at 1 mA, which represents a safe and effective suprathreshold value as stated by the INMSG.

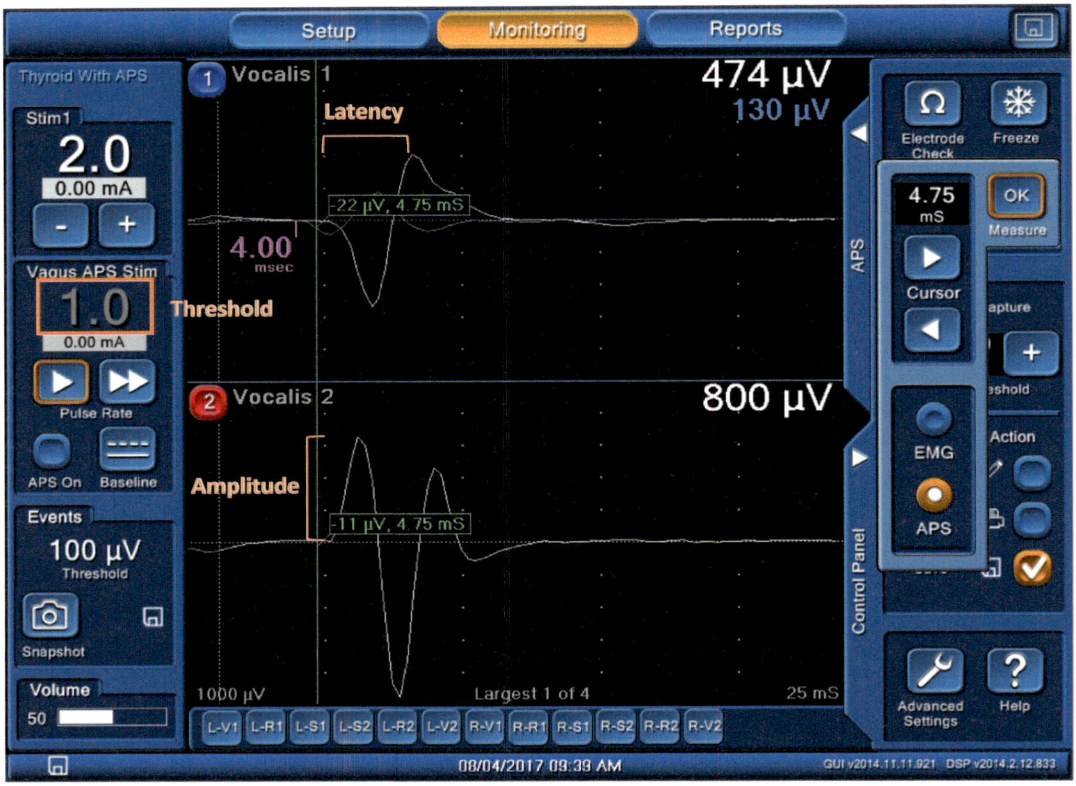

Fig. 7.3 An example of an evoked EMG waveform of the recurrent laryngeal nerve with labeled waveform parameters

IV. Signal Loss

A signal loss occurs when the evoked waveform amplitude is less than 100 μV with supra-threshold stimulation current of 1 or 2 mA [18]. The electrophysiologic signal change should be correlated intraoperatively with a laryngeal twitch assessment and direct visualization of glottic movement. If no response is found on EMG, twitch, or glottic exams, this may be interpreted as a true nerve injury, and the surgical team is advised to identify site of injury and weigh decisions on timing of contralateral surgery [18].

V. Baseline

The INMSG recommends a set of baseline normative EMG data, including stimulation current of between 1 and 2 mA and initial EMG waveform with amplitude of at least 500 μV, combined with a robust laryngeal twitch with monopolar stimulation [18]. In addition, it is important to check the impedance value of each electrode, which should be less than 5 kiloohms on either side [18]. A high impedance value could imply poor electrode contact with the vocal cord and should signal a need to adjust the endotracheal tube position.

Continuous Intraoperative Nerve Monitoring

Despite increasingly widespread use, intermittent IONM has several limitations in its efficacy. First, it is only able to provide assessment of nerve and vocal cord function at the time of stimulation. During the interval between stimulations, the nerve is not being monitored, and may be susceptible to undetected intraoperative injury. Thus, intermittent IONM may detect nerve injuries after they have already occurred. Aside from transection injuries, nerve injury can result from thermal, traction, clamping forces with traction forces the most frequent mechanism of injury [24, 25]. Second, evaluation of RLN function is limited to lesions distal to the site of direct stimulation, which can give false-negative results of a more proximal neural injury [26]. An estimated 10% of surgeons were able to identify an intraoperative vagal or RLN nerve injury, while most nerve injuries were discovered after causative force has occurred [25, 27]. Continuous intraoperative nerve monitoring (C-IONM) techniques developed from the need for a preventative tool against imminent nerve injury and to stimulate the nerve from a very proximal location.

The principle of C-IONM involves continuous assessment of functional integrity along the vagal-RLN axis by near constant yet continuous (every 6 s) ipsilateral vagal stimulation. This allows for almost immediate recognition of nerve injury and provides an opportunity for correction of harmful surgical maneuvers [24]. In 2000, the first application of continuous recurrent laryngeal nerve monitoring was reported in Germany by Lamadé and colleagues [28]. They used a continuous transtracheal intraoperative monitoring technology in primary and revision thyroid surgeries with zero reported cases of permanent nerve injury [28]. Modern-day CIONM methodology involves complete circumferential exposure of the ipsilateral vagal nerve and placement of automatic periodic stimulation (APS) electrodes around the nerve trunk [19] (Fig. 7.4). Like in intermittent IONM, an ETT-based surface electrode is used and placed to facilitate electrode contact with the glottic folds.

The vagal nerve is preferred over the RLN in C-IONM for several reasons. First, it has a larger caliber which provides easier intraoperative identification and higher tolerance to manipulation and mechanical injury [29]. Second, it is not directly in the surgical field and decreases the risk of electrode lead displacement during dissection [29]. Compared to direct RLN stimulation, indirect RLN stimulation via the vagus nerve provides more accurate prognostic information of postoperative vocal cord function [30].

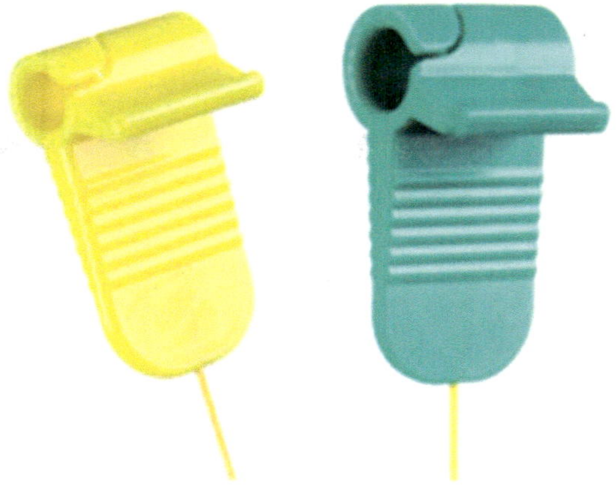

Fig. 7.4 Example of an automatic periodic stimulation electrode used in C-IONM. (Courtesy of Medtronic)

The protective effect of C-IONM lies in its ability to detect timely changes in EMG properties, which forewarns of impending nerve damage. For instance, traction injuries are preceded by changes in the amplitude and latency of the EMG signal, collectively known as a combined event. This is characterized by EMG changes of at least 50% decrease in amplitude from baseline and at least a 10% increase in latency from baseline [24, 31]. A combined event is both sensitive and specific for impending RLN injury, as other mechanical forces such as change in endotracheal tube positioning and laryngeal traction have been associated with only amplitude changes on EMG, without changes in latency [31]. Studies have noted increased risk of vocal cord palsy with combined events that persist for at least 40 s [32, 33] which suggests that the functional sequelae of combined events may be duration-dependent. Thus, there could be a window of opportunity to intervene and ease up on specimen retraction before the onset of sustained nerve damage and that highlights the importance of early identification of nerve injury. These EMG findings are reversible in cases or retraction when these forces are relaxed [32, 33].

One of the criticisms of C-IONM includes potential side effects of continuous vagal stimulation due to its effects on the autonomic sympathetic tone resulting in cardiovascular changes [34, 35]. However, multiple studies have reported on the systemic safety and efficacy of repetitive vagal stimulation in pediatric and adults [36–38]. Repetitive stimulation up to 16 h at 1–2 mA and 6 s stimulus intervals have been found not to result in neurologic adverse effects in animal models [3].

Minimally Invasive Video-Assisted Thyroidectomy/Parathyroidectomy and Remote Access Robotic Thyroidectomy

To improve postoperative cosmetic outcome, remote access robotic and minimally invasive video-associated thyroidectomy and parathyroidectomy (TOETVA/TOEPVA/MIVAT/P) were introduced [39, 40]. Visualization of the RLN is technically more difficult in these techniques given the smaller operative space and more limited angles of view, and there has been increasing interest in use of nerve monitoring techniques in these settings. Terris and colleagues were the first to investigate the feasibility of IONM in MIVAT, using the standard IONM setup as described above in accordance to the INSMG guidelines, with a reported reduction in rate of temporary RLN palsy, although nonsignificant [41, 42]. In addition, Kandil and colleagues used IONM in 47 patients who underwent MIVAT with 77 RLNs at risk and found no difficulty with intraoperative stimulation through the small operating wound, a low rate of RLN injury (1.29% rate of temporary RLN paresis), and no intraoperative complications or conversions to an open approach [40].

Similarly, IONM use in remote access robotic thyroidectomy has also been investigated with favorable outcomes. A systematic review of 8 studies and 522 RLN dissections concluded that IONM technology was useful as an adjunct for nerve identification in these challenging procedures [43]. Despite its utility, IONM use and robotic thyroidectomy procedures do involve a steep learning curve, which may limit the initial efficacy. For instance, Ji and colleagues used IONM in robotic thyroidectomy via the transoral and facelift approaches and found significant differences in success rates between the first 15 (7/15 or 47%) and subsequent procedures (41/43 or 95.3%) [43]. Other considerations include positioning of the EMG endotracheal tube, which can be susceptible to displacement particularly in the transoral approaches, and necessitate vigilant monitoring. Thus, IONM appears to be a safe and effective technique in MIVAT and serves as a useful adjunct for identifying the RLN intraoperatively in difficult surgical exposures.

Does Use of IONM Decrease Rate of Nerve Injury?

Over the past few decades, there has been a significant increase in use of IONM as an adjunct to the gold standard of direct nerve visualization to avoid vocal cord injury in endocrine neck surgery. In the United States, over 80% of otolaryngologists and 50% of general surgeons report using IONM in thyroidectomy [44, 45]. However, literature on the functional outcomes of nerve visualization alone versus IONM have stated conflicting results. Some studies have reported significant decreases in prevalence of transient vocal cord palsy in favor of nerve monitoring [46–48]. In particular, the use of IONM in higher-risk thyroidectomy cases such as revision, invasive malignancies, and retrosternal goiters has been shown to decrease post-op RLN paresis [49, 50]. In contrast, the Cochrane Review included 594 publications comparing visualization alone and IONM and found no significant difference in the rates of temporary or permanent cord paralysis [51]. However, these study conclusions should be interpreted with caution due to lack of an adequately powered study. Given the overall low incidence vocal cord injury, Dralle and colleagues estimated that 9 million benign goiters and 40 thousand malignancy cases would be required in each treatment arm to detect a statistically significant difference [52]. In addition, the heterogeneity in nerve monitoring methodology also plays a role in the variability of results. Despite the lack of evidence to support improved postoperative outcomes, the INMSG and German

Association of Endocrine Surgery recommend use of IONM to prevent nerve injury in all thyroid and parathyroid cases and to date. To date, no committee recommends against the use of IONM in any setting.

Conclusion

Although knowledge of anatomy and proper surgical expertise are fundamental in nerve preservation, intraoperative nerve monitoring via the aforementioned techniques is a valuable adjunct in endocrine neck surgeries, particularly in cases with higher risk of nerve injury. IONM has a role in neural mapping, identification of anatomic variants placing the RLN or vagal nerve at higher risk for injury, and assessment of functional integrity to help make intraoperative decisions about timing of contralateral surgery.

References

1. Kim H, Tufano R, Chai Y, et al. Intraoperative neural monitoring in thyroid surgery: role and responsibility of surgeon. J Endocr Surg. 2018;18(1):49–50.
2. Hayward N, Grodski S, Yeung M, Johnson WR, Serpell J. Recurrent laryngeal nerve injury in thyroid surgery: a review. ANZ J Surg. 2013;83(1–2):15–21.
3. Schneider R, Randolph G, Dionigi G, et al. International neural monitoring study group guideline 2018 part I: staging bilateral thyroid surgery with monitoring loss of signal. Laryngoscope. 2018;128:S1–17.
4. Chiang F, Lu I, Kuo W, et al. The mechanism of recurrent laryngeal nerve injury during thyroid surgery – the application of intraoperative neuromonitoring. Surgery. 2008;143:743–9.
5. Bergenfelz A, Jansson S, Kristoffersson A, et al. Complications to thyroid surgery: results as reported in a database from a multicenter audit comprising 2660 patients. Langenbecks Arch Surg. 2008;393:667–73.
6. Lahey F, Hoover W. Injuries to the recurrent laryngeal nerve in thyroid operations. Ann Surg. 1938;108(4):545–62.
7. Haugen B, Alexander E, Bible K, et al. 2015 american thyroid association management guidelines for adult patients with thyroid nodules and differentiated thyroid cancer. Thyroid. 2016;26(1):1–133.
8. Shedd D, Durham C. Electrical identification of the recurrent laryngeal nerve: I. Response of the canine larynx to electrical stimulation of the recurrent laryngeal nerve. Ann Surg. 1966;163(1):1–9.
9. Miller MC, Spiegel JR. Identification and monitorin of the recurrent laryngeal nerve during thyroidectomy. Surg Oncol Clin N Am. 2008;17:121–44.
10. Hvidegaard T, Vase P, Jorgensen K, Blichert-Toft M. Identification and functional recording of the recurrent laryngeal nerve by electrical stimulation during neck surgery. Laryngoscope. 1983;93:370–3.
11. Kratz R. The identification and protection of the laryngeal motor nerves during thyroid and laryngeal surgery: a new microsurgical technique. Laryngoscope. 1983;83(1):59–78.
12. Premachandra D, Radcliffe G, Stearns M. Intraoperative identification of the recurrent laryngeal nerve and demonstration of its function. Laryngoscope. 1990;100(1):94–6.
13. Tanigawa K, Inou Y, Iawata S. Protection of recurrent laryngeal nerve during neck surgery: a new combination of neutracer, laryngeal mask airway, and fiberoptic bronchoscope. Anesthesiology. 1991;74:966–7.
14. Hillerman CL, Tarpey J, Phillips DE. Laryngeal nerve identification during thyroid surgery – feasibility of a novel approach. Can J Anaesth. 2003;50:189–92.
15. Pott L, Swick J, Stack B Jr. Assessment of recurrent laryngeal nerve during thyroid surgery with laryngeal mask airway. Arch Otolaryngol Head Neck Surg. 2007;133:266–9.
16. Flisberg K, Lindholm T. Electrical stimulation of the human recurrent laryngeal nerve during thyroid operation. Acta Otolarygol Suppl. 1969;263:63–7.
17. Rea L, Kahn A. Clinical evoked electromyography for current laryngeal nerve preservation: use of an endotracheal tube electrode in a postcricoid surface electrode. Laryngoscope. 1998;108:1418–20.
18. Randolph G, Dralle H, Abdullah H, et al. Electrophysiologic recurrent laryngeal nerve monitorign during thyroid and parathyroid surgery: international standards guideline statement. Laryngoscope. 2011;121:S1–16.
19. Schneider R, Machens A, Lorenz K, Dralle H. Intraoperative nerve monitoring in thyroid surgery – shifting current paradigms. Gland Surg. 2020;9:S120–8.
20. Scott AR, Chong PS, Harnick CJ, Randolph GW. Spontaneous and evoked laryngeal electromyoghraphy of the thyroarytenoid muscle: a canine model for intraoperative recurrent laryngeal nerve monitoring. Ann Rhinol Laryngol. 2010;119:54–63.
21. Chu KS, Wu SH, Lu IC, et al. Feasibility of intraoperative neuromonitoring during thyroid surgery after administration of nondepolarizing neuromuscular blocking agents. World J Surg. 2009;33:1408–13.
22. Yu T, Wang F, Meng L, Li J, Miao G. Early detection of recurrent laryngeal nerve damage using intraoperative nerve monitoring during thyroidectomy. J Int Med Res. 2019;48:1–11.
23. Blitzer A, Crumley RL, Dailey SH, et al. Recommendations of the Neuro-laryngology Study Group on laryngeal electromyography. Otolaryngol Head Neck Surg. 2009;140:782–93.

24. Schneider R, Randolph GW, Sekulla C, et al. Continuous intraoperative vagus nerve stimulation for identification of imminent recurrent nerve injury. Head Neck. 2012;35:1591–8.
25. Bergenfeltz A, Jansson S, Martensson H, et al. Scandinavian quality register for thyroid and parathyroid surgery: audit of surery for primary hyperparathyroidism. Langenbecks Arch Surg. 2006;392:445–51.
26. Dionigi G, Wu C, Lombardi D, et al. The current state of recurrent laryngeal nerve monitoring for thyroid surgery. Curr Otorhinolaryngol Rep. 2014;2:44–54.
27. Lo CY, Kwok KF, Yuen PW. A prospective evaluation of recurrent laryngeal nerve paralysis during thyroidectomy. Arch Surg. 2000;135:204–7.
28. Lamadé W, Meyding-Lamade U, Buchhold C, et al. First continuous. Nerve monitoring in thyroid gland surgery. Chirurg. 2000;71:551–7.
29. Singer M. Safety and feasibility of a novel recurrent laryngeal nerve monitoring technique. Laryngoscope. 2018;128:S1–8.
30. Thomusch O, Sekulla C, Machens A, et al. Validity of intra-operative neuromonitoring signals. In thyroid surgery. Langenbecks Arch Surg. 2004;389: 499–503.
31. Kandil E, Mohsin K, Murcy M, Randolph G. Continuous vagal monitoring value in prevention of vocal cord paralysis following thyroid surgery. Laryngoscope. 2018;128:2429–32.
32. Phelan E, Potenza A, Slough C, et al. Recurrent laryngeal nerve monitoring during thyroid surgery: normative vagal and recurrent laryngeal nerve electrophysiological data. Otolaryngol Head Neck Surg. 2012;147(4):640–6.
33. Marin Arteaga A, Peloni G, Leuchter I, et al. Modification of the surgical strategy for the dissection of the recurrent laryngeal nerve using continuous intraoperative nerve monitoring. World J Surg. 2018;42(2):444–50.
34. Terris DJ, Chaung K, Duke WS. Continuous vagal nerve monitoring is dangerous and should not routinely be done during thyroid surgery. World J Surg. 2015;39(10):2471–6.
35. Choi S, Son Y. Intraoperative neuromonitoring for thyroid surgery: the proven benefits and limitations. Clin Exp Otorhinolaryngol. 2019;12(4):335–6.
36. White WM, Randolph GW, Hartnick CJ, Cunningham MJ. Recurrent laryngeal nerve monitoring during thyroidectomy and related cervical procedures in the pediatric population. Arch Otolaryngol Head Neck Surg. 2009;135:88–94.
37. Randolph GW. Surgical anatomy of the recurrent laryngeal nerve. In: Randolph GW, editor. Surgery of the thyroid and parathyroid glands. Philadelphia: Saunders; 2003. p. 300–49.
38. Schneider R, Machens A, Sekulla C, Lorenz K, Weber F, Dralle H. Twenty-year experience of paediatric thyroid surgery using intraoperative nerve monitoring. Cr J Surg. 2018;105(8):996–1005.
39. Miccoli P, Berti P, Materazzi G, Minuto M, Barellini L. Minimally invasive video-assisted thytroidectomy: five years of experience. J Am Coll Surg. 2004;199(2):243–8.
40. Kandil E, Wassef S, Alabbas H, Freidlander P. Minimally invasive video-assisted thyroidectomy and parathyroidectomy with intraoperative recurrent laryngeal nerve monitoring. Int J Otolaryngol. 2009;2009:739798.
41. Terris D, Anderson S, Watts T, Chin E. Laryngeal nerve monitoring and minimally invasive thyroid surgery. Arch Otolaryngol Head Neck Surg. 2007;133(12):1254–7.
42. Dionigi G, Kim H, Wu C, et al. Neuromonitoring in endoscopic and robotic thyroidectomy. Updates Surg. 2017;69(2):171–9.
43. Ji Y, Ko S, Song C, et al. Feasibility and efficacy of intraoperative neural monitoring in remote access robotic and endoscopic thyroidectomy. Oral Oncol. 2020;103:1–6.
44. Singer MC, Rosenfeld RM, Sundaram K. Laryngeal nerve monitoring: current utilization among head and neck surgeons. Otolaryngol Head Neck Surg. 2012;146:895–9.
45. Ho Y, Carr MM, Goldenberg D. Trends in intraoperative neural monitoring for thyroid and parathyroid surgery amongst otolaryngologists and general surgeons. Eur Arch Otorhinolaryngol. 2013;270:2525–30.
46. Bárczynski M, Konturek A, Cichon S. Randomized clinical trial of visualization versus neuromonitoring of recurrent laryngeal nerves during thyroidectomy. Br J Surg. 2009;96:240–6.
47. Zheng S, Xu Z, Wei Y, Zeng M, He J. Effect of intraoperative neuromonitoring on recurrent laryngeal nerve paly rates after thyroid surgery – a meta-analysis. J Formos Med Assoc. 2013;112:463–72.
48. Vasileiadis I, Karatzas T, Charitoudis G, et al. Association of intraoperative neuromonitoring with reduced recurrent laryngeal nerve injury in patients undergoing total thyroidectomy. JAMA Otolaryngol Head Neck Surg. 2016;142:994–1001.
49. Wong KP, Mak KL, Wong CK, Lang BH. Systematic review and meta-analysis on intra-operative neuromonitoring in high-risk thyroidectomy. Int J Surg. 2017;38:21–30.
50. Chuang YC, Huang SM. Protective effect of intraoperative nerve monitoring against recurrent laryngeal nerve injury during re-exploration of the thyroid. World J Surg Oncol. 2013;11:94.
51. Cirocchi R, Arezzo A, D'Andrea V, et al. Intraoperative neuromonitoring versus visual nerve identification for prevention of recurrent laryngeal nerve injury in adults undergoing thyroid surgery (Review). Cochrane Database Syst Rev. 2019;1:1–81.
52. Dralle H, Sekulla C, Heart J, et al. Risk factors of paralysis and functional outcome after chuanrecurrent laryngeal nerve monitoring in thyroid surgery. Surgery. 2004;136:1310–22.

Monitoring of the Superior Laryngeal Nerve

8

Claudio R. Cernea, Erivelto M. Volpi, and Marcin Barczynski

Introduction

The EBSLN is a branch of the superior laryngeal nerve, which originates from the X cranial nerve [1]. It is the motor nerve of the CTM. This muscle approximates the cricoid and the thyroid cartilage, stretching the vocal fold and increasing its tension, and performing an opponent action to the thyroarytenoid muscle. This lengthening and tensioning of the vocal fold is essential for the production of high-frequency sounds, especially among female individuals and voice professionals.

Surgical Anatomy

Many authors proposed several anatomical classifications for the relationship of EBSLN with the superior pedicle and the upper pole of the thyroid gland and the CTM. However, the most widely accepted and employed is the Cernea classification used in this chapter [2].

The EBSLN crosses the superior thyroid vessels on its way to the CTM, usually more than 1 cm above the upper border of the superior thyroid pole. However, in about 14% [3] to 20% [4], this crossing may happen well below the upper border of the superior thyroid pole. This is the type 2b EBSLN, according to the classification proposed by Cernea et al. [5] (Fig. 8.1). Clearly, this anatomical relationship increases the risk of nerve injury during ligation and cutting of the superior thyroid vessels.

How to Avoid Injury to the EBSLN During Thyroidectomy

The surgeon must exert caution when dissecting the superior thyroid pole, in order to avoid inadvertent injury of the EBSLN. It is important to emphasize that, even with the use of magnifying loupes (strongly advisable), it may be quite difficult to identify this nerve, which is usually much thinner than the recurrent laryngeal nerve. The distal portion of the EBSLN frequently enters the CTM within the limits of the sternothyroid-laryngeal triangle, described by Moosman and DeWeese [7]. However, from the surgical point of view, it is more important to be

C. R. Cernea
Department of Surgery, University of São Paulo School of Medicine, São Paulo, São Paulo, Brazil

E. M. Volpi
CETRUS Medical Education Center, Sao Paulo, Sao Paulo, Brazil

M. Barczynski (✉)
Department of Endocrine Surgery, Third Chair of General Surgery, Jagiellonian University Medical College, Krakow, Poland
e-mail: marcin.barczynski@uj.edu.pl

© The Author(s), under exclusive license to Springer Nature Switzerland AG 2022
J. Scharpf, G. W. Randolph (eds.), *Intraoperative Cranial Nerve Monitoring in Otolaryngology-Head and Neck Surgery*, https://doi.org/10.1007/978-3-030-84916-0_8

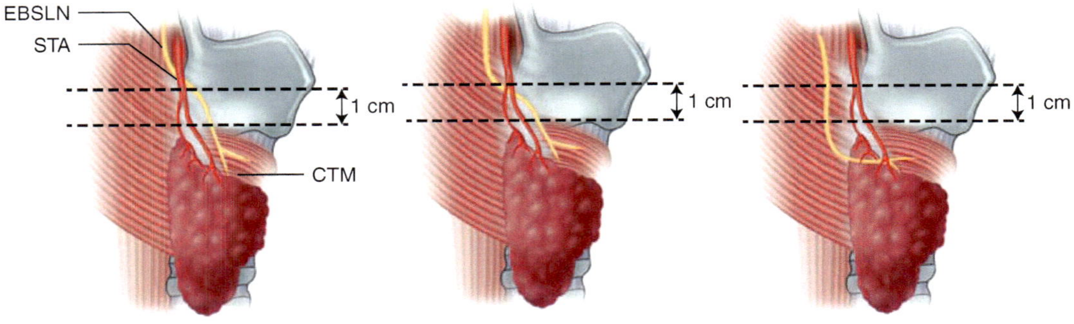

Fig. 8.1 Cernea's external branch of the superior laryngeal nerve (EBSLN) surgical anatomic classification. (From Barczynski et al. [6])

able to identify the EBSLN at the area of the superior thyroid pole.

How to Diagnose the EBSLN Paralysis?

In male individuals, the symptoms of EBSLN paralysis may be mild. However, in female patients and in voice professionals, usually, there are symptomatic voice changes: vocal fatigue, difficulty to phonate in high-frequency tones, and lowering of the vocal register. Even at laryngoscopy, it may be quite difficult to detect this paralysis, as the features are far subtler than those that accompany paralysis of the inferior laryngeal nerve. The more common signs of EBSLN paralysis are discrete bowing of the affected vocal fold, posterior glottic rotation toward the side of the paralysis, inferior displacement of the affected vocal fold, and asymmetry of the vocal fold mucosal wave [8]. When injury of the EBSLN occurs, several parameters of the phonation may be affected: lowering of the voice register is the most usual consequence. The gold standard of the diagnosis of an EBSLN paralysis is the percutaneous electromyography of the CTM [4].

Intraoperative Monitoring of the EBSLN

Relevance of EBSLN Intraoperative Monitoring

During dissection of the superior thyroid pole, the identification of the EBSLN without any kind of magnification can be difficult. In fact, it has been reported that only one third of the nerves can be positively identified in this way [6]. Thus, according to the recommendations of the guideline of the International Neural Monitoring Study Group, the surgeon is advised to use some form of nerve stimulation in order to enhance his or her capability to effectively identify the EBSLN [6].

Does EBSLN Intraoperative Monitoring Reduce the Frequency of Nerve Injury?

There are several reports in the literature suggesting that it is advisable to use intraoperative nerve monitoring of the EBSLN during dissection of the superior pole of the thyroid gland, in order to minimize the risk of inadvertent injury.

Barczyński et al. [9] reported a randomized trial comparing 105 patients submitted to thyroidectomy identifying the EBSLN without any monitoring with 105 patients in whom EBSLN intraoperative monitoring was performed. The conclusion was that the nerve identification was less frequent in the first group (34.5%), compared to the second group (83.8%). In addition, there was a marked reduction of EBSLN injury in the second group, when compared to the first group (5% vs. 1%, respectively; $p = 0.02$).

Uludag et al. [10] also compared two groups of patients who underwent dissection of the superior thyroid pole: in Group 1, there was no attempt to identify the EBSLN, whereas in Group 2, intraoperative monitoring mapping of the EBSLN was undertaken. Nerve injury was documented in 8.6% of patients in Group 1, compared to 0.9% in Group 2 ($p = 0.015$).

Dionigi et al. [11] prospectively evaluated the frequency of injury of the EBSLN in 400 patients submitted to thyroidectomy in the three types of nerve according to Cernea's classification [1]. They found evidence of nerve injury of 4.9%, 11.2%, and 18.5%, respectively, among types 1, 2a, and 2b EBSLN ($p = 0.01$). They proposed the addition to routine evaluation of the EBSLN before and after the dissection of the superior thyroid pole (S1 and S2, respectively) to the algorithm already recommended by the International Neural Monitoring Study Group in 2011 [12].

Lee et al. [13] published a large series of patients submitted to thyroidectomy, divided into two groups: in Group 1, they prospectively analyzed 490 thyroidectomies in which intraoperative monitoring of the EBSLN was employed; Group 2 included 500 operations without the use of intraoperative nerve monitoring, performed by the same surgeon. The use of nerve monitoring markedly improved the identification, especially among individuals with type 2b EBSLN.

Naytah et al. [14], in a recent meta-analysis, showed that injury of EBSLN occurs in up to 58% of patients who underwent thyroidectomies, and the use of IONM resulted in a significant increase in EBSLN identification, decreasing the incidence of post-thyroidectomy voice disorders.

Frequency of Use of EBSLN Intraoperative Nerve Monitoring

According to Barczyński et al. [15], the EBSLN intraoperative nerve monitoring during the dissection of the superior thyroid pole is more often employed by more experienced surgeons (61.4%), when compared with low-volume surgeons (15.8%), and this difference is significant ($p < 0.001$). This interesting finding supports the usefulness of intraoperative nerve monitoring of the EBSLN during thyroidectomy.

Normative Features of EBSLN Intraoperative Monitoring

In 2013, Potenza et al. [16] presented normative features of EBSLN intraoperative monitoring and suggested that it may be used in order to facilitate the quantitative analysis of the physiologic status of the nerve during dissection of the superior thyroid pole. They performed a prospective nonrandomized study of 72 patients submitted to thyroidectomy. All individuals underwent pre- and postoperative laryngoscopy, and those with abnormalities in the preoperative valuation were excluded. Initial intraoperative electrical stimulation in the region of the superior thyroid pole was done with 2 mA, in order to map the EBSLN, and was reduced to 1 mA after the nerve was identified. In all cases, the stimulation caused a CTM twitch. On the other hand, a typical glottis waveform was observed in 78.1% of the EBSLN. The mean amplitude of the EBSLN complex was 269.9 (±178.6), compared with the mean RLN amplitude of 782.2 (±614.4) observed in the same side. There was no significant difference between the response of the EBSLN when stimulated with 1 mA (280.8 [±216.9] and those nerves stimulated with 2 mA (261.8 [±142.4] ($p = 0.7041$). Regarding the results before and after the dissection of the superior thyroid pole, the mean amplitude of EMG response of the EBSLN obtained initially was 270.1 (±190.7), while the mean post-dissection response was 260.4 (±177.9). No significant difference was found between initial and final amplitudes of response ($p = 0.4689$).

In addition, in 2014, Darr et al. [17] reported, based on a prospective study undertaken in a cohort of 22 patients, that novel endotracheal tube (with an additional pair of superficial electrodes located on an anterior aspect of the tube) allows for quantifiable EBSLN EMG activity in 100% of cases. The clinical applicability of this observation is still under international and multi-institutional evaluation.

Final Messages

1. The EBSLN, especially the type 2b, is at risk during the dissection of the superior thyroid pole.
2. It is advisable to employ intraoperative monitoring not only of the recurrent laryngeal nerve but of the EBSLN as well, in order to facilitate its recognition and to reduce the risk of inadvertent injury, particularly when operating on female individuals and voice professionals.
3. Stimulation of the EBSLN will cause a CTM twitch, readily visible within the operative field, whereas nearly 80% of the intact stimulated EBSLN will result in measurable wave during intraoperative monitoring although higher rates have been reported with certain neural monitoring tubes. It is important to document the physiologic integrity of the nerve after the completion of the superior thyroid pole dissection; ideally, the obtained amplitude should be similar to the pre-dissection values.

References

1. Cernea CR, Brandão LG, Hisham AN. Surgical anatomy of the superior laryngeal nerve. In: Randolph GW, editor. Surgery of thyroid and parathyroid gland. Philadelphia: Elsevier Saunders; 2018. p. 316–25.
2. Wang K, Cai H, Kong D, et al. The identification, preservation, and classification of the external branch of the superior laryngeal nerve in thyroidectomy. World J Surg. 2017;41:2521–9. https://doi.org/10.1007/s00268-017-4046-z.
3. Cernea CR, Ferraz AR, Nishio S, et al. Surgical anatomy of the external branch of the superior laryngeal nerve. Head Neck. 1992;14:380–3. https://doi.org/10.1002/hed.2880140507.
4. Cernea CR, Ferraz AR, Furlani J, et al. Identification of the external branch of the superior laryngeal nerve during thyroidectomy. Am J Surg. 1992;164:634–9. https://doi.org/10.1016/s0002-9610(05)80723-8.
5. Furlan JC, Cordeiro AC, Brandão LG. Study of some "intrinsic risk factors" that can enhance an iatrogenic injury of the external branch of the superior laryngeal nerve. Otolaryngol Head Neck Sur. 2003;128(3):396–400.
6. Barczyński M, Randolph GW, Cernea CR, et al. External branch of the superior laryngeal nerve monitoring during thyroid and parathyroid surgery: International Neural Monitoring Study Group standard guidelines. Laryngoscope. 2013;123(suppl 4):S1–S14.
7. Moosman DA, DeWeese MS. The external laryngeal nerve as related to thyroidectomy. Surg Gynecol Obstet. 1968;129:1011–6.
8. Wenig BL. Superior laryngeal nerve injury from thyroid surgery. Head Neck. 1995;17:36–40.
9. Barczyński M, Konturek A, Stopa M, Honowska A, Nowak W. Randomized controlled trial of visualization versus neuromonitoring of the external branch of the superior laryngeal nerve during thyroidectomy. World J Surg. 2012;36(6):1340–7.
10. Uludag M, Aygun N, Kartal K, et al. Contribution of intraoperative neural monitoring to preservation of the external branch of the superior laryngeal nerve: a randomized prospective clinical trial. Langenbecks Arch Surg. 2017;402(6):965–76.
11. Dionigi G, Kim HY, Randolph GW, et al. Prospective validation study of Cernea classification for predicting EMG alterations of the external branch of the superior laryngeal nerve. Surg Today. 2016;46(7):785–91.
12. Randolph GW, et al. Electrophysiologic recurrent laryngeal nerve monitoring during thyroid and parathyroid surgery: international standards guideline statement. Laryngoscope. 2011;121(Suppl 1):S1–16.
13. Lee J, Fraser S, Glover A, Sidhu S. Prospective evaluation of the utility of routine neuromonitoring for an established thyroid surgical practice. ANZ J Surg. 2017;87(10):E138–42.
14. Naytah M, Ibrahim I, da Silva S. Importance of incorporating intraoperative neuromonitoring of the external branch of the superior laryngeal nerve in thyroidectomy: a review and meta-analysis study. Head Neck. 2019;41(6):2034–41. https://doi.org/10.1002/hed.25669.
15. Barczyński M, Randolph GW, Cernea C. International Neural Monitoring Study Group in Thyroid and Parathyroid Surgery. International survey on the iden-

tification and neural monitoring of the EBSLN during thyroidectomy. Laryngoscope. 2016;126(1):285–91.
16. Andre S, Potenza A, Phelan EA, Claudio R, Cernea CR, et al. Normative intra-operative electrophysiologic waveform analysis of superior laryngeal nerve external branch and recurrent laryngeal nerve in patients undergoing thyroid surgery. World J Surg. 2013;37:2336–42.
17. Darr EA, Tufano RP, Ozdemir S, Kamani D, Hurwitz S, Randolph G. Superior laryngeal nerve quantitative intraoperative monitoring is possible in all thyroid surgeries. Laryngoscope. 2014;124(4):1035–41.

Intraoperative Cranial Nerve Monitoring in Otolaryngology – Head and Neck Surgery

9

Rick Schneider, Leonardo Rangel, and Antonio Bertelli

Introduction

Intraoperative neuromonitoring (IONM) was introduced in thyroid surgery 50 years ago [11]. Since that time, the technology has improved considerably, especially in the last decade [36]. Standardized intermittent intraoperative neuromonitoring (iIONM) of the recurrent laryngeal nerve (RLN) and the vagus nerve has been adopted as an adjunct to gold-standard nerve visualization in many centers of the world [34].

Continuous intraoperative neuromonitoring (cIONM) enables real-time evaluation of the RLN by placing a probe on the vagus nerve. The vagal probe repeatedly and continuously stimulates the vagus nerve and subsequently the RLN during surgery depending on the setup frequency. IIONM tests nerve integrity only while the surgeon touches the nerve or surrounding tissues with the probe. Most of the time, the nerve is not being stimulated, and when paralysis occurs, it is already installed. This means that for the majority of intraoperative time "what the nerve has to say is not heard" [41]. Damage to the RLN usually happens between two different stimulations, and after loss of signal (LOS) during iIONM, the nerve function is not reversible. During cIONM, the surgeon is alerted by the equipment if some maneuver is causing nerve damage or stress, so the surgeon can identify and change the operation strategy. CIONM can turn an irreversible and installed paralysis detected with iIONM into a reversible and potentially avoidable paralysis. Amplitude and latency are continuously analyzed by the software of the monitoring device allowing continuous interpretation of these important data. Therefore, cIONM is the only form of neuromonitoring which can avoid nerve damage during surgery.

Rationale for Use

IONM during thyroid surgery has been used as an adjunct to the standard visual nerve identification to preserve RLN function. Recent studies demonstrate more than 90% adoption in Germany and 40% in the USA [42]. IIONM was initially indicated for cases where some difficulty in preserving RLN could be predicted such as revision surgery, associated thyroiditis, intrathoracic goiters, malignant disease, and bilateral thyroid surgery. Presently, within the evolution of IONM from

R. Schneider (✉)
Department of Visceral, Vascular and Endocrine Surgery, Martin Luther University Halle-Wittenberg, Halle (Saale), Germany
e-mail: rick.schneider@uk-halle.de

L. Rangel
State University of Rio de Janeiro, Rio de Janeiro, Brazil
e-mail: leonardo.rangel@uerj.br

A. Bertelli
Department of Surgery, Head and Neck Surgery Division, Santa Casa de Sao Paulo Medical School, Sao Paulo, Sao Paulo, Brazil

© The Author(s), under exclusive license to Springer Nature Switzerland AG 2022

J. Scharpf, G. W. Randolph (eds.), *Intraoperative Cranial Nerve Monitoring in Otolaryngology-Head and Neck Surgery*, https://doi.org/10.1007/978-3-030-84916-0_9

intermittent to continuous, many surgeons use iIONM routinely and indicate cIONM for the most difficult cases such as the initial indications for iIONM, and few centers use cIONM routinely.

An investigation conducted by Schneider et al. regarding IONM of the RLN during thyroid surgery revealed a higher sensitivity for cIONM compared with iIONM for early postoperative vocal cord (VC) palsy, although the difference was not statistically significant ($P = 0.09$). In patients operated on with cIONM, there was no permanent VC palsy in the 1314 nerves at risk, whereas four unilateral permanent VC palsies were seen in patients who had iIONM (0.4% of 965 nerves; $P = 0.019$) [38].

CIONM has the potential to monitor the entire RLN and vagus nerve functional integrity continuously during thyroid surgery alerting the surgeon to any hazardous maneuver and making nerve restoration possible.

Operating Instructions and Standardized Approach

Prior to RLN visual identification, the surgeon must locate the vagus nerve and carefully dissect it 360° around for 1 cm to place the vagal electrode correctly (Fig. 9.1). Some electrodes for cIONM don't require 360° dissection, but those electrodes are more likely to displace during gland manipulation. IIONM helps the surgeon find the vagus nerve inside the carotid sheath, and at the same time, the whole system can be tested. A positive response with amplitude >500 μV is the ideal baseline. In patients in whom the initial baseline is inferior to 500 μV, tube positioning should be checked and corrected until a > 500 μV response is obtained. Usually continuous vagal stimulation is set up as 1.0 Hz, 100 μs, 1 mA. In addition to continuous vagal stimulation, the handheld probe (iIONM) should be used for directed dissection of RLN [38].

Safety

The routine dissection and visual identification of the RLN are proven to be effective methods to ensure VC function [13]. RLN visualization is the gold standard to avoid its injury, although the leading cause of nerve injury is not transection. Since the introduction of IONM, surgical skills have honed rapidly to understand nerve injury's common causes (traction and thermal) [29].

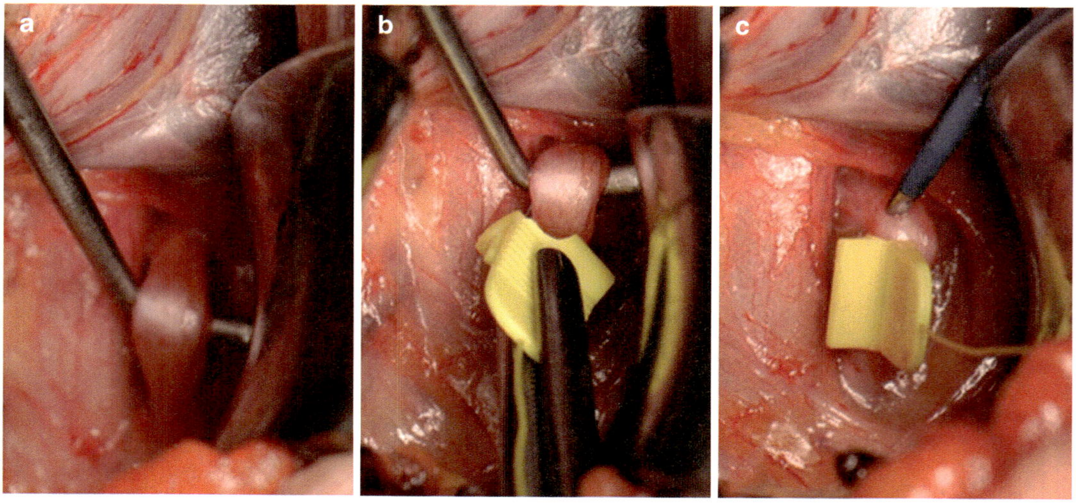

Fig. 9.1 Placement of a monopolar Automatic Periodic Stimulation (APS®, Medtronic, Minneapolis, USA) electrode on the vagus nerve. (**a**) Retraction of the vagus nerve after circular dissection of a short nerve segment. (**b**) Resting of the APS® electrode on the nerve, with an anatomic forceps keeping the enclosure tabs open. (**c**) Released APS® electrode resting on the vagus nerve and stimulation with handheld probe above the APS® electrode probe to exclude dissection or electrode related lesions

The principle for continuous stimulation of the vagus nerve described before needs to meet safety; otherwise, it is useless. The concerns of side effects emerged from its use in psychiatry and neurology [29]. Most of them are meaningless under general anesthesia (stimulation-induced voice alterations, dysphagia, or altered breathing patterns). Nevertheless, cardiac arrhythmias or hemodynamic alterations should be taken under consideration – the two key elements relating to the cIONM safety rely on vagus dissection and repeatedly nerve stimulation. The usual current of 1 to 2 mA for vagus stimulation is supramaximal exclusively for the efferent motor A fibers and myelinated autonomic B fibers. These clinical findings are aligned with the basic research that demonstrates no increase in EMG signal with increased stimulation above the 0.8 to 1 mA threshold [29].

Additionally, the frequency of stimulation for cIONM is generally 1 to 3 Hz. Data show that frequencies lower than 30 Hz are not associated with adverse effects (central nervous system, cardiac, pulmonary, or gastrointestinal). Friedrich et al. [13] conducted a prospective controlled trial comparing cIOMN and iIONM with vagus dissection and vessel loop position. They observed an increased parasympathetic activity during the procedure without any heart rate, blood pressure, or TNF-alpha, thus proving the procedure's safety.

The second key element for a safe cIONM is the gentle vagus nerve dissection. The anatomy between the vagus nerve, the internal jugular vein, and carotid artery is paramount. Before observing the vagus nerve, we need to map its location with the IONM probe [4]. A 360°-degree dissection is necessary for the most common electrodes. Avoiding compression, excessive dissection, and energy instruments are mandatory since we need to install the cIONM electrode and preserve the vagus nerve function. The amount of nerve dissection is minimal; thus, it is only the necessary to fit the electrode. Once the device is in place, caution is needed to avoid unwanted traction on the electrode's cord during the procedure. The vagus nerve's preferred approach is dissecting the carotid sheath between sternocleidomastoid and infrahyoid muscles, thus leaving the central field exclusively for the thyroid/parathyroid surgery. Finally, cIONM is a surgical skill and, as such, has a learning curve associated with it. Pragacz et al. [23] demonstrated that when comparing the first 50 cases to the following 50, the number of identified nerves was higher, surgical time was reduced, and the number of injured nerves was reduced. Zhao et al. [47] studied the IONM learning curve in thyroid cancer surgery, showing a reduction in the time necessary to identify the RLN between the eleventh and sixteenth cases performed.

Intraoperative Damage Control: Impending Nerve Injury and Intraoperative Recovery of EMG Signal

Impending Nerve Injury and Artificial Electromyographic Tracing

In order to facilitate the interpretation of the clinically important quantitative electromyogram (EMG), the so-called adverse "combined" EMG events were defined, which indicate an impending injury of the RLN. These concordant EMG changes consist of a decrease in both signal amplitude of more than 50% compared to the initial baseline value and increase in the latency of more than 10% compared to the baseline value (Fig. 9.2a) [36]. In a recent proof-of-concept study of 52 patients (52 nerves at risk), inappropriate traction led to RLN injury. In another series of 102 patients, combined events, 73% of which were reversible, found positive and negative predictive values of 33% and 97%, respectively [22]. Isolated changes in amplitude or latency were unassociated with VC palsy. As established in an international multicenter study of 115 patients (115 nerves at risk) with persistent LOS, 80% of LOS events were caused by neural traction [33]. An institutional review of 101 patients monitored under continuous vagus stimulation found that 68% of combined events resolved after halting the causative surgical maneuver [20]. Another large study with 788 patients (1314 nerves at risk) found that 80% of combined events did not

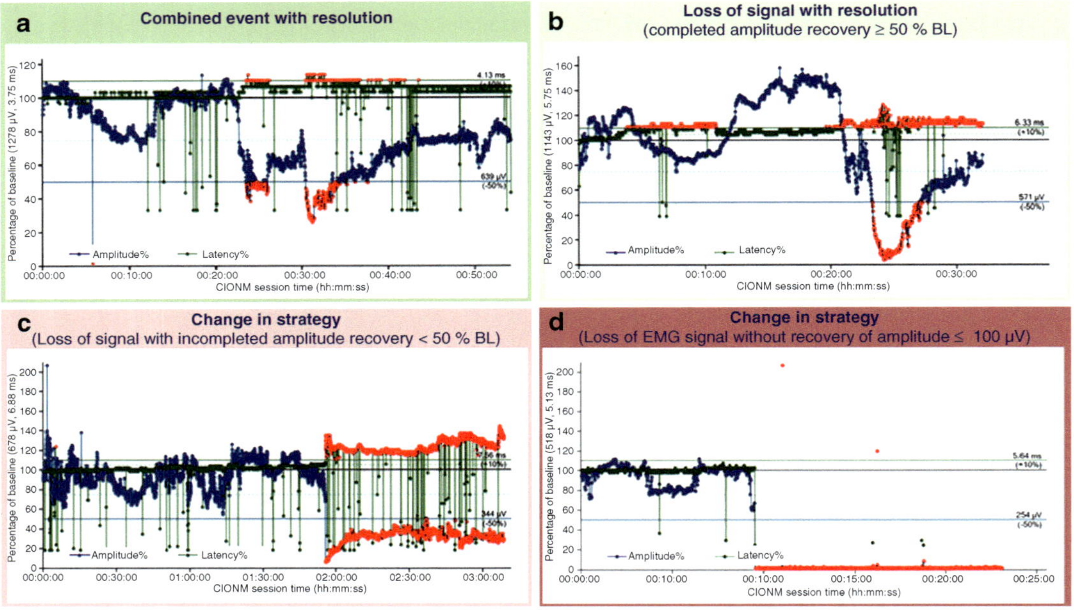

Fig. 9.2 EMG changes under CIONM in planned bilateral thyroidectomy, prompting damage control or a change in strategy; the blue curve denotes nerve amplitude, whereas the green curve indicates latency. (**a**) 'Combined event' (amplitude <50% of baseline with latency >10% of baseline) produced by traction on the RLN, suggesting impending nerve injury, reversed by promplty releasing it, and intact postoperative vocal cord function. (**b**) Complete intraoperative EMG recovery (amplitude ≥50% of baseline) after loss of signal with intact postoperative vocal cord function, enabling total thyroidectomy to continue. (**c**) Incomplete intraoperative EMG recovery (amplitude <50% of baseline) after loss of signal with transient postoperative vocal cord palsy, calling for postponing completion thyroidectomy. (**d**) Definitive loss of signal without intraoperative recovery and transient postoperative vocal cord paralysis, calling for postponing completion thyroidectomy

result in LOS upon release of the related maneuver to the RLN [38]. As most recently shown in an investigation with 455 nerves at risk, interruption of harmful retraction led to functional recovery of all distressed nerves, but only if LOS was yet incomplete [17].

Depending on the type and time course of nerve injury, varying changes in amplitude and latency can be seen. In contrast to more acute injuries to the RLN with more severe damage such as transection, cautery, clamping, etc. in which the nerve monitoring signal is lost immediately, slower injury scenarios such as mild ongoing traction or compression are the most preventable by cIONM, but only if the surgeon is receptive to the real-time data being provided by vagus stimulation [37]. EMG changes can be subdivided into two successive EMG phases with amplitude depression first and then latency elevation with further amplitude depression. Surgical strategy is geared at avoiding transitioning from milder injury (phase 1) into more serious injury (phase 2) which is not necessarily reversible by promptly releasing distressed nerves [27, 29, 34].

For stable and reliable EMG signals, the baseline amplitude must reach ≧500 µV [36]. Nevertheless, mindful use of CIONM requires experience and observation of the EMG screen to enable the differentiation and interpretation of artificial EMG tracing from clinically relevant quantitative EMG signals. Isolated amplitude decreases to less than 50% from baseline or latency increases to less than 110% of baseline may be artificial, believed to arise from tube malrotation or tracheal shifting with impaired contact between the recording endotracheal tube surface electrodes and VC as a result of thyroid manipulation and traction or be considered "subclincal adverse EMG events." Besides temporary loss of EMG tracing caused by bipolar coagulation, electrode dislocation may occur after inadvertent pulling on the conduction wire, or an electrode to vagus mismatch may result in poor stimulation characteristics or prompt the electrode to detach. In contrast to dangerous traction-related EMG changes, non-dangerous artefacts typically resolve after repositioning of the thyroid into its original position [25, 27, 34, 36].

Intraoperative Recovery of EMG Signal

With the implementation of cIONM, there are practically no more unsupervised intervals during nerve monitoring, so that once a transient signal loss has been completed with intraoperative amplitude recovery, the completion surgery on the other side can be continued as planned. A recent multicenter study found that intraoperative amplitude recovery of ≥50% relative to baseline reliably predicts normal early postoperative VC function in all patients after transient segmental or global loss of signal (Fig. 9.2b). This single threshold predicts normal early postoperative VC function accurately after segmental LOS, the more acute and more severe form of nerve injury, but may underestimate normal early postoperative VC function slightly after global LOS, the more gradual and less serious form of nerve injury [32, 37]. Because of the warning of imminent nerve injury with an adverse condition that may be amenable to a reversed nerve injury as neuropraxia, continuous neuromonitoring increases the accuracy of prediction of VC function [38].

Typically, after LOS, the segmental nerve injury resolves within 8 minutes and the global injury within 16 minutes, so that waiting longer than 20 minutes for an amplitude recovery above 50% of the initial baseline value is not effective [32, 37].

Change in Surgical Strategy: Staged Thyroidectomy

When LOS persists or intraoperative recovery of EMG amplitude on the first side of resection is less than 50% in the planned bilateral thyroidectomy, a staged procedure should be established to protect these patients from a serious postoperative complication of bilateral VC paralysis (Figs. 9.2c, d and 9.3) [6, 12, 21, 26, 28, 34]. An intraoperative waiting time longer than 20 minutes is not recommended if t he nerve amplitude has not recovered or is only <50% of the baseline. A persistent LOS on this first side of the resection warrants postponing the contralateral

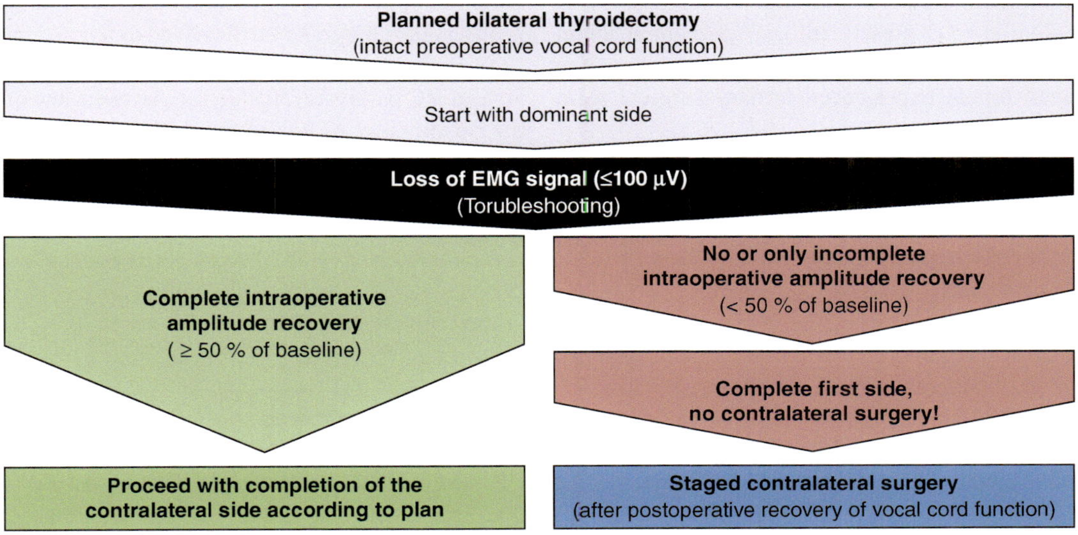

Fig. 9.3 Algorithm of intraoperative management of bilateral thyroid disease after loss of EMG signal on the first side of resection with no, incomplete, or complete recovery with continuous intraoperative neuromonitoring

thyroidectomy, since 95% of patients with segmental LOS type 1 and 70% of patients with global type 2 have early postoperative VC paralysis [32, 35, 37].

As recently reported by various authors on the basis of the cIONM data, staging can safely be decided intraoperatively in the case of persistent LOS on the first side in order to protect these patients from the serious postoperative complication of bilateral RLN paralysis. It was concluded that cIONM was extremely helpful in protecting the RLN from stretch injury in dissections of very large thyroid glands, including large substernal goiter [17, 20].

After VC function has been restored, a second-staged thyroidectomy should follow as a logical consequence. An early period within the first 3 days or at the earliest 3 months after the initial operation, taking into account complete nerve restoration, is considered the optimal and, above all, safe time for the completion operation [9, 10, 14, 26, 35, 37]. In a series of 803 consecutive thyroid surgeries, 95% of the completion surgeries were completed within 6 months of the first procedure, minimizing the risk of the second procedure [44].

If the nerve function of the RLN does not recover within 6 months after the first operation, a multidisciplinary approach is required, depending on the genesis of the underlying disease. If completion surgery is absolutely necessary, it is essential to expressly inform the patient about the possibility of a tracheotomy and about the need for an experienced tertiary surgical team [24, 26, 35].

Superiority of Continuous over Intermittent Intraoperative Nerve Monitoring

In a most recently reported multivariable analysis of 6029 patients (10,232 nerves at risk), continuous IONM independently reduced early postoperative VC palsy 1.8-fold (odds ratio 0.56) and permanent VC palsy 29.4-fold (odds ratio 0.03) compared with intermittent IONM. In addition, the superiority of continuous over intermittent nerve stimulation in thyroid surgery is supported by the following: the magnitude of effect associated with the use of continuous IONM; the consistency of these size effects across a broad variety of benign and malignant thyroid disease and surgical procedures; the lower severity and significantly better prognosis of early postoperative VC palsy with cIONM; and the biological plausibility with no unsupervised periods of dissection, resulting in greater sensitivity of cIONM in identifying imminent RLN injury [30].

The predictive accuracy of continuous stimulation with 99.5% is very high and represents a perfect basis for intraoperative decision-making in favor of or against contralateral surgery. The lowest rate of false positive (0.4%) may further decrease the number of unnecessary staged procedures, in particular when the concept of complete amplitude recovery (>50% of intial baseline) after transient LOS is considered in cIONM-guided thyroidectomy [30, 38]. Therefore, an extended management algorithm is proposed after LOS during continuous stimulation in thyroid surgery [28]. Furthermore, cIONM might further decrease the rate of false-negative findings (0.2%) and the risk for potential bilateral VC palsy, since it overcomes the fundamental risk of intermittent IONM not to register transient LOS during thyroid surgery, and end up with a presumed "intact" EMG (but weaker as the initial amplitude), but an early postoperative VC palsy is observed. This could be dissolved as a transient LOS with incomplete recovery with a risk for 70% of VC paralysis [30, 37, 38]. An overview of the performance of IONM for prediction of postoperative vocal cord palsy is given in Table 9.1.

In a recently published paper on pediatric thyroid surgery in 504 children with intraoperative nerve monitoring with 20 years of experience, no permanent VC paralysis was found in any age group with cIONM [31].

Future Perspectives

CIONM of the vagus nerve for thyroid and parathyroid surgery is already a well-established technique. The technology has improved, mostly due to the new electrode shapes, which allowed

Table 9.1 Literature review: prediction of early postoperative and permanent vocal cord palsy by type of intraoperative nerve monitoring in thyroid surgery

Author, year	NAR; n	Sensitivity; %	Specificity; %	PPV; %	NPV; %	Early postoperative VCP; n (%)	Permanent VCP; n (%)
Intermittent intraoperative nerve monitoring							
Calò et al. 2014 [3]	2068	91.3	99.4	77.8	99.8	23 (1.1)	6 (0.3)
De Falco et al. 2014 [7]	600	83.3	99.5	62.5	99.8	5 (0.8)	4 (0.7)
Melin et al. 2014 [21]	3426	85.4	99.0	68.0	99.6	82 (2.4)	–‡
Barczynski et al. 2014 [2]	500	90.0	95.0	78.3	99.6	13 (2.6)	7 (1.4)
Anuwong et al. 2016 [1]	768	–‡	–‡	–‡	–‡	35 (4.5)	8 (1.0)
Cavicchi et al. 2018 [5]	1264	90.0	99.2	78.3	99.7	40 (3.16)	3 (0.2)
Yu et al. 2019 [45]	374	90.0	99.2	75.0	99.7	7 (1.9)	3 (0.8)
Sedlmeier et al. 2019 [39]	409	76.7	97.8	80.5	97.3	43 (10.5)	6 (1.5)
Schneider et al. 2020 [30]	5024	52.4	99.2	61.9	98.8	124 (2.5)	29 (0.6)
Continuous intraoperative nerve monitoring							
van Slyke et al. 2013 [43]	180	100	100	100	100	4 (2.2)	1 (0.6)
Jonas and Boskovic 2014 [16]	1184	–‡	–‡	–‡	–‡	34 (2.9)	1 (0.1)
Anuwong et al. 2016 [1]	626	–‡	–‡	–‡	–‡	20 (3.1)	0 (0)
Mangano et al. 2016 [19]	400	–‡	–‡	–‡	–‡	15 (3.7)	0 (0)
Kandil et al. 2018 [17]	455	–‡	–‡	–‡	–‡	15 (3.3)	0 (0)
De la Quintana et al. 2018 [8]	400	100	97.7	47	100	8 (2.0)	0 (0)
Yu et al. 2019 [45]	173	100	99.4	66.7	100	2 (1.2)	0 (0)
Hamilton et al. 2019 [15]	256	100	85.0	18.0	100	8 (3.1)	6 (2.3)
Sedlmeier et al. 2019 [39]	204	100	90.2	47.6	100	10 (2.9)	2 (1.0)
Schneider et al. 2020 [30]	5208	88.5	99.6	79.3	99.8	78 (1.5)	1 (0.02)

NAR nerves at risk, *NPV* negative predictive value, *PPV* positive predictive value, *VCP* vocal cord palsy, No information

easy installation, and consistent registers. Nevertheless, thyroid surgery is evolving with endoscopic or robotic accesses becoming frequent (Fig. 9.4). However, regardless of the surgical technique, one common setback is the need to dissect the carotid sheath [18, 48].

Zhao et al. addressed the transcutaneous stimulation of the vagus nerve. They described the use of noninvasive vagus monitoring and proved its feasibility until the point of CO_2 insufflation when they lost signal. The group outlined that the cIONM probe should be stable in position, easily applicable, and removable in open, endoscopic, and robotic thyroidectomy and demand low stimulation current and have signal stability. However, further studies are necessary to refine this method for endoscopic approaches [48].

Zhang et al. [46] described one prototype for continuous endotracheal stimulation of the RLN. It consisted of two distal electrodes that deliver a mean of 2.5 mA resulting in over 1000 μV bilateral register. The authors did not find any statistical difference between the handheld probe and the trachea. Sinclair et al. [40] described another endotracheal initiative, using a regular TriVantage NIM® tube. However, instead of using the electrodes to register the potentials, the authors stimulated the electrodes of one side and captured the signal on the contralateral pair using the laryngeal adductor reflex. This last technique equires more sophisticated equipment and analysis [40].

Lastly, thyroid nodule management will incorporate the directed thermal therapies. Advanced cases will only be possible if nerve integrity is guaranteed once ultrasound images cannot individualize the RLN. This is a promising field of research.

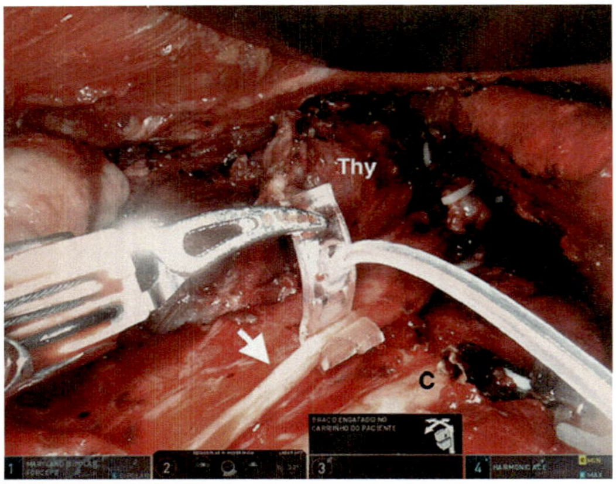

Fig. 9.4 Placement of a bipolar DELTA®-Electrode (Inomed, Emmendingen, Germany) on the vagus nerve during robotic (Da Vinci Xi® platform, Intuitive, USA) neck dissection using retroauricular approach (Thy, right thyroid lobe; C, right common carotid artery; arrow, right vagus nerve)

References

1. Anuwong A, Lavazza M, Kim HY, Wu CW, Rausei S, Pappalardo V, et al. Recurrent laryngeal nerve management in thyroid surgery: consequences of routine visualization, application of intermittent, standardized and continuous nerve monitoring. Updat Surg. 2016;68:331–41.
2. Barczyński M, Konturek A, Pragacz K, Papier A, Stopa M, Nowak W. Intraoperative nerve monitoring can reduce prevalence of recurrent laryngeal nerve injury in thyroid reoperations: results of a retrospective cohort study. World J Surg. 2014;38:599–606.
3. Calò PG, Pisano G, Medas F, Pittau MR, Gordini L, Demontis R, et al. Identification alone versus intraoperative neuromonitoring of the recurrent laryngeal nerve during thyroid surgery: experience of 2034 consecutive patients. J Otolaryngol Head Neck Surg. 2014;43:16–23.
4. Caruso E, Pino A, Pontin A, Pinto G, Damiano C, Catalfamo A, et al. Limitations of continuous neural monitoring in thyroid surgery. Sisli Etfal Hastan Tip Bul. 2019;53:81–3.
5. Cavicchi O, Burgio L, Cioccoloni E, Piccin O, Macrì G, Schiavon P, et al. Intraoperative intermittent neuromonitoring of inferior laryngeal nerve and staged thyroidectomy: our experience. Endocrine. 2018;62:560–5.
6. Christoforides C, Papandrikos I, Polyzois G, Roukounakis N, Dionigi G, Vamvakidis K. Two-stage thyroidectomy in the era of intraoperative neuromonitoring. Gland Surg. 2017;6:453–63.
7. De Falco M, Santangelo G, Del Giudice S, Gallucci F, Parmeggiani U. Double probe intraoperative neuromonitoring with a standardized method in thyroid surgery. Int J Surg. 2014;12:S140–4.
8. De la Quintana BA, Iglesias Martínez A, Salutregui I, Agirre Etxabe L, Arana González A, Yurrebaso SI. Continuous monitoring of the recurrent laryngeal nerve. Langenbeck's Arch Surg. 2018;403:333–9.
9. Dralle H, Sekulla C, Lorenz K, Nguyen Thanh P, Schneider R, Machens A. Loss of the nerve monitoring signal during bilateral thyroid surgery. Br J Surg. 2012;99:1089–95.
10. Erbil Y, Bozbora A, Ademoglu E, et al. Is timing important in thyroid reoperation? J Otolaryngol Head Neck Surg. 2008;37:56–64.
11. Flisberg K, Lindholm T. Electrical stimulation of the human recurrent laryngeal nerve during thyroid operation. Acta Otolaryngol Suppl. 1969;263:63–7.
12. Fontenot TE, Randolph GW, Setton TE, Alsaleh N, Kandil E. Does intraoperative nerve monitoring reliably aid in staging of total thyroidectomies? Laryngoscope. 2015;125:2232–5.
13. Friedrich C, Ulmer C, Rieber F, Kern E, Kohler A, Schymik K, et al. Safety analysis of vagal nerve stimulation for continuous nerve monitoring during thyroid surgery. Laryngoscope. 2012;122:1979–87.
14. Glockzin G, Hornung M, Kienle K, et al. Completion thyroidectomy: effect of timing on clinical complications and oncologic outcome in patients with differentiated thyroid cancer. World J Surg. 2012;36:1168–73.
15. Hamilton N, Morley H, Haywood M, Arman S, Mochloulis G. Continuous intraoperative nerve monitoring in thyroidectomy using automatic periodic stimulation in 256 at-risk nerves. Ann R Coll Surg Engl. 2019;101:432–5.
16. Jonas J, Boskovic A. Intraoperative neuromonitoring (IONM) for recurrent laryngeal nerve protection: comparison of intermittent and continuous nerve stimulation. Surg Technol Int. 2014;24:133–8.
17. Kandil E, Mohsin K, Murcy MA, Randolph GW. Continuous vagal monitoring value in prevention of vocal cord paralysis following thyroid surgery. Laryngoscope. 2018;128:2429–32.
18. Ling Y, Zhao J, Zhao Y, Li K, Wang Y, Kang H. Role of intraoperative neuromonitoring of recurrent laryngeal nerve in thyroid and parathyroid surgery. J Int Med Res. 2020;48:300060520952646.
19. Mangano A, Kim HY, Wu CW, Rausei S, Hui S, Xiaoli L, et al. Continuous intraoperative neuromonitoring in thyroid surgery: safety analysis of 400 consecutive electrode probe placements with standardized procedures. Head Neck. 2016;38 Suppl1:e1568–74.
20. Marin Arteaga A, Peloni G, Leuchter I, Bedat B, Karenovics W, Triponez F, et al. Modification of the surgical strategy for the dissection of the recurrent laryngeal nerve using continuous intraoperative nerve monitoring. World J Surg. 2018;42:444–50.
21. Melin M, Schwarz K, Pearson MD, Lammers BJ, Goretzki PE. Postoperative vocal cord dysfunction despite normal intraoperative neuromonitoring: an unexpected complication with the risk of bilateral palsy. World J Surg. 2014;38:2597–602.

22. Phelan E, Schneider R, Lorenz K, et al. Continuous vagal IONM prevents RLN paralysis by revealing initial EMG changes of impending neuropraxic injury: a prospective, multicenter study. Laryngoscope. 2014;124:1498–505.
23. Pragacz K, Barczynski M. Evaluation of the learning curve for intraoperative neural monitoring of the recurrent laryngeal nerves in thyroid surgery. Pol Przegl Chir. 2015;86:584–93.
24. Sadowski SM, Soardo P, Leuchter I, Robert JH, Triponez F. Systematic use of recurrent laryngeal nerve neuromonitoring changes the operative strategy in planned bilateral thyroidectomy. Thyroid. 2013;23:329–33.
25. Schneider R, Lorenz K, Machens A, et al. Continuous intraoperative neuromonitoring (CIONM) of the recurrent laryngeal nerve. In: Randolph GW, editor. The recurrent and superior laryngeal nerves. 1st ed. Springer; 2016. p. 169–83.
26. Schneider R, Lorenz K, Sekulla C, et al. Surgical strategy during intended total thyroidectomy after loss of EMG signal on the first side of resection. Chirurg. 2015;86:154–63.
27. Schneider R, Machens A, Randolph G, et al. Evolution and progress of continuous intraoperative neural monitoring. Annals of Thyroid. 2018;3:29.
28. Schneider R, Machens A, Randolph G, Kamani D, Lorenz K, Dralle H. Impact of continuous intraoperative vagus stimulation on intraoperative decision making in favor of or against bilateral surgery in benign goiter. Best Pract Res Clin Endocrinol Metab. 2019;33:101285.
29. Schneider R, Machens A, Randolph GW, Kamani D, Lorenz K, Dralle H. Opportunities and challenges of intermittent and continuous intraoperative neural monitoring in thyroid surgery. Gland Surg. 2017;6:537–45.
30. Schneider R, Machens A, Sekulla C, Lorenz K, Elwerr M, Dralle H. Superiority of continuous over intermittent intraoperative nerve monitoring in preventing vocal cord palsy. Br J Surg. 2020. Online ahead of print.
31. Schneider R, Machens A, Sekulla C, Lorenz K, Weber F, Dralle H. Twenty-year experience of paediatric thyroid surgery using intraoperative nerve monitoring. Br J Surg. 2018;105:996–1005.
32. Schneider R, Randolph G, Dionigi G, et al. Prediction of postoperative vocal fold function after intraoperative recovery of loss of signal. The International Neuromonitoring Study Group's PREC Study. Laryngoscope. 2019;129:525–31.
33. Schneider R, Randolph G, Dionigi G, et al. Prospective study of vocal fold function after loss of the neuromonitoring signal in thyroid surgery: The International Neural Monitoring Study Group's POLT Study. Laryngoscope. 2016;126:1260–6.
34. Schneider R, Randolph GW, Barczynski M, et al. Continuous intraoperative neural monitoring of the recurrent nerves in thyroid surgery: a quantum leap in technology. Gland Surg. 2016;5:607–16.
35. Schneider R, Randolph GW, Dionigi G, et al. International neural monitoring study group guideline 2018 part I: staging bilateral thyroid surgery with monitoring loss of signal. Laryngoscope. 2018;128 Suppl3:S1–S17.
36. Schneider R, Randolph GW, Sekulla C, et al. Continuous intraoperative vagus nerve stimulation for identification of imminent recurrent laryngeal nerve injury. Head Neck. 2013;35:1591–8.
37. Schneider R, Sekulla C, Machens A, et al. Dynamics of loss and recovery of the nerve monitoring signal during thyroidectomy predict early postoperative vocal fold function. Head Neck. 2016;38:E1144–51.
38. Schneider R, Sekulla C, Machens A, et al. Postoperative vocal fold palsy in patients undergoing thyroid surgery with continuous or intermittent nerve monitoring. Br J Surg. 2015;102:1380–7.
39. Sedlmeier A, Steinmüller T, Hermanns M, Nawka T, Weikert S, Sedlmaier B, et al. Continuous versus intermittent intraoperative neuromonitoring in complex benign thyroid surgery: a retrospective analysis and prospective follow-up. Clin Otolaryngol. 2019;44:1071–9.
40. Sinclair CF, Téllez MJ, Tapia OR, Ulkatan S, Deletis V. A novel methodology for assessing laryngeal and vagus nerve integrity in patients under general anesthesia. Clin Neurophysiol. 2017;128:1399–405.
41. Stankovic P, Wittlinger J, Georgiew R, et al. Continuous intraoperative neuromonitoring (cIONM) in head and neck surgery - a review. HNO. 2020;68:86–92.
42. Sturgeon C, Sturgeon T, Angelos P. Neuromonitoring in thyroid surgery: attitudes, usage patterns, and predictors of use among endocrine surgeons. World J Surg. 2009;33:417–25.
43. Van Slyke S, Gillardin JP, Brusselaers N, Vermeersch H. Initial experience with S-shaped electrode for continuous vagal nerve stimulation in thyroid surgery. Langenbeck's Arch Surg. 2013;398:717–22.
44. Wu CW, Sun H, Zhang G, Kim HY, Catalfamo A, Portinari M, Carcoforo P, Randolph GW, Chai YJ, Dionigi G. Staged thyroidectomy: a single institution perspective. Laryngosc Investig Otolaryngol. 2018;3:326–32.
45. Yu Q, Liu K, Zhang S, Li H, Xie C, Wu Y, et al. Application of continuous and intermittent intraoperative nerve monitoring in thyroid surgery. J Surg Res. 2019;243:325–31.
46. Zhang D, Wang T, Zhao Y, Sun H, Pino A, Kim HY, et al. Pre-prototype stimulating and recording endotracheal tube for continuous monitoring of the recurrent laryngeal nerve during thyroid surgery. J Investig Surg. 2020:1–11.
47. Zhao N, Bai Z, Teng C, Zhang Z. Learning curve for using intraoperative neural monitoring technology of thyroid cancer. Biomed Res Int. 2019;8904736.
48. Zhao Y, Li C, Zhang D, Li S, Wang T, Dionigi G, et al. Continuous neural monitoring in endoscopic thyroidectomy: feasibility experimental study for transcutaneous vagal nerve stimulation. J Laparoendosc Adv Surg Tech A. 2020;30:1095–101.

Emerging Trends for Vagus/ Recurrent Laryngeal Nerve Monitoring

10

Vaninder K. Dhillon and Catherine F. Sinclair

Introduction

Intraoperative nerve monitoring (IONM) has been utilized for over five decades by a multitude of surgical specialists including spine surgeons, neurosurgeons, vascular surgeons, and otolaryngologists. Uses have included localization of neural structures, determination of nerve functional status, and early detection of intraoperative injury, allowing for immediate corrective measures. In thyroid and parathyroid surgery, injury to the recurrent laryngeal (RLN) and external branch of the superior laryngeal (EBSLN) nerves can lead to substantial changes in voice, swallowing, and breathing with resultant increased postoperative patient morbidity and, occasionally, mortality [1]. These nerves are in close proximity to the thyroid and parathyroid glands during surgical dissection, and injury to the main trunk or branches of these nerves can lead to vocal fold paralysis as well as partial neural dysfunction. These dysfunctional states are best identified by direct visualization of the larynx and pharynx using laryngoscopy or videostroboscopy [2].

Quoted rates of nerve injury after thyroid and parathyroid surgery have been traditionally reported as low (3–5%) [3]. However the true rate of injury is likely much higher, especially for the EBSLN where the actual incidence of injury remains unknown but has been reported to approach 58% [4, 5]. These inconsistencies in reported injury rates is multifactorial and related to lack of standardization of pre- and postoperative laryngeal examination practices and inadequate recognition of subtle laryngeal dysfunction states that affect voice, swallow, and breathing. Laryngeal dysfunction can be difficult to diagnose postoperatively unless the larynx is directly examined because patients may be relatively asymptomatic or have voice, swallow, or breathing complaints that require specialist assessment and testing [2].

Two types of nerve monitoring include intermittent (IIONM) and continuous (CIONM) nerve monitoring. Intermittent nerve monitoring, which is the predecessor to continuous monitoring, involves intermittent direct stimulation of the vagus or RLN nerve with a handheld probe [6]. Intermittent nerve monitoring does not allow for corrective behaviors at the time of identification of injury, but it does allow for the following: (1)

V. K. Dhillon
Division of Laryngology and Endocrine Head and Neck Surgery, Johns Hopkins University, Department of Otolaryngology-Head and Neck Surgery, Bethesda, MD, USA
e-mail: vdhillo2@jhmi.edu

C. F. Sinclair (✉)
Department of Otolaryngology-Head and Neck Surgery, Icahn School of Medicine at Mount Sinai, New York, NY, USA
e-mail: Catherine.sinclair@mountsinai.org

© The Author(s), under exclusive license to Springer Nature Switzerland AG 2022
J. Scharpf, G. W. Randolph (eds.), *Intraoperative Cranial Nerve Monitoring in Otolaryngology-Head and Neck Surgery*, https://doi.org/10.1007/978-3-030-84916-0_10

RLN localization; (2) identifying whether a loss of signal (LOS) from nerve injury has occurred, and (3) determining whether staged surgery is warranted in the case of an ipsilateral LOS during a bilateral procedure [6]. By contrast, continuous IONM (CIONM) can potentially identify impending nerve injury in real time, allowing the surgeon to take remedial actions before the occurrence of a neurophysiologic injury and thus theoretically prevent RLN nerve injury before it occurs [3, 7].

IONM outcomes have traditionally focused on rates of temporary and permanent vocal fold paralysis (VFP). Temporary VFP is immobility of the vocal fold in question with recovery of mobility on direct visualization typically within 3–6 months. Permanent VFP refers to vocal fold immobility that does not recover after 12 months. VFP can be unilateral or bilateral depending on whether one or both of the recurrent laryngeal nerves are subject to injury. The challenge in demonstrating the benefit of nerve monitoring in prevention of nerve injury is the standardization of technique intraoperatively, pre- and postoperative laryngeal examination, and reporting of methodology. In addition, surgeons must have realistic expectations of what the different forms of IONM (IIONM versus CIONM) can achieve and report appropriate outcome measures. In 2006, the International Nerve Monitoring Study Group (INMSG) published guidelines on RLN [6] and EBSLN [8] nerve monitoring standards for thyroid and parathyroid surgery with the hopes of standardizing the protocol for monitoring and improving quality standards and adherence to good technique. Since the initial publication of the group's guidelines, several papers documenting normative electromyography (EMG) data of the vagus nerve, RLN, and EBSLN have been published [9–11]. Furthermore, updated guidelines have focused on pitfalls of nerve monitoring and how to stage bilateral thyroid surgery when there is a loss of signal and have commented on the role of nerve monitoring in invasive thyroid cancer with nerve involvement [12, 13].

The ability of clinical trials to demonstrate a clear benefit of IONM over no monitoring is limited by heterogeneity as well as lack of adequate power in study design [14–23]. Dralle et al. discussed the required power for a study to differentiate between visual identification alone and IONM, one that would require 9 million nerves at risk (NAR) in benign goiter patients and 40,000 NAR in thyroid cancer patients per arm to detect statistical significance [24]. Furthermore, the results demonstrated by many non-randomized controlled studies have shown mixed results in terms of efficacy of recurrent laryngeal nerve monitoring. Barczyński et al. compared the outcomes of 1000 patients with intermittent IONM (IIONM) versus 1000 patients without IIONM in a prospective study. They reported a lesser prevalence of transient but not permanent nerve damage in the IIONM group compared to visualization alone [25]. Other studies have found no difference between nerve palsy rates using IIONM versus visualization [26] and improved permanent nerve palsy rates using continuous IONM (CIONM) compared to visualization alone or IIONM [12, 27].

Intermittent Nerve Monitoring Technologies

There are a number of existing techniques for nerve monitoring, some of which are still in development. Most techniques are variations of "intermittent" IONM, meaning that nerve stimulation occurs in a surgeon-driven manner at various time points during a surgical procedure. The different intermittent technologies focus on one of the two main aspects of monitoring: recording *and* stimulation (Fig. 10.1). The most widely popularized and proven method for recording vocal fold electromyographic signals utilizes an electromyographic endotracheal tube (EMG-ETT) to record contractile responses from the vocal fold adductor muscles in response to direct RLN or vagus nerve stimulation. These endotracheal tubes (ETT) utilize surface electrodes that sit between vocal folds. The contractile response is detected by the electrodes and appears as a waveform on the recording equipment. Amplitude and latency of this waveform are used to assess

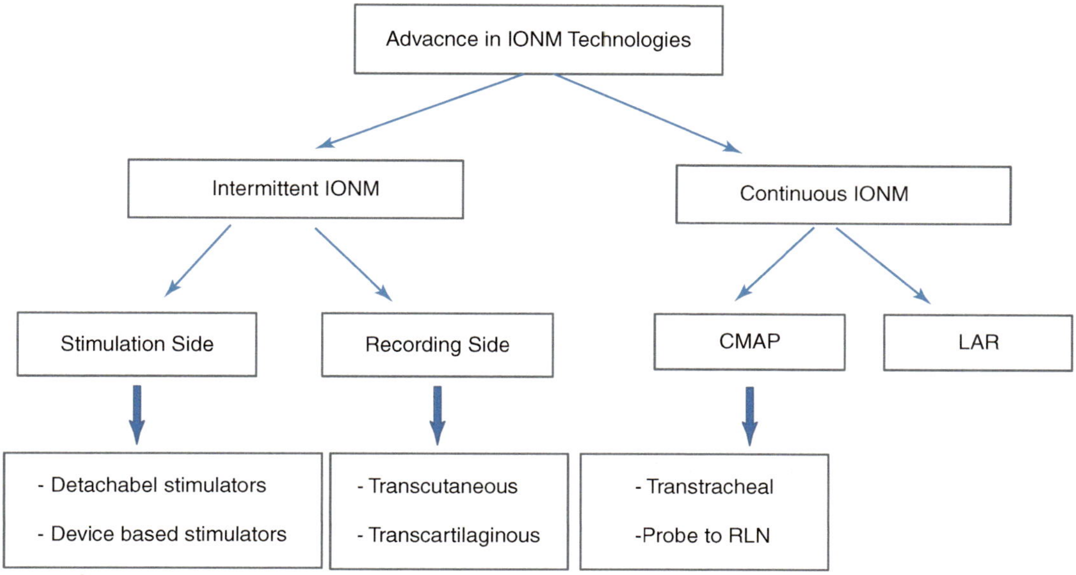

Fig. 10.1 New technologies in IONM. Legend: IONM intraoperative nerve monitoring, CMAP compound muscle action potential, LAR laryngeal adductor reflex, RLN recurrent laryngeal nerve

nerve function sporadically during the surgery. ETT electrode style, dimensions, location, and type may vary depending on the brand of endotracheal tube. EMG-ETT has been shown to be the most feasible and least invasive method for recording vocal fold responses to laryngeal nerve stimulation and has similar stimulation thresholds to intramuscular or endoscopically placed electrodes [6]. However, the ETT can rotate or be displaced during surgical manipulation of the thyroid or parathyroid glands which can cause false-positive or false-negative results. The surgeon must take an active role in ensuring the tube is correctly placed prior to commencement of the surgical procedure as significant craniocaudal displacement has been demonstrated during neck extension following intubation [6].

Recently, alternative methods for recording the EMG response from the vocal fold adductor muscles have been proposed including anterior laryngeal electrodes (ALE) which are placed on the thyroid cartilage or skin to monitor the glottic contractile response [28]. EMG waveforms from such surface electrodes have been compared to EMG-ETT waveforms and acceptable amplitudes reported. However, although proponents of this technique claim it bypasses concerns around ETT misplacement, malrotation, or manipulation, the surface electrodes themselves have the potential to become displaced intraoperatively. These studies have utilized wide-neck incisions for placement of the electrodes [28], and the ability to correctly place and retain such electrodes when utilizing a small neck incision remains to be validated. Also, EMG waveforms have lower amplitudes than ETT readings and can be adversely affected by patient age and cartilage ossification. This technique requires further clinical validation but could be a cheaper alternative to EMG-ETT in low-resource environments due to the lower cost.

The other aspect of intermittent IONM for which new technologies have been proposed relates to the methodology for nerve stimulation (Fig. 10.1). The most common technique for nerve stimulation is a handheld probe with which the surgeon touches the nerve when they desire to check functional status. Probes may be monopolar or bipolar and differ somewhat in appearance depending on the manufacturer. Alternatives to the handheld probe have been recently proposed whereby a stimulation device is incorporated *into* other instrumentation or energy devices utilized during surgery [29–31]. A detachable magnetic monitoring device attached to dissecting instrumentation is one such permutation which has shown promise in being able to stimulate the surgical field constantly while the dissecting instrument is being actively utilized by the surgeon [31]. Provided the surgeon is dissecting directly on the nerve, this technique has the ability to provide real-time signal. However, the signal will cease once dissection ceases, and thus this technique does not provide continuous assessment of nerve functional status and cannot detect nerve injury that may result at other times during the surgery (e.g., from gland retraction). Studies on these devices to date have demonstrated that this nerve monitoring technology is effective and safe as an attachable connection to established instrumentation [32].

Continuous Nerve Monitoring Technologies

CIONM of the RLN was first reported by Lamade who utilized electrodes on the cuff of an ETT to transtracheally stimulate the RLN in the neck. EMG vocal fold responses are then recorded on the normal ETT electrodes at the level of the glottis [33]. More recently, Zhang et al. have again reported this technique as being able to provide continuous RLN stimulation in pigs [34]. The main limitation of this technique in humans is that the RLN in humans runs at a more oblique angle than in pigs (especially on the right), and thus the currents required to stimulate the nerve are high. In addition, the entire course of the RLN is unable to be assessed by this technique such that injuries occurring proximal to the point of RLN stimulation will not be detected [34]. Also, for patients requiring RLN mobilization as part of a central neck dissection, it is unclear whether this technology would continue to provide adequate EMG waveforms as the trachea would fail to closely approximate the nerve.

Continuous RLN stimulation using a handheld probe or cuff electrode placed adjacent to the nerve has also been proposed; however, these techniques are limited by the need for an assistant to hold the probe constantly on the nerve and/or the need to dissect the nerve out to place the monitoring cuff, a procedure that could itself cause nerve injury [35].

A completely different technique for CIONM was discovered in 2016 and has since been developed into a methodology that is gaining popularity worldwide among neurosurgeons, neurophysiologists, and neck endocrine surgeons [36]. This technology utilizes the laryngeal adductor reflex (LAR) to monitor RLN and vagus nerve function continuously during surgical procedures. The laryngeal adductor reflex is a primitive brainstem response that causes bilateral vocal fold adduction in response to supraglottic laryngeal mucosal stimulation. Supraglottic stimulation causes afferent impulses to travel up the internal branch of the superior laryngeal nerve to the brainstem. Efferent impulses travel via the vagus nerve and RLNs to the larynx where laryngeal adductor muscles are activated to contract. The resultant contractile response can be detected on an EMG-ETT and is composed of two EMG waves – an early R1 wave and a later R2 wave. This LAR physiologic contractile response that is elicited in the vocal fold adductor muscles is unique and different from the stimulated compound muscle action potential (CMAP) response elicited by direct RLN or vagus nerve stimulation as described above and is subject to its own standards [37–40]. A recent prospective case-historical control study demonstrated significant reduced rates of transient VFP with LAR-CIONM compared with no monitoring. Permanent VFP rates were unchanged [27]. Benefits of this technique include its simplicity (requires only an EMG-ETT), ability to monitor sensory/brainstem/motor function of the vagus nerve (allowing it to be utilized in posterior fossa and vagus schwannoma surgeries), good correlation with CMAP responses elicited by direct nerve stimulation, ability to obtain opening traces prior to skin incision (thus ensuring true baseline traces are obtained before any nerve dissection is initiated), ability for contraction of the contralateral vocal fold in the bilateral laryngeal reflex response to act as a control against tube rotation or displacement, and strong correlation with postoperative laryngoscopic outcomes. Disadvantages of this technique are that it currently requires total intravenous anesthesia, is dependent on the EMG-ETT for both stimulation and recording of the response and is therefore exquisitely sensitive to alterations in ETT position intraoperatively, and in its current form has lower EMG amplitudes than traditional CMAP methodologies for IONM. These disadvantages will likely be overcome once an ETT with electrode positioning appropriate and dedicated to LAR-CIONM is released; however, until that time, this technology can only be accurately and reliably performed in centers with experienced intraoperative neurophysiology support.

Controversies

One controversy in the IONM world is whether CIONM has advantages over IIONM alone. There have been few studies to date directly comparing CIONM to IIONM. One large observational study [41] evaluated the utilization of intermittent IONM and CMAP-CIONM in parallel, with a gradual transition to CMAP-CIONM alone by the end of the series. This study found improved rates of permanent, but not transient, vocal fold paralysis with CMAP-CIONM. However, there was no breakdown of results by individual surgeon, and thus the impact of CMAP-CIONM at the individual level was unclear. In addition, by performing intermittent IONM and CIONM in parallel, rates of nerve injury with intermittent IONM alone may have been falsely depressed due to cognitive bias where knowledge gleaned from CIONM cases was subconsciously applied to intermittent IONM cases. Other studies have found improved rates of transient but not permanent RLN palsy with CMAP-CIONM, and some have found no difference between modalities [14–23]. The single study comparing LAR-CIONM to IIONM found improved rates of transient, but not permanent, VFP [27, 37].

Another controversy regarding IONM relates to whether or not it is actually able to alter nerve palsy rates compared to nerve visualization alone [14–23]. Studies to date present conflicting results with regard to this question. The main issue with all studies reporting on *intermittent* IONM versus no monitoring is that IIONM is not able to *prevent* nerve injury by virtue of its methodology. This form of nerve monitoring is best thought of as a stimulation technique which provides functional neural information at an isolated point in time. It is useful for determining when staged surgery is appropriate and for nerve localization. However, its ability to actually prevent nerve injury is limited to nonexistent. By contrast, continuous IONM can potentially prevent nerve injury provided the time course of injury is such that it can be detected by gradual EMG waveform decline. As such, vocal fold paralysis as an outcome measure of IONM success should predominantly be utilized when reporting on CIONM techniques.

Conclusion

New techniques in IONM continue to emerge with the primary goal of enhancing ability to prevent nerve injury intraoperatively. Advances in nerve monitoring aim to improve patient outcomes by maintaining functional integrity of the nerve at risk. These emerging new technologies will continue to evolve and will likely become more feasible and accessible and cheaper and troubleshoot existing technical problems. The future for vagal and RLN IONM looks bright.

References

1. Nouraei SA, Allen HK, Middleton SE, et al. Vocal palsy increases the risk of lower respiratory tract infection in low risk low-morbidity patients undergoing thyroidectomy for benign disease: a big data analysis. Clin Otolaryngol. 2017;42(6):1259–66.
2. Dhillon VK, Randolph GW, Stack B, et al. Immediate and partial neural dysfunction after thyroid and parathyroid surgery: need for recognition, laryngeal exam and early treatment. An AHNS consensus statement. Head Neck. 2020;42(12):3779–94.
3. Sinclair CF, Kamani D, Randolph GW. The evolution and progression of standard procedures for

intraoperative nerve monitoring. Gland surgery. Ann Thyroid. 2019;4(1):1–12.
4. Jeannon JP, Orabi AA, Bruch GA, et al. Diagnosis of recurrent laryngeal nerve palsy after thyroidectomy: a systematic review. Int J Clin Pract. 2009;63:624–9.
5. Francis DO, Pearce EC, Ni S, et al. Epidemiology of vocal fold paralyses after total thyroidectomy for well- differentiated thyroid cancer in a medicare population. Otolaryngol Head Neck Surg. 2014;150: 548–57.
6. Randolph GW, Dralle H, Abdullah H, et al. Electrophysiologic recurrent laryngeal nerve monitoring during thyroid and parathyroid surgery: international standards guideline statement. Laryngoscope. 2011;121(Suppl 1):S1–16.
7. Phelan E, Schneider R, Lorenz K, et al. Continuous vagal IONM prevents recurrent laryngeal nerve paralysis by revealing initial EMG changes of impending neuropraxic injury: a prospective, multicenter study. Laryngoscope. 2014;124(6):1498–505.
8. Barczyński M, Randolph GW, Cernea CR, et al. External branch of the superior laryngeal nerve monitoring during thyroid and parathyroid surgery: International Neural Monitoring Study Group standards guideline statement. Laryngoscope. 2013;123(Suppl 4):S1–14. https://doi.org/10.1002/lary.24301.
9. Potenza AS, Phelan EA, Cernea CR, et al. Normative intra-operative electrophysiologic waveform analysis of superior laryngeal nerve external branch and recurrent laryngeal nerve in patients undergoing thyroid surgery. World J Surg. 2013;37:2336–42.
10. Sritharan N, Chase M, Kamani D, et al. The vagus nerve, recurrent laryngeal nerve, and external branch of the superior laryngeal nerve have unique latencies allowing for intraoperative documentation of intact neural function during thyroid surgery. Laryngoscope. 2015;125:E84–9.
11. Phelan E, Potenza A, Slough C, et al. Recurrent laryngeal nerve monitoring during thyroid surgery: normative vagal and recurrent laryngeal nerve electrophysiological data. Otolaryngol Head Neck Surg. 2012;147:640–6.
12. Schneider R, Randolph GW, Dionigi D, et al. international neural monitoring study group guideline 2018: part I: staging bilateral thyroid surgery with monitoring loss of signal. Laryngoscope. 2018;00:1–17.
13. Wu CW, Diongini G, Barczynski M, et al. International neuromonitoring study group guidelines 2018: part II: optimal recurrent laryngeal nerve management for invasive thyroid cancer-incorporation of surgical, laryngeal and neural electrophysiologic data. Laryngoscope. 2018;00:1–10.
14. Calò PG, Pisano G, Medas F, Pittau MR, et al. Identification alone versus intraoperative neuromonitoring of the recurrent laryngeal nerve during thyroid surgery: experience of 2034 consecutive patients. J Otolaryngol Head Neck Surg. 2014;43:16–23.
15. Pisanu A, Porceddu G, Podda M, Cois A, Uccheddu A. Systematic review with meta-analysis of studies comparing intraoperative neuromonitoring of recurrent laryngeal nerves versus visualization alone during thyroidectomy. J Surg Res. 2014;188(1):152–61. https://doi.org/10.1016/j.jss.2013.12.022.
16. Alesina PF, Rolfs T, Hommeltenberg S, et al. Intraoperative neuromonitoring does not reduce the incidence of recurrent laryngeal nerve palsy in thyroid reoperations: results of a retrospective comparative analysis. World J Surg. 2012;36(6):1348–53. https://doi.org/10.1007/s00268-012-1548-6.
17. Cirocchi R, Arezzo A, D'Andrea V, Abraha I, Popivanov GI, Avenia N. Intraoperative neuromonitoring versus visual nerve identification for prevention of recurrent laryngeal nerve injury in adults undergoing thyroid surgery. Cochrane Database Syst Rev. 2019;1:CD012483. https://doi.org/10.1002/14651858.CD012483.
18. Henry BM, Graves MJ, Vikse J, et al. The current state of intermittent intraoperative neural monitoring for prevention of recurrent laryngeal nerve injury during thyroidectomy: a PRISMA-compliant systematic review of overlapping meta-analyses. Langenbecks Arch Surg. 2017;402(4):663–73. https://doi.org/10.1007/s00423-017-1580-y.
19. Thomusch O, Sekulla C, Machens A, Neumann HJ, Timmermann W, Dralle H. Validity of intraoperative neuromonitoring signals in thyroid surgery. Langenbecks Arch Surg. 2004;389:499–503.
20. Beldi G, Kinsbergen T, Schlumpf R. Evaluation of intraoperative recurrent nerve monitoring in thyroid surgery. World J Surg. 2004;28:589–91.
21. Chan WF, Lang BH, Lo CY. The role of intraoperative nerve monitoring of recurrent laryngeal nerve during thyroidectomy: a comparative study on 1000 nerves at risk. Surgery. 2006;140:866–72.
22. Tomoda C, Hirokawa Y, Uruno T, et al. Sensitivity and specificity of intraoperative recurrent laryngeal nerve stimulation test for predicting vocal cord palsy after thyroid surgery. World J Surg. 2006;30:1230–3.
23. Barczynski M, Konturek A, Cichon S. Randomized clinical trial of visualization versus nerve monitoring of recurrent laryngeal nerves during thyroidectomy. Br J Surg. 2009;96:240–6.
24. Dralle H, Sekulla C, Haerting J, et al. Risk factors of paralysis and functional outcome after recurrent laryngeal nerve monitoring in thyroid surgery. Surgery. 2004;136:1310–22.
25. Barczyński M, Konturek A, Pragacz K, et al. Intraoperative nerve monitoring can reduce prevalence of recur- rent laryngeal nerve injury in thyroid reoperations: results of a ret-rospective cohort study. World J Surg. 2014;38:599–606.
26. Cirocchi R, Arezzo A, D'Andrea V, et al. Intraoperative neuromonitoring versus visual nerve identification for prevention of recurrent laryngeal nerve injury in adults undergoing thyroid surgery. Cochrane Database Syst Rev. 2019;1(1):CD012483. https://doi.org/10.1002/14651858.CD012483.
27. Sinclair CF, Tellez MJ, Ulkatan S. Continuous laryngeal adductor reflex versus intermittent nerve

monitoring in neck endocrine surgery. Laryngoscope. 2020;131(1):230–6.
28. Liddy W, et al. Anterior laryngeal electrodes for recurrent laryngeal nerve monitoring during thyroid and parathyroid surgery: new expanded options for neural monitoring: ALEs for RLN monitoring. Laryngoscope. 2018;128(12):2910–5.
29. Wu CW, Chai YJ, Dionigi G, Chiang FY, Liu X, Sun H, Randolph GW, Tufano RP, Kim HY. Recurrent laryngeal nerve safety parameters of the Harmonic Focus during thyroid surgery: porcine model using continuous monitoring. Laryngoscope. 2015;125:2838–45.
30. Dionigi G, Chiang FY, Kim HY, Randolph GW, Mangano A, Chang PY, Lu IC, Lin YC, Chen HC, Wu CW. Safety of LigaSure in recurrent laryngeal nerve dissection-porcine model using continuous monitoring. Laryngoscope. 2016;127(7):1724–9.
31. Sung ES, et al. Development of a novel detachable magnetic nerve stimulator for intraoperative neuromonitoring. World J Surg. 2018;42:137–42.
32. Chin SC, et al. Feasibility and safety of nerve stimulator attachment to energy-based devices: a porcine model study. Int J Surg. 2017;48:155–9.
33. Friedrich C, Ulmer C, Rieber C, et al. Safety analysis of vagal nerve stimulation for continuous nerve monitoring during thyroid surgery. Laryngoscope. 2012;122:1979–87.
34. Zhang D, Li S, Dionigi G, et al. Feasibility of continuous intraoperative neural monitoring during transoral endoscopic thyroidectomy vestibular approach in a porcine model. J Laparoendosc Adv Surg Tech A. 2018;29(12):1592–7.
35. Schneider R, Randolph GW, Barcynskzi M, et al. Continuous intraoperative neural monitoring of the recurrent nerves in thyroid surgery: a quantum leap in technology. Gland Surg. 2016;5(6):607–16.
36. Sinclair CF, Tellez MJ, Ulkatan S. Noninvasive, tube-based, continuous vagal nerve monitoring using the laryngeal adductor reflex: feasibility study of 134 nerves at risk. Head Neck. 2018;40(11):2498–506.
37. Sinclair CF, Tellez MJ, Tapia OR, Ulkatan S. Contralateral R1 and R2 components of the Laryngeal Adductor Reflex in humans under general anesthesia. Laryngoscope. 2017;127(12):E443–8.
38. Sinclair CF, Tellez MJ, Tapia OR, Ulkatan S. A novel methodology for assessing laryngeal and vagus nerve integrity in patients under general anesthesia. Clin Neurophysiol. 2017;128(7):1399–407.
39. Sinclair CF, Tellez MJ, Ulkatan S. Sensory receptor mapping in humans illuminates the mechanisms of laryngeal adductor reflex control. Laryngoscope. 2018;128(11):E365–70.
40. Sinclair CF, Tellez MJ, Blitzer A, Ulkatan S. Unearthing a consistent bilateral R1 component of the laryngeal adductor reflex in awake humans. Laryngoscope. 2018;128(11):2581–7.
41. Schneider R, et al. Opportunities and challenges of intermittent and continuous intraoperative neural monitoring in thyroid surgery. Gland Surg. 2017;6(5):537–45.

Troubleshooting System Integrity

11

Douglas M. Bennion and Nitin A. Pagedar

Introduction

More than a century ago in Berlin, Dr. Fedor Krause described the first reported use of intraoperative nerve monitoring during an acoustic nerve neurectomy performed on a woman with disabling tinnitus. He applied monopolar stimulation to the facial nerve and noted that "the weakest possible current of the induction apparatus resulted in contractions of the facial region." He immediately recognized the consequences of nonspecific tissue spread of the current, an ongoing limitation of nerve monitoring: "The irritation of the displaced acusticus caused the right shoulder to be elevated twice in succession. The accessories situated below had undoubtedly been reached by the current, because it was…bathed in liquor that had trickled down" [1]. The refinement of intraoperative nerve stimulation and monitoring from this rudimentary foundation has resulted in a broad array of tools and techniques to assist surgeons in preserving cranial nerve integrity and function during operations ranging from routine to complex. The first reported recording of recurrent laryngeal nerve electromyographic (EMG) activity was obtained by needle insertion through the cricothyroid membrane into the vocalis muscle during thyroid surgery in 1970 [2]. From these early beginnings, the use of intraoperative nerve monitoring has expanded to include all cranial nerves (excepting olfactory) in performing a wide range of otolaryngology-head and neck surgical procedures including neck dissection, thyroidectomy, parathyroidectomy, parotidectomy, resection of carotid body tumors, various otologic and neurotologic surgeries, and many more.

Suboptimal functioning of nerve monitoring systems has been a consistent source of frustration for the head and neck surgeon, with an early report detailing an attempt to consolidate equipment into a single unit with controls designed to eliminate "a common, annoying problem with EMG monitoring in the operating room – namely, background electrical noises, including the electrocautery and stimulus artifact that falsely trigger the loudspeaker," creating false alarms that "can be both annoying and misleading to the surgeon" [3]. Indeed, a 2007 survey of 685 practicing otolaryngologists 20 years later revealed that 20% preferred not to use recurrent laryngeal nerve (RLN) monitoring in thyroid surgery due to the unreliability and excessive number of false positives [4], and this despite having advanced through the use of transoral wire hook electrodes placed in the vocal folds [5] to the use of surface EMG electrodes embedded within the endotracheal tube as first reported in 1996 [6]. In this

D. M. Bennion · N. A. Pagedar (✉)
Department of Otolaryngology – Head and Neck Surgery, University of Iowa, Iowa City, IA, USA
e-mail: douglas-bennion@uiowa.edu; nitin-pagedar@uiowa.edu

© The Author(s), under exclusive license to Springer Nature Switzerland AG 2022
J. Scharpf, G. W. Randolph (eds.), *Intraoperative Cranial Nerve Monitoring in Otolaryngology-Head and Neck Surgery*, https://doi.org/10.1007/978-3-030-84916-0_11

chapter, we will present an approach to the use of recurrent laryngeal nerve monitoring in thyroid and parathyroid surgery designed to alleviate some of this frustration. We first briefly review the mechanism of nerve injury and practice patterns for use of nerve monitoring systems, including discussion of the intraoperative points during which use of the nerve monitor may be of greatest utility in avoiding injury and decision-making for staging of contralateral resection. We conclude with a practical outline for understanding and troubleshooting the intraoperative nerve monitor.

Mechanisms of RLN Injury

While voice complaints following thyroid surgery, which occur in 30–87% of patients, are often attributed to intubation trauma and irritation, the contribution of recurrent laryngeal nerve injuries cannot be discounted, with rates of injury thought to be close to 10% [7, 8]. Temporary vocal cord paralysis rate has been reported to be 9.8% in a recent systematic review [7] and 9% in a Medicare cohort [8]. Slightly better rates of temporary cord paralysis in 6% and permanent paralysis in 3% of patients have also been previously reported [9]. Patients may additionally suffer injury to the superior laryngeal nerve [10], resulting in a more subtle loss of voice projection and higher pitches, usually more noticeable to professional voice users.

Regarding intraoperative RLN injury, a study of 115 nerves with monitoring loss of signal revealed that injury was due to traction in 83%, and three out of every five of these localized the neuropraxic segment to the suspensory ligament of the thyroid [11]. Other publications also suggest that virtually all traction injuries localize to that site [12]. Visual evidence of nerve injury was only observed in 14% of 281 nerves identified intraoperatively to have loss of signal, emphasizing the lack of sensitivity of visual neural inspection, with the percentages of initial and permanent RLN paralysis by injury mechanism presented in Table 11.1 [13].

Table 11.1 Rates of initial and permanent rates of recurrent laryngeal nerve (RLN) paralysis by injury mechanism

Injury mechanism	Initial rate of RLN paralysis (%)	Rate of permanent RLN paralysis (%)
Traction of the nerve	98	1.4
Thermal injury	72	28
Compression	100	0
Clamping	50	50
Ligature entrapment	100	100
Suction-related injury	100	0
Transection	100	100

Trends in Nerve Monitoring for Thyroid Surgery

Over the last 20 years, there has been a widespread adoption of intraoperative RLN monitoring during thyroid surgery. In a 2007 survey study, 28.6% of otolaryngologists reported using intraoperative monitoring for all thyroidectomies, whereas 60% of respondents reported using RLN monitoring rarely or never, with those surgeons having been trained in its use being 3× more likely to have adopted it [4]. More recent survey data show a large shift in practice patterns, with 80% of otolaryngologists reporting routine use of nerve monitoring during most operations [14]. Over this time, there has been a trend toward bilaterality in thyroid surgery [15], the rate having nearly doubled from 1993 to 2007 in one study [16] and tripled in another [17]. This is despite recommendations to perform unilateral surgery in low-risk cancers up to 4 cm as articulated in the most recent 2015 ATA guidelines [18]. It is in the performance of bilateral thyroid lobectomies that patients assume the risk of bilateral cord paralysis.

While uncommon, bilateral vocal cord paralysis can be devastating and is associated with a 50% risk of requiring acute airway intervention, whether tracheostomy or other acute airway surgery [11]. Importantly, the rate of bilateral cord paralysis was as high as 17% if loss of signal was undetected or disregarded despite detection compared to 0% if second side aborted or performed as a staged procedure in a retrospective review of more than 1300 patients with suggested benign bilateral thyroid disease [19]. Additional studies confirm that continuation to the second side after initial LOS resulted in a similarly unacceptably high rate of bilateral VCP, 16% versus 0% [20]. A salient cost-utility analysis evidenced that nerve monitoring with loss of signal incorporation into the surgical strategy allowing for staged surgery is cost-effective, even when using the most conservative estimates for rates of contralateral nerve paralysis [21].

Intraoperative Troubleshooting of the Nerve Monitor

The efficacy and cost-effectiveness of intraoperative recurrent laryngeal nerve monitoring in thyroid surgery rest on reliable implementation of the system in the operating room. Many factors contribute to the successful use of nerve monitoring, and methods in practice are variable. There are multiple reasons for this, including equipment-related issues, especially endotracheal tube displacement, different amplitudes used as the cutoff for defining loss of signal, inconsistent time to postoperative evaluation with prior spontaneous recovery in an unknown number of patients, and variability in adherence to troubleshooting algorithms.

The International Neural Monitoring Study Group (INMSG) has published guidelines that recommend obtaining an initial normative baseline waveform with amplitude of 500 μV or greater using a stimulation current of 1–2 mA along with a good laryngeal twitch assessment at the beginning of surgery. These guidelines suggest that a loss of amplitude of >50% concordant with latency increase of >10% implies that the nerve is at elevated risk of postoperative dysfunction and recommend immediate cessation of the surgical maneuver associated with the onset of these EMG changes [12]. The finding of concurrent latency and amplitude changes, also described as concordant amplitude decrease and latency increase, or "combined event," is an important early marker of impending neuropraxic injury [22], especially if repetitively occurring [23]. This is a distinctly different signal change as compared to loss of amplitude without change in latency, which is observed with endotracheal tube displacement [24].

With these general considerations in mind, we turn to troubleshooting of nerve monitoring difficulties, with the commonly used Medtronic Nerve Integrity Monitor NIM-Response® system as a working example. We find it helpful to conceptualize the intraoperative nerve monitoring system as a simple circuit (Fig. 11.1) [25], including a power source, a conducting system through which the current flows, a load or resistor across which a change in voltage can be detected using a voltmeter, and a ground through which residual current is returned and that provides an electrically neutral point of comparison. In the case of intraoperative recurrent laryngeal nerve monitoring, the power enters the circuit in several ways: intentionally by use of monopolar or bipolar stimulation of relevant tissues or unintentionally by electrocautery or other mechanical stimulation of the nerve. The conducting "wire" of this circuit depends on the point of stimulation but typically involves a small amount of soft tissue with any associated blood or irrigation fluid, followed by transmission along the nerve itself, either through the main vagal trunk if stimulating proximally or directly into the recurrent nerve if stimulating distally. The load or resistors in this circuit are the motor endplates at the neuromuscular junctions within the vocalis and other laryngeal muscles that produce electrochemical stimulation affecting muscle depolarization and contraction in response to nerve action potentials. The change in intramuscular voltage is measured by a pair of appropriately placed recording electrodes, one (+) cathode and one (−) anode for the right side (red) and one each for the left side (blue) of the larynx (total of four recording electrodes). The intramuscular voltage difference detected between the cathode and anode during this signal transduction is depicted as the multi-

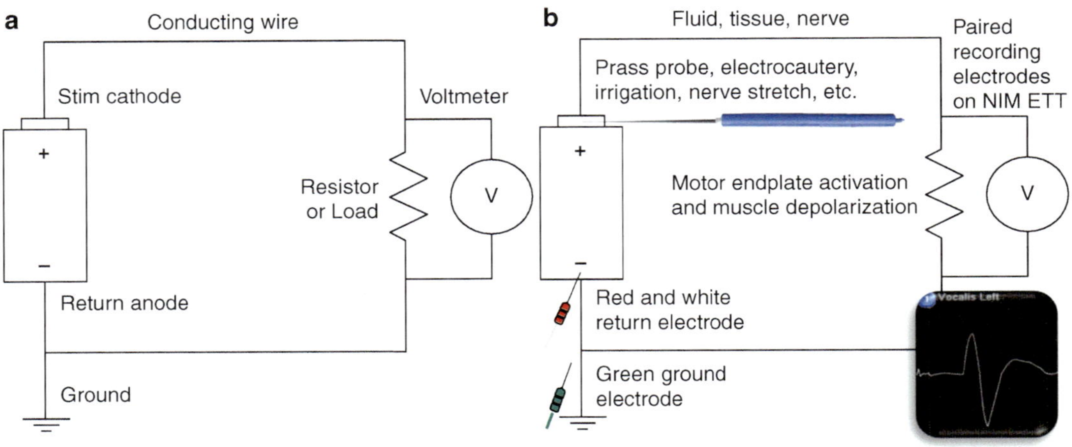

Fig. 11.1 Diagram representing intraoperative recurrent laryngeal nerve monitoring system as a circuit (published with permission from the Iowa Head and Neck Protocols) [25]. (**a**) Simple circuit shown with power source, including cathode and anode, from which current is derived, conducting wire, resistor or load, voltmeter, and ground. (**b**) Representation of the nerve monitoring system in its context as a circuit. Current is either purposefully generated with use of monopolar (e.g., Prass probe) or bipolar stimulating probes or unintentionally generated via electrocautery spread, nerve irritation through stretch, irrigation, or other noxious stimuli. The conductor in this circuit includes overlying fluids, fascia, muscle, fat, or other tissue and the nerve itself, with current being transmitted at the neuromuscular junction as an electrical potential within the motor endplate. This results in vocalis muscle depolarization which is detected by the paired recording electrodes positioned on either side of the endotracheal tube (a pair of red electrodes positioned along the right vocalis muscle and another pair of blue electrodes on the left). The voltage difference between each recording cathode and anode pair is depicted as an EMG motor unit action potential on the NIM monitor, left vocalis (blue) and right vocalis (red), respectively. Finally the remaining current is returned to the red and white return anode, usually placed in the subcutaneous tissues overlying the sternum, along with the green ground electrode

phasic EMG wave observed on the monitor. The electrical potential difference recorded in this way is also compared to the ground electrode (green), usually placed in electrically neutral skin overlying the bone. An additional stimulus return anode electrode (red plug with white wire) is placed more distally in the same area with the electrode tips several centimeters apart to serve as a sink for the return of current that is applied during the use of the monopolar nerve stimulator.

In conceptualizing the system as a circuit in this way, it becomes apparent that the waveforms depicted on the monitoring screen are not nerve action potentials, as commonly misunderstood. Rather, they represent motor unit action potentials, which are the summation of intramuscular potentials of the individual motor fibers of a motor unit during muscle contraction. These EMG waveforms should typically have peak to peak amplitudes of ~0.5 mV and duration of 8–14 ms, include 3–4 phases, and have a 7–10 msec latency in a healthy nerve and muscle (Fig. 11.2). The action potential phase of signal transduction along the nerve fibers themselves occurs much more quickly and is automatically excluded from the monitoring display via an adjustable delay feature. Without this automatic exclusion, the action potential signal would be detected as stimulation artifact. Additional sources of artifactual noise include pacemaker signal, entangling of the recording and stimulating cables leading to a short in the circuit, absence of a muting detector on the nerve stimulator wiring, or the current discharge that occurs with striking together of two metal instruments (galvanic coupling) [26]. Additional factors affect the stimulus intensity required for detectable current conduction through the circuit. Impairment of the nerve (e.g., involvement with tumor) or the neu-

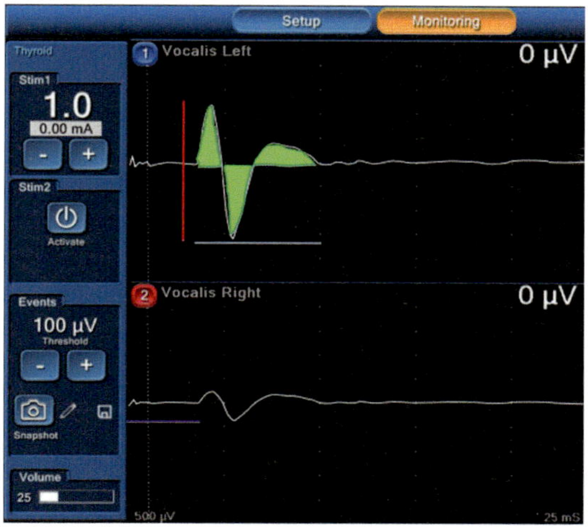

Fig. 11.2 Nerve integrity monitoring display with amplitude (red bar), duration (blue bar), phase (green), and latency (purple bar) of a typical EMG motor unit action potential

romuscular junction (e.g., muscle relaxation) will raise the resistance to current flow and therefore increase the stimulus intensity required to reach the depolarization threshold. Use of a monopolar probe, such as the Prass probe, requires higher intensity than bipolar probe stimulation. Greater distance between the probe and the nerve will similarly result in higher required intensity for activation. Finally, the pulse width of the stimulus plays a role, with widths of 50–100 µs preferentially triggering Aα motor fibers. This is not a parameter that commonly requires adjustment.

In the operating room, there are several essential anesthetic factors to consider related to the NIM endotracheal tube (ETT). First, no topical anesthetic should be applied to the vocal cords or tube. The use of long-acting neuromuscular blocking agents is contraindicated, though short-acting agents can be considered if communicated clearly between the surgeon and anesthesiologist. The largest size ETT that can be safely accommodated by the patient's airway should be used to maximize contact between the recording electrodes and the vocalis muscle. We recommend the use of video laryngoscopy during intubation to visualize the placement of the tube by the anesthesia provider in correct orientation (e.g., avoidance of rotation of the tube) and depth (wide blue cross hatch at the level of the vocal cords), ideally done with the neck extended in position for surgery. Securing tape should be placed such that it does not apply rotational forces on the tube. During setup of the remaining portions of the NIM system, the recording, stimulating, ground, and return electrode wires should briefly be examined to rule out exposed wiring, and secure insertion to the white Patient Interface box should be ensured. Recording and stimulating wires should cross at 90-degree angles when necessary and should not be allowed to intertwine. Electrical shorts may result from exposed wiring or from contact of the electrode needle tips, which should ideally be 5 cm apart with the green ground electrode closest to the surgical field. The electrocautery and bipolar cords should be placed through the Muting Detector, which serves to temporarily silence the audio and visual functioning of the monitor during electrocautery unit discharge. The Muting Detector should not be used on the cautery grounding pad wire. The neural monitoring unit display should be checked by the surgeon prior to scrubbing in to verify the appropriate impedances, absence of errors, and volume, threshold, and stimulation settings. While commonly performed after NIM setup is complete, the "tap test" is neither a physiologic nor reliable method for confirming proper electrode placement and functioning of the system.

For intraoperative optimization of the nerve monitoring system, commonly involved components and practical troubleshooting comments are outlined in flow diagrams for absent event tone when stimulating a visible RLN (Fig. 11.3) and for excessive noise or continuous train signal (Fig. 11.4). These algorithms are organized such that the most common and easily checked factors are addressed first, followed by less common and potentially more disruptive troubleshooting maneuvers. The flow diagrams were compiled using the authors' experience, instructions provided by the device manufacturer's guide and published algorithms [27]. In the scenario in which stimulation of the RLN results in visible or palpable laryngeal twitch without triggering an event tone, troubleshooting should begin directly with assessment of the NIM setup and proceed to

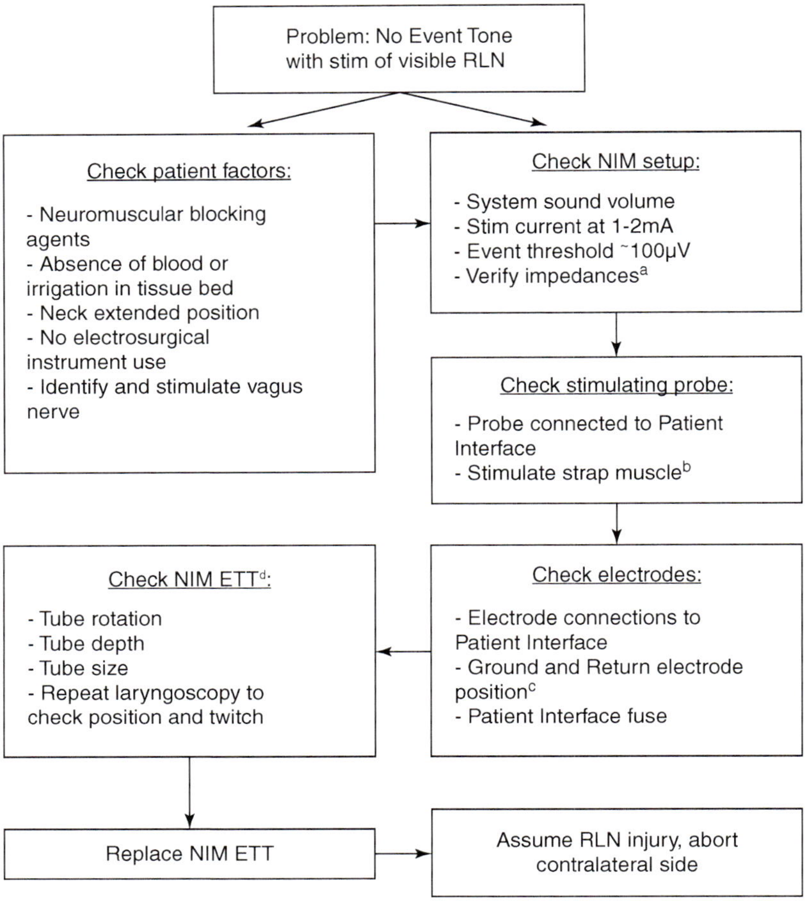

Fig. 11.3 Loss of signal troubleshooting flow diagram (published with permission from the Iowa Head and Neck Protocols) [25]. When stimulus of a visible RLN does not result in signal, factors related to the patient and surgical field can be explored while simultaneously having operating room staff check the NIM setup before proceeding with additional troubleshooting as outlined. ETT endotracheal tube, NIM nerve integrity monitor. (**a**) Suggested <5kΩ on each channel and <2kΩ difference between channels. If not, reposition tube, and then replace if needed. If the neural monitoring unit indicates high impedance (>7.5kΩ), check the connection at the patient interface (white) box, and consider repositioning the NIM ETT. (**b**) For the stimulation probe, since output is pulsatile 4 per seconds, dragging over the tissue rather than hopping with the tip will give a more reliable result. (**c**) Ground electrode should be placed in the skin near the bone without a muscle (e.g., sternum), with system ground (green) closer to the larynx than stimulus return (red/white), 5 cm apart. (**d**) Avoid rotation of tube during intubation, as right-handed anesthesiologists tend to rotate the tube about 30 degrees clockwise inadvertently, typically requiring counterclockwise rotation typically for correction. Avoid tape on the lips as this tends to apply torque/rotational force that can displace the electrodes from optimal contact with the vocal cords. If needed, direct or video laryngoscopy may be used to visually verify the ETT and evaluate for cord twitch with nerve stimulation. Verify no pooling of saliva which can result in salt bridging of current between electrodes

checking the electrodes and the endotracheal tube and replacing the tube if needed, skipping over an assessment of patient factors and the stimulating probe. Of note, the situation in which there is a loss of event tone can be managed with more confidence if the vagus nerve has been identified and stimulated prior to any potential manipulation of the recurrent laryngeal nerve. While not all surgeons routinely perform vagal nerve stimulation, this represents one well-studied aspect of nerve monitoring, with a normal signal providing a negative predictive value

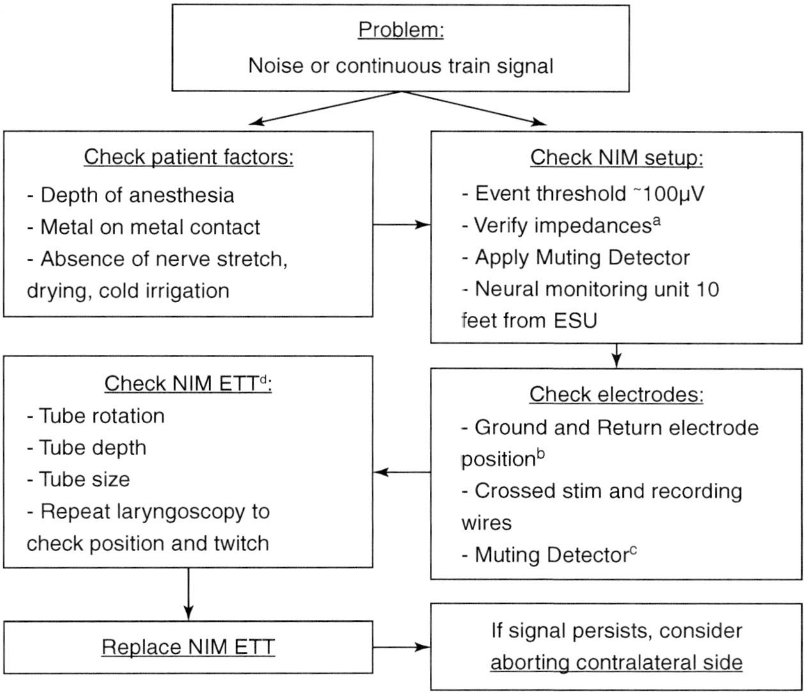

Fig. 11.4 Noise or continuous train signal troubleshooting flow diagram (published with permission from the Iowa Head and Neck Protocols) [25]. When unexpected noise or continuous signal is elicited, begin with assessment of patient/surgical field factors along with the NIM setup with assistance from the circulating nurse before proceeding as outlined. ESU electrosurgical cautery unit, ETT endotracheal tube, NIM nerve integrity monitor. (**a**) Suggested <5kΩ on each channel and <2kΩ difference between channels. If not, reposition tube, and then replace if needed. Higher overall impedance bilaterally is preferred over large differential between sides as this leads to increased artifact and noise. If low impedance detected (<0.1kΩ), remove and replace with new NIM ETT. (**b**) Ground electrode should be placed in the skin near the bone without a muscle (e.g., sternum), with system ground (green) closer to the larynx than stimulus return (red/white), 5 cm apart. Place ground and stimulus return on opposite side from pacer. (**c**) Monopolar and bipolar cautery wires may be additionally looped through the Muting Detector for low electrosurgical unit settings. (**d**) If needed, direct or video laryngoscopy may be used to visually verify the ETT and evaluate for cord twitch concurrent with unexpected signal. Verify no pooling of saliva which can result in salt bridging of current between electrodes

(i.e., maintenance of signal indicating no nerve injury) of 90–100% in multiple series in the literature. Unfortunately, reported positive predictive values (i.e., loss of signal indicating actual nerve injury) vary to a much greater extent, from 12% to 88% [28]. Vagal nerve stimulation before any RLN manipulation, especially in cases of surprise variant or pathologic anatomy, allows the troubleshooting algorithm for absent event tone to be more effective, therefore minimizing the chances of false-positive loss of signal. The generally accepted criterion is the reduction of EMG amplitude to under a 100 μV threshold, which is highly associated with subsequent vocal fold immobility with only a fraction achieving intraoperative recovery. Ultimately, if efforts fail to restore normal signal, the decision should be made to abort and stage contralateral lobe resection after cord function can be assessed in follow-up.

Conclusion

For head and neck and endocrine surgeons, intraoperative nerve monitoring is a tool of great utility that is sometimes frustrated by the technical failures and nuance that were noted by Dr. Krause in his first use of the nascent technology more than 100 years ago. Conceptualizing what may at first appear to be a complex system as a simple circuit may aid in understanding how each of the electrical components can both help and hinder the surgeon in attaining her goal of safe and efficacious thyroid and parathyroid surgery. Our experience has been that consistent application of the nerve monitoring system in even routine cases provides the benefit of experience in anticipating common problems, troubleshooting them when they arise, and more confidently recognizing when the system is in fact working to provide the critical warning that nerve integrity may be compromised. Greater experience with the use of the system has yielded greater confidence in safe thyroid and parathyroid surgery for patients.

References

1. Krause F. Surgery of the brain and spinal cord based on personal experiences (3 vols). In: Translated by Haubold H, Thorek M. New York: Rebman Co; 1910–1912.
2. Flisberg K, Lidholm T. Electrical stimulation of the human recurrent laryngeal nerve during thyroid operation. Acta Otolaryngol. 1970;69(263):63–7.
3. Metson R, Thornton A, Nadol JB Jr, Fee WE Jr. A new design for intraoperative facial nerve monitoring. Otolaryngol Head Neck Surg. 1988;98(3):258–61. PubMed PMID: 3127791. Epub 1988/03/01. eng.
4. Horne SK, Gal TJ, Brennan JA. Prevalence and patterns of intraoperative nerve monitoring for thyroidectomy. Otolaryngol Head Neck Surg. 2007;136(6):952–6. PubMed PMID: 17547986. Epub 2007/06/06. eng.
5. Lipton RJ, McCaffrey TV, Litchy WJ. Intraoperative electrophysiologic monitoring of laryngeal muscle during thyroid surgery. Laryngoscope. 1988;98(12):1292–6. PubMed PMID: 3200073. Epub 1988/12/01. eng
6. Eisele DW. Intraoperative electrophysiologic monitoring of the recurrent laryngeal nerve. Laryngoscope. 1996;106(4):443–9. PubMed PMID: 8614219. Epub 1996/04/01. eng
7. Jeannon JP, Orabi AA, Bruch GA, Abdalsalam HA, Simo R. Diagnosis of recurrent laryngeal nerve palsy after thyroidectomy: a systematic review. Int J Clin Pract. 2009;63(4):624–9. PubMed PMID: 19335706. Epub 2009/04/02. eng
8. Francis DO, Pearce EC, Ni S, Garrett CG, Penson DF. Epidemiology of vocal fold paralyses after total thyroidectomy for well-differentiated thyroid cancer in a Medicare population. Otolaryngol Head Neck Surg. 2014;150(4):548–57. PubMed PMID: 24482349. PMCID: PMC4229384. Epub 2014/02/01. eng.
9. Steurer M, Passler C, Denk DM, Schneider B, Niederle B, Bigenzahn W. Advantages of recurrent laryngeal nerve identification in thyroidectomy and parathyroidectomy and the importance of preoperative and postoperative laryngoscopic examination in more than 1000 nerves at risk. Laryngoscope. 2002;112(1):124–33. PubMed PMID: 11802050. Epub 2002/01/22. eng
10. Teitelbaum BJ, Wenig BL. Superior laryngeal nerve injury from thyroid surgery. Head Neck. 1995;17(1):36–40. PubMed PMID: 7883547. Epub 1995/01/01. eng
11. Schneider R, Randolph G, Dionigi G, Barczyński M, Chiang FY, Triponez F, et al. Prospective study of vocal fold function after loss of the neuromonitoring signal in thyroid surgery: The International Neural Monitoring Study Group's POLT study. Laryngoscope. 2016;126(5):1260–6. PubMed PMID: 26667156. Epub 2015/12/17. eng
12. Schneider R, Randolph GW, Dionigi G, Wu CW, Barczynski M, Chiang FY, et al. International neural monitoring study group guideline 2018 part I: staging bilateral thyroid surgery with monitoring loss of signal. Laryngoscope. 2018;128 Suppl 3:S1–s17. PubMed PMID: 30289983.Epub 2018/10/06. eng
13. Dionigi G, Wu CW, Kim HY, Rausei S, Boni L, Chiang FY. Severity of recurrent laryngeal nerve injuries in thyroid surgery. World J Surg. 2016;40(6):1373–81. PubMed PMID: 26817650. Epub 2016/01/29. eng
14. Singer MC, Rosenfeld RM, Sundaram K. Laryngeal nerve monitoring: current utilization among head and neck surgeons. Otolaryngol Head Neck Surg. 2012;146(6):895–9. PubMed PMID: 22399282. Epub 2012/03/09. eng
15. Davies L, Morris LG, Haymart M, Chen AY, Goldenberg D, Morris J, et al. American Association of Clinical Endocrinologists and American College of Endocrinology Disease State Clinical Review: The Increasing Incidence of Thyroid Cancer. Endocr Pract. 2015;21(6):686–96. PubMed PMID: 26135963. PMCID: PMC4923940. Epub 2015/07/03. eng
16. Ho Y, Carr MM, Goldenberg D. Trends in intraoperative neural monitoring for thyroid and parathyroid surgery amongst otolaryngologists and general surgeons. Eur Arch Otorhinolaryngol. 2013;270(9):2525–30. PubMed PMID: 23371538.Epub 2013/02/02. eng
17. Gourin CG, Tufano RP, Forastiere AA, Koch WM, Pawlik TM, Bristow RE. Volume-based trends in thyroid surgery. Arch Otolaryngol Head Neck Surg. 2010;136(12):1191–8. PubMed PMID: 21173367. Epub 2010/12/22. eng
18. Haugen BR, Alexander EK, Bible KC, Doherty GM, Mandel SJ, Nikiforov YE, et al. 2015 American Thyroid Association Management Guidelines for Adult Patients with Thyroid Nodules and Differentiated Thyroid Cancer: The American Thyroid

Association Guidelines Task Force on Thyroid Nodules and Differentiated Thyroid Cancer. Thyroid. 2016;26(1):1–133. PubMed PMID: 26462967. PMCID: PMC4739132. Epub 2015/10/16. eng
19. Goretzki PE, Schwarz K, Brinkmann J, Wirowski D, Lammers BJ. The impact of intraoperative neuromonitoring (IONM) on surgical strategy in bilateral thyroid diseases: is it worth the effort? World J Surg. 2010;34(6):1274–84. PubMed PMID: 20143072. Epub 2010/02/10. eng
20. Melin M, Schwarz K, Lammers BJ, Goretzki PE. IONM-guided goiter surgery leading to two-stage thyroidectomy--indication and results. Langenbeck's Arch Surg. 2013;398(3):411–8. PubMed PMID: 23179319. Epub 2012/11/28. eng
21. Al-Qurayshi Z, Kandil E, Randolph GW. Cost-effectiveness of intraoperative nerve monitoring in avoidance of bilateral recurrent laryngeal nerve injury in patients undergoing total thyroidectomy. Br J Surg. 2017;104(11):1523–31. PubMed PMID: 28707698. Epub 2017/07/15. eng
22. Schneider R, Randolph GW, Sekulla C, Phelan E, Thanh PN, Bucher M, et al. Continuous intraoperative vagus nerve stimulation for identification of imminent recurrent laryngeal nerve injury. Head Neck. 2013;35(11):1591–8. PubMed PMID: 23169450. Epub 2012/11/22. eng
23. Phelan E, Schneider R, Lorenz K, Dralle H, Kamani D, Potenza A, et al. Continuous vagal IONM prevents recurrent laryngeal nerve paralysis by revealing initial EMG changes of impending neuropraxic injury: a prospective, multicenter study. Laryngoscope. 2014;124(6):1498–505. PubMed PMID: 24307596. Epub 2013/12/07. eng
24. Barber SR, Liddy W, Kyriazidis N, Cinquepalmi M, Lin BM, Modi R, et al. Changes in electromyographic amplitudes but not latencies occur with endotracheal tube malpositioning during intraoperative monitoring for thyroid surgery: implications for guidelines. Laryngoscope. 2017;127(9):2182–8. PubMed PMID: 27861939. Epub 2016/11/20. eng
25. Hoffman HT (ed). Thyroidectomy and thyroid lobectomy. Iowa Head and Neck Protocols. Updated 2020. https://medicine.uiowa.edu/iowaprotocols/thyroidectomy-and-thyroid-lobectomy. Accessed 1 Dec 2020.
26. Pearlman RC, Isley MR, Ganley JC. Electrical artifact during intraoperative electromyographic neuromonitoring. Am J Electroneurodiagnostic Technol. 2008;48(2):107–18. PubMed PMID: 18680898. Epub 2008/08/07. eng.
27. Randolph GW, Dralle H, Abdullah H, Barczynski M, Bellantone R, Brauckhoff M, et al. Electrophysiologic recurrent laryngeal nerve monitoring during thyroid and parathyroid surgery: international standards guideline statement. Laryngoscope. 2011;121 Suppl 1:S1–16. PubMed PMID: 21181860. Epub 2010/12/25. eng
28. Schneider R, Machens A, Lorenz K, Dralle H. Intraoperative nerve monitoring in thyroid surgery-shifting current paradigms. Gland Surg. 2020;9(Suppl 2):S120–s8. PubMed PMID: 32175252. PMCID: PMC7044089. Epub 2020/03/17. eng

Loss of Neural Signal in Thyroid and Parathyroid Surgery

12

Simon A. Holoubek and David J. Terris

Introduction

Injury to the recurrent laryngeal nerve (RLN) remains a not uncommon complication during thyroid and parathyroid surgery. Laryngeal nerve monitoring (LNM) is often employed in an effort to prevent injury and to provide valuable information to the surgeon. Intraoperative processing of the information and particularly in the event of dysfunction requires thoughtful and stepwise behavior. These steps actually begin with an informed patient, and therefore preoperative discussion is critical for laying the proper groundwork and patient expectations should a loss of signal (LOS) occur.

Preoperative Discussion

A discussion about the potential for LOS is reasonable to include in the informed consent process of patients for whom the RLN is at risk during surgery. This conversation may include divulging the frequency of nerve injury and the anticipated course of action in the event that LOS occurs. The potential options that a surgeon can discuss with the patient include completing the surgery as planned, accomplishing a more conservative resection on the contralateral lobe that carries a very low (nearly zero) risk of nerve injury, or even aborting the surgery (in order to stage it).

While the potential need for additional surgical interventions is often raised when surgery is planned, the particular context of surgery involving the RLNs makes this an especially reasonable topic for discussion.

Finally, the limitations of nerve monitoring are usually shared with the patient. Although intended to help prevent nerve injury, the principal value probably rests in the intraoperative information it provides regarding anticipated postoperative TVF function. Even this information has a small but meaningful error rate which may lead, for example, to the staging of an operation that could have been completed safely. The monitoring is generally intended to confirm nerve function once it has already been revealed by dissection, rather than blindly seeking it. A wet environment may cause a false-negative stimulation, while stimulation distal to an injury may provide a false-positive stimulation. Transient injury may be detected, but it is not possible to predict the duration of the dysfunction.

S. A. Holoubek · D. J. Terris (✉)
Department of Otolaryngology – Head and Neck Surgery, Augusta University, Augusta, GA, USA
e-mail: sholoubek@augusta.edu; dterris@augusta.edu

© The Author(s), under exclusive license to Springer Nature Switzerland AG 2022

J. Scharpf, G. W. Randolph (eds.), *Intraoperative Cranial Nerve Monitoring in Otolaryngology-Head and Neck Surgery*, https://doi.org/10.1007/978-3-030-84916-0_12

Technical Considerations of Nerve Monitoring

The use of LNM does not eliminate nerve injury, but rather serves to confirm nerve integrity. This information requires processing by the surgeon to determine subsequent action. The optimal implementation of LNM generally starts with a thorough preoperative assessment of laryngeal function. This is most easily accomplished by an endoscopic laryngeal examination, which is important to be able to distinguish between preexisting nerve dysfunction and intraoperative injury.

The International Neural Monitoring Study Group proposed a series of guidelines regarding laryngeal nerve monitoring and an algorithm for proceeding in the event of LOS [1, 2]. While a rigid sequence of steps is advocated, it probably represents an overly burdensome series of maneuvers for routine surgeries. Instead, most practicing surgeons pursue a more streamlined and practical approach.

There are a variety of options for LNM. We utilize a hybrid system which combines a nerve integrity monitor interface (Medtronic, Jacksonville, FL) with custom-designed nondisposable stimulating instruments (Neurovision, Ventura, CA) (Fig. 12.1). These instruments allow for simultaneous dissection and stimulation, which results in far-reduced numbers of instrument exchanges and leads to efficient, rhythmic surgery.

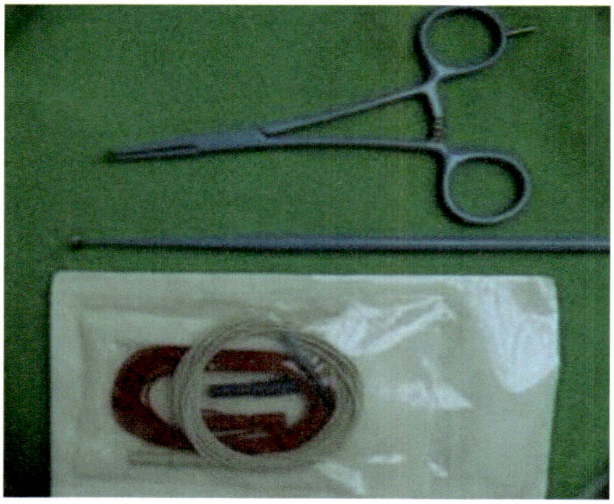

Fig. 12.1 Hybrid nerve monitoring

Setup of the system can be done by the surgeon or a circulating nurse or with the assistance of an intraoperative neural monitoring technician. Intubation with a GlideScope allows for direct visualization of the TVFs and assures the proper positioning of the laryngeal EMG endotracheal tube placement between the folds. The tube is secured lateral to the tongue and teeth so that coughing and gagging are less likely to cause displacement of the endotracheal tube (Fig. 12.2a). The respiratory tubing can then be secured to the side of the bed with slack to prevent pulling which can turn the head and alter the anatomy (Fig. 12.2b). LNM grounding wires are secured in a redundant fashion with tape to prevent inadvertent removal (Fig. 12.2c).

In difficult surgeries, especially when bilateral surgery is anticipated, the integrity of the system may be verified by stimulating the ipsilateral vagus nerve (at a setting of 2.5 mA). After the RLN has been positively identified, it is usually stimulated, at a setting of 1.0 mA. After all dissection is complete, either the RLN or vagus nerve is usually stimulated again to verify functional integrity (this step may be omitted for unilateral surgery).

While similar principles apply to parathyroid surgery, in our practice, vagal nerve stimulation is even more common than with thyroid surgery, because it is rarely necessary to identify the RLN in a routine modern parathyroidectomy. Nevertheless, despite the very low risk of even temporary RLN dysfunction during parathyroid surgery, if contralateral dissection is to be pursued, then ipsilateral vagal nerve stimulation will essentially ensure the absence of bilateral nerve dysfunction.

Loss of Signal: Intraoperative Troubleshooting

A consistent approach is helpful when troubleshooting intraoperative findings of nerve monitoring. Early vagal nerve stimulation (while not regularly performed) may help differentiate equip-

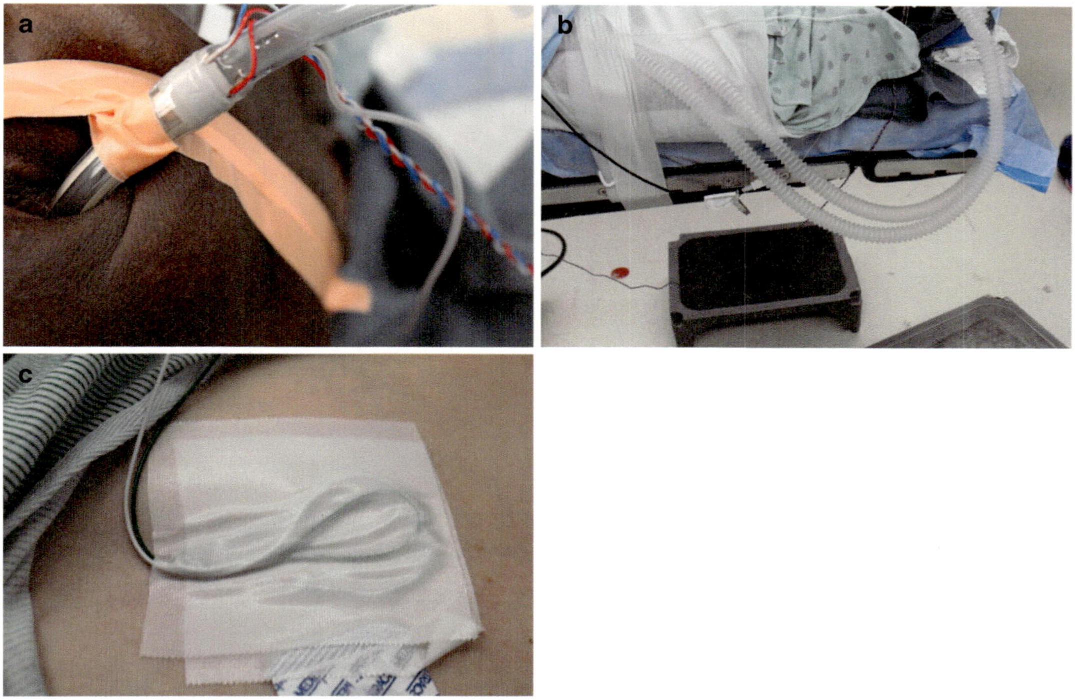

Fig. 12.2 Securing the LNM components
A. tube
B. circuit
C. grounding leads

ment malfunction from true LOS. If there is apparent malfunctioning of the system, early steps to discern the cause include ensuring all electrodes are plugged into the console and connected as intended. The endotracheal tube should be evaluated to determine if it has become displaced.

If there is still no signal when stimulating the RLN after initially confirming appropriate signal, the ipsilateral vagus should be stimulated as it provides an easy point of access for proximal verification of nerve function (Fig. 12.3). If there is no signal with stimulation of the ipsilateral vagus nerve, an attempt to elicit a laryngeal twitch can be done to differentiate between equipment failure and true LOS (Fig. 12.4). This is done with palpation posterior to the larynx while simultaneously stimulating the RLN or vagus nerve [3]. This is a straightforward maneuver that is easily learned and should become part of an endocrine surgeon's repertoire.

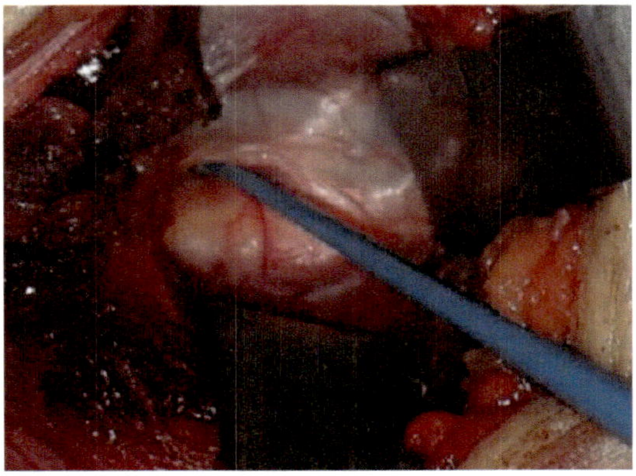

Fig. 12.3 Indirect stimulation of vagus nerve (carotid sheath)

Inability to elicit a laryngeal twitch (especially combined with a positive stimulation of the contralateral vagus nerve confirming proper endotracheal tube positioning) reinforces the

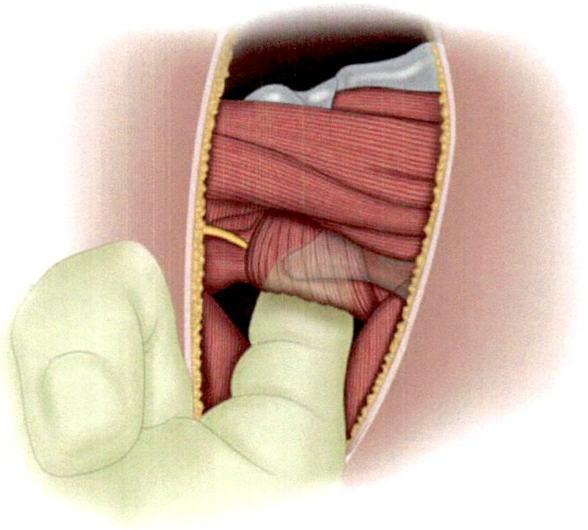

Fig. 12.4 Laryngeal twitch

conclusion that the patient has at least a temporary RLN dysfunction.

Loss of Signal: Management Strategies

Management strategies will differ based on why LOS has occurred. Thermal and traction injuries are common causes of temporary nerve dysfunction in the presence of an anatomically intact RLN. In this situation, virtually, all nerves will recover within 2–3 months postoperatively [4]. Because some nerves manifest ultra-transient dysfunction and may recover intraoperatively [5], it is reasonable to wait a short period of time (15–30 minutes) to see if recovery occurs. In the absence of rapid recovery, staging the operation until the nerve has recovered reduces the potential for bilateral RLN injury and is one option to consider. A staged completion thyroidectomy may be safely accomplished as soon as nerve recovery is demonstrated. This decision of whether to stage the operation must consider the value of the reduction of the risk of bilateral injury weighed against (and balanced with) the risk of undergoing a second operation, with attendant anesthesia risks and inconvenience for the patient.

An alternative to staging the operation is to cautiously proceed to the contralateral lobe and accomplish a conservative resection. If the nerve can be visualized proximal to the ligament of Berry and also distally, just proximal to the inferior constrictor muscle, then a small (0.5 gram or so) remnant of thyroid tissue can be spared by dividing the tissue ventral to the ligament. This maneuver will reduce the likelihood of temporary dysfunction which can sometimes occur with meticulous dissection of the entire length of the RLN.

Because of the potential need to stage the operation, planning the operative approach when undertaking bilateral surgery takes on added importance. In a case that will involve bilateral exploration of the neck, the more clinically important side should be operated on first. For example, when a total thyroidectomy is done for cancer, it is best to start by removing the lobe with the malignancy. For benign disease, starting with the larger or more symptomatic side is recommended. For symmetrical Graves' disease, starting on the right side is preferable; if the nerve is injured and the contralateral lobe requires surgery, it is safer to do this on the left side where the RLN is more predictable in its course.

In the event that the RLN has been transected, the options for management differ. Intraoperative primary repair of the transected nerve should generally be pursued. While normal function will not be achieved, restoration of innervation will reduce atrophy of the vocalis muscle and therefore improve long-term postoperative muscle tone [6]. The repair is performed with one or two well-placed interrupted 7–0 Prolene sutures under magnification with care taken to avoid tension.

For some conditions, such as benign disease and small malignancies, a decision may be made to forgo further surgery because the risk for bilateral nerve injury may be more serious than any benefit that accrues from accomplishing a total thyroidectomy [7, 8]. In contrast, if radioactive iodine is judged to be unequivocally necessary, then it may be preferable (even in the event of a transected nerve) to proceed to the contralateral side to accomplish a total or near-total thyroid resection to avoid a second operation with attendant granulation tissue or scar tissue.

Confirmed Laryngeal Dysfunction: Management Strategies

When a nerve has been transected, even with a successful repair, early intervention may be appropriate. Injection medialization of a TVF provides bulk and helps move the paralyzed fold toward the midline so that approximation with the functioning contralateral fold can be achieved [9]. The vocal fold injection can be done as an awake office procedure in which a 23- or 25-gauge needle is used to inject one of a number of substances (may include a hyaluronic acid compound, calcium hydroxylapatite, or autologous fat), or it can be done under a brief general anesthetic. This approach is also appropriate in the uncommon event that a nerve fails to recover even when it was seen to be anatomically intact at the completion of a procedure. Timing varies, but if recovery has not been observed after 6–12 months, definitive intervention may be considered.

When a nerve has been resected as part of an oncologic resection, or is otherwise not amenable to a repair, transfer of the ansa cervicalis (also called ansa hypoglossi) to the distal stump of the RLN is an excellent option. This may be done at the time of the thyroidectomy or at a later date. The ansa cervicalis can be quickly and easily identified with blunt dissection in the plane between the sternohyoid and sternothyroid muscles. The ansa is transected low and mobilized medially; a neurorrhaphy with the distal RLN remnant is accomplished with two interrupted 7–0 Prolene sutures under magnification [10]. Sacrifice of the ansa cervicalis goes unnoticed in most patients, as it provides motor innervation to strap muscles and the omohyoid.

Parathyroid surgery bears special mention here. Because of the gentle nature of the dissection required to expose the parathyroid glands (which is almost entirely blunt), it may be reasonable to explore the contralateral thyroid bed even in the presence of an ipsilateral nerve dysfunction, especially when on abnormal gland is anticipated in the inferior location, which is ventral to the RLN.

Confirmed Laryngeal Dysfunction: Impact on Discharge

While many surgeons routinely admit patients following a straightforward thyroidectomy or parathyroidectomy, there are now a number of studies confirming the safety of outpatient thyroidectomy [11–13]. Even in the patient that suffers a confirmed temporary or permanent unilateral TVF paralysis, outpatient management can be pursued as long as the patient meets usual criteria [11]. Counseling includes avoidance of thin liquids because of the risk for aspiration. A consultation for assessment of swallowing can be sought but is rarely necessary. Steroid administration may decrease symptoms.

In the event of bilateral LOS, inpatient admission is often needed as these patients may manifest respiratory compromise depending on the position of their TVFs. These patients warrant careful follow-up as they may require re-intubation or even tracheostomy. Empiric steroids are suggested to decrease edema of the TVFs postoperatively.

Superior Laryngeal Nerve Injury

Consideration of the physiologic ramifications of nerve injury appropriately focuses predominantly on the RLN. However, it is well recognized that damage to the external branch of the superior laryngeal nerve (EBSLN) can also have a profound impact on the quality of life of selected individuals; this impact is especially pronounced when combined RLN and EBSLN injuries occur.

The EBSLN innervates the cricothyroid muscle [14]. This muscle controls tension of the ipsilateral TVF and is particularly important when both TVFs are approximated. Isolated EBSLN injury will go unnoticed by most patients; however, singers and professional voice users will be aware of the loss of vocal register (especially in the higher ranges) as well as early vocal fatigue [14].

When injury to the EBSLN is combined with an ipsilateral RLN injury, patients have significantly more symptoms than with RLN dysfunction alone. These include cough, aspiration of liquids, and dysphonia [15]. These consequences underscore the importance of preservation of the SLN.

Conclusions

Thyroid and parathyroid surgery pose a risk of injury to the RLN or the EBSLN. When LOS occurs, it is important to distinguish between true LOS and equipment malfunction. In the event of true LOS in planned bilateral surgery, management options include staging the operation to reduce the potential for bilateral RLN injury or proceeding cautiously to the contralateral lobe and accomplishing a conservative resection.

When unilateral laryngeal dysfunction is confirmed, there are a number of management options, and importantly these patients can be safely discharged as routine same-day surgery cases. Bilateral LOS is associated with the potential for airway compromise, sometimes justifies the need for admission for observation, and may require an artificial airway.

References

1. Schneider R, Randolph GW, Dionigi G, et al. International neural monitoring study group guideline 2018 part I: staging bilateral thyroid surgery with monitoring loss of signal. Laryngoscope. 2018;128 Suppl 3:S1–S17.
2. Wu CW, Dionigi G, Barczynski M, et al. International neuromonitoring study group guidelines 2018: part II: optimal recurrent laryngeal nerve management for invasive thyroid cancer-incorporation of surgical, laryngeal, and neural electrophysiologic data. Laryngoscope. 2018;128 Suppl 3:S18–27.
3. Randolph GW, Kobler JB, Wilkins J. Recurrent laryngeal nerve identification and assessment during thyroid surgery: laryngeal palpation. World J Surg. 2004;28(8):755–60. https://doi.org/10.1007/s00268-004-7348-x. PMID: 15457354.
4. Schneider R, Randolph G, Dionigi G, et al. Prediction of postoperative vocal fold function after intraoperative recovery of loss of signal. Laryngoscope. 2019;129(2):525–31.
5. Sitges-Serra A, Gallego-Otaegui L, Fontané J, Trillo L, Lorente-Poch L, Sancho J. Contralateral surgery in patients scheduled for total thyroidectomy with initial loss or absence of signal during neural monitoring. Br J Surg. 2019;106(4):404–11.
6. Chou FF, Su CY, Jeng SF, Hsu KL, Lu KY. Neurorrhaphy of the recurrent laryngeal nerve. J Am Coll Surg. 2003;197(1):52–7.
7. Haugen BR, Alexander EK, Bible KC, et al. American Thyroid Association Management Guidelines for Adult Patients with Thyroid Nodules and Differentiated Thyroid Cancer: The American Thyroid Association Guidelines Task Force on Thyroid Nodules and Differentiated Thyroid Cancer. Thyroid. 2015;26(1):32–5.
8. Holoubek SA, Yan H, Khokar AH, et al. Aggressive variants of papillary thyroid microcarcinoma are associated with high-risk features, but not decreased survival. Surgery. 2020;167(1):19–27.
9. Yung KC, Likhterov I, Courey MS. Effect of temporary vocal fold injection medialization on the rate of permanent medialization laryngoplasty in unilateral vocal fold paralysis patients. Laryngoscope. 2011;121(10):2191–4.
10. Yuan Q, Hou J, Liao Y, Zheng L, Wang K, Wu G. Selective vagus-recurrent laryngeal nerve anastomosis in thyroidectomy with cancer invasion or iatrogenic transection. Langenbeck's Arch Surg. 2020;405(4):461–8.
11. Segel JM, Duke WS, White JR, Waller JL, Terris DJ. Outpatient thyroid surgery: safety of an optimized protocol in more than 1,000 patients. Surgery. 2016;159(2):518–23.
12. Snyder SK, Hamid KS, Roberson CR, et al. Outpatient thyroidectomy is safe and reasonable: experience with more than 1,000 planned outpatient procedures. J Am Coll Surg. 2010;210(5):575–82, 582–4.
13. Terris DJ, Snyder S, Carneiro-Pla D, et al. American Thyroid Association Surgical Affairs Committee Writing Task Force. American Thyroid Association statement on outpatient thyroidectomy. Thyroid. 2013;23(10):1193–202.
14. Reeve T, Thompson NW. Complications of thyroid surgery: how to avoid them, how to manage them, and observations on their possible effect on the whole patient. World J Surg. 2000;24(8):971–5.
15. Kennedy TL. Surgical complications of thyroidectomy. Oper Tech Otolaryngol Head Neck Surg. 2003;14:74–9.

13 Recurrent Laryngeal Nerve Monitoring and Decision-Making in Advanced Thyroid Cancer

Garren M. I. Low, Richard J. Wong, and Mark Zafereo

Advanced Thyroid Cancer

Locoregionally advanced or invasive thyroid cancer generally constitutes disease that has extended beyond the thyroid gland [i.e., extrathyroidal extension (ETE)] or cervical lymph nodes (extranodal extension). The extension of malignancy beyond the confines of the thyroid gland or recurrence of thyroid disease in a previously operated surgical bed complicates tumor extirpation. This heightens the stakes with regard to two important ever-present surgical goals: to completely remove disease and to preserve patient quality of life by minimizing injury to surrounding structures. The recurrent laryngeal nerve and resultant vocal fold function are relatively more often threatened in patients with advanced or recurrent thyroid cancer [1–6]. Due to the overall prevalence of disease, biologically aggressive DTC makes up the majority of overall thyroid cancer cases which threaten the nerve. Other thyroid cancer types such as medullary thyroid cancer, poorly differentiated thyroid cancer, and anaplastic thyroid cancer more commonly present with extrathyroidal or extranodal extension and nerve invasion but make up a minority of advanced thyroid cancer cases.

Preoperative Recurrent Laryngeal Nerve Evaluation

While preoperative vocal fold evaluation is recommended in all thyroid cancer cases, it should especially be emphasized in patients with locoregionally advanced and/or recurrent thyroid cancer. There are several governing bodies that provide guidance in the management of these cancers, including the American Thyroid Association (ATA) [7], the American Head and Neck Society (AHNS) [8–10], and the International Neural Monitoring Study Group (INMSG) [11–13]. Each of these guidelines individually recommend a standard preoperative evaluation of patients with invasive thyroid cancer.

History of voice changes, dysphagia, stridor, or shortness of breath can all be indicative of true vocal fold (TVF) dysfunction. Even in

G. M. I. Low
Department of Otorhinolaryngology-Head and Neck Surgery, University of Texas Health Sciences Center at Houston, Houston, TX, USA

R. J. Wong
Department of Surgery, Memorial Sloan-Kettering Cancer Center, New York, NY, USA
e-mail: wongr@mskcc.org

M. Zafereo (✉)
Department of Head and Neck Surgery, University of Texas MD Anderson Cancer Center, Houston, TX, USA
e-mail: MZafereo@mdanderson.org

© The Author(s), under exclusive license to Springer Nature Switzerland AG 2022
J. Scharpf, G. W. Randolph (eds.), *Intraoperative Cranial Nerve Monitoring in Otolaryngology-Head and Neck Surgery*, https://doi.org/10.1007/978-3-030-84916-0_13

the presence of documented vocal fold mobility, a history of vocal weakness and particularly vocal fatigue after voice use should at least raise the possibility that a recurrent laryngeal nerve may be affected by tumor. A well-performed mirror laryngoscopy can be sufficient to visualize function of the vocal folds in some patients; however, a mirror examination may not provide sufficient evaluation of vocal cord mobility, largely due to oropharyngeal anatomy and gag reflex. Many studies have demonstrated that vocal fold evaluation transnasal flexible laryngoscopy is well tolerated by patients, has a fast learning curve for the surgeon, and provides superior visualization of the TVFs [10, 14]. In locoregionally advanced and recurrent thyroid cancer cases, the surgeon should particularly heed and document any minor asymmetry in vocal fold movement noted on flexible laryngoscopy. While slight asymmetry of vocal cord movement may be physiologic (i.e., the patient's normal baseline), this asymmetry can be indicative of relatively early tumor invasion of the nerve causing a relative weakness.

For locoregionally advanced and recurrent thyroid cancer, radiographic evaluation of the thyroid and neck with both high-definition ultrasound and cross-sectional imaging with CT neck or MRI with contrast is highly recommended. While the recurrent laryngeal nerve cannot be visualized on cross-sectional imaging, CT or MRI is particularly helpful in (1) determining extent of extrathyroidal and/or extranodal disease invading the tracheoesophageal groove(s); (2) evaluating superior mediastinal disease near the subclavian artery (right) or aortic arch (left) which may affect the respective recurrent nerves; (3) assessing extranodal lateral neck or retropharyngeal disease which could potentially affect the vagus nerve(s); and (4) evaluating tracheal, esophageal, or laryngeal invasion with implications for the dissection and management of the recurrent nerves [10, 15]. This information helps provide a clear picture of disease burden and extent of invasion, which can then be used for both surgical planning and preoperative patient discussion.

Preoperative Planning

Standard informed consent must be tailored to the specifics of the patient's disease and circumstances. In particular, the effect of any degree of preoperative unilateral TVF dysfunction, or disease burden that threatens the nerve which in turn increases postoperative risk of unilateral or bilateral TVF function, must be discussed with the patient. The possibility of tracheostomy in the setting of postoperative bilateral TVF dysfunction, the possibility of staging second side surgery based on intraoperative loss of signal, and the relative risks given preoperative specifics of the patient's disease should be addressed [16].

In all cases of invasive thyroid cancer, nerve monitoring is recommended, whether continuous or intermittent. Preoperative planning is largely informed by preoperative function of the TVFs. If one TVF is completely immobile preoperatively, the obvious implication is that protection of the contralateral nerve during surgery will be paramount. In this situation, a nuanced conversation must take place with the multidisciplinary team caring for the patient. Neoadjuvant targeted therapies can be utilized in situations where a patient presents initially with a single functioning nerve. This can cytoreduce the tumor, enhance chance for nerve preservation, and buy time so that the patient can enjoy current quality of life with one or both functioning nerves [17, 18]. Additionally, the relative availability of postoperative adjuvant therapies such as targeted therapy, radioactive iodine, and external beam radiation therapy can inform the aggressiveness of the surgeon's intraoperative approach with a tumor intimately involved with a recurrent laryngeal nerve.

Intraoperative Recurrent Laryngeal Nerve Monitoring

Either intermittent or continuous monitoring can be utilized for intraoperative recurrent laryngeal nerve monitoring [19]. Intermittent nerve monitoring can be used with a Neural Integrity Monitor (NIM) electromyogram (EMG) endotracheal tube and a nerve stimulator run through the NIM monitor. This type of nerve monitoring can assist in identifying the recurrent laryngeal nerve and its branches. It is important to remember that intermittent nerve stimulation can only provide data that the nerve is intact distal to the point of stimulus [20].

Continuous monitoring, such as a system connected and providing a low baseline stimulation to the ipsilateral vagus nerve, offers additional benefits [21]. Of most importance, continuous monitoring provides the ability to identify real-time loss of signal associated with intraoperative nerve injury [11, 22]. As it is generally recognized that the vast majority of nerve injuries (especially temporary) are associated with stretch injury rather than actual nerve severance, and as cases of recurrent and advanced thyroid cancer are more likely to be associated with stretch injury, continuous nerve monitoring should at least be considered in such cases. Additionally, continuous nerve monitoring provides information on integrity of the length of the vagus nerve leading into the recurrent laryngeal nerve, as opposed to evaluation of the nerve only distal to the point of stimulus. This low level of continuous monitoring has been shown to have little risk of iatrogenic vagal neuropraxia and has been recommended by the International Neuromonitoring Study Group for select cases [13].

As continuous nerve monitoring involves placing an electrode on the vagus nerve, there are additional considerations including risk of direct harm to the vagus nerve associated with placing the electrode, although this risk has been demonstrated to be extremely low. It is also important to note that while continuous nerve monitoring provides real-time feedback with regard to signals of neural injury, there are cases when injury happens too quickly to be caught even by continuous monitoring [23]. It is also important to note that continuous nerve monitoring has not been proven to reduce nerve injury as compared to intermittent, so the choice of nerve monitoring remains largely a matter of surgeon practice patterns and preference [24].

Segmental tracheal resection represents a unique situation wherein, if intermittent nerve monitoring is employed, the nerve typically cannot effectively be monitored during the tracheal anastomosis aspect of the surgery, as it is during this time that the endotracheal tube is pulled back (such that the electrodes will no longer be touching the vocal cords) and the patient is intubated directly into the distal trachea. However, after the anastomosis is complete and the NIMs endotracheal tube is re-advanced into the trachea, intermittent nerve monitoring via the NIMs tube typically remains effective. In all cases, whether intermittent or continuous nerve monitoring is employed, it is important that the surgeon remember that digital palpation of the posterior cricoarytenoid muscle is an effective measure of intermittent nerve function in the event of equipment failure or doubt about the accuracy of the nerve monitor.

Intraoperative Decision-Making with Nerve Monitoring

At the onset of surgery, the integrity of the endotracheal tube positioning and nerve monitor circuit should be carefully assessed. The proper tube depth of insertion, tube torque, and grounding should be initially confirmed. During surgery, initially establishing that the circuit is intact through obtaining a true positive stimulation of the recurrent laryngeal nerve or vagus nerve confirms that the system is reliable. The desired probe stimulation levels (0.5–3 mA) as well as the threshold amplitudes (100–200 uV) are set for desired sensitivity depending on the proximity of the nerve. For conditions where the integrity of the system remains in question, stimulating the nerve while palpating the posterior cricoarytenoid muscle will yield a palpable twitch. Stimulation of the superior laryngeal nerve, which may course within or lateral to the cricothyroid muscle, will result in a visible cricothyroid twitch and allow the superior pole vessels to be ligated and divided safely.

Loss of signal (LOS), as identified either by dropped signal during continuous nerve monitoring or failure of stimulus at a nerve location that previously tested as intact, is an ominous sign for nerve management [12, 13, 25, 26]. Though many nerves can regain complete function after LOS, the intraoperative surgical plan must be reconsidered once the surgeon is provided with evidence of at least neuropraxia [27, 28]. Despite known neuropraxia, it is important to continue to protect the palsied nerve. Even if there is incomplete recovery of the nerve, there is significant physiologic benefit from remaining tone [29–32].

The nuances of each patient's clinical circumstances and tumor heavily influence intraoperative decision-making. If intraoperative LOS occurs on the first side in a bilateral case, this plays heavily into any decisions regarding the second side [32]. Possible alterations in surgical plan after LOS can include proceeding to the second side as planned based on clinical urgency or staging the second side of the surgery after anticipated nerve recovery. The extent of dissection of the nerve on the contralateral side may also be impacted by LOS on the initial side. Every attempt should be made to minimize or obviate the risk of bilateral vocal cord paralysis, particularly in a situation where the contralateral side can be safely staged and resected at a later date after nerve recovery of the initial side. These decisions are informed by a myriad of factors. In patients who are young, are likely to be good candidates for effective adjuvant therapy such as RAI, and have PTC, elderly patients with preoperatively increased risk for aspiration, and who have preoperative pulmonary disease, have distant metastases, or are voice professionals, a nerve-sparing approach may be more heavily favored, even at the expense of not achieving an R0 resection. In patients with aggressive histopathologic subtypes and iodine refractory disease, who are intraoperatively found to have nerve invasion at the entry to the larynx, and/or who have normal contralateral nerve function, a more aggressive approach toward nerve sacrifice may be more appropriate [13].

In approaching a recurrent nerve that is encased by tumor, microdissection of the nerve should proceed with nerve monitoring from both proximal and distal to the tumor encasement. This 360-degree approach to microdissecting nerve encasement is favored when possible (Fig. 13.1). The use of loupe or microscope magnification, microsurgical scissors, fine mosquito dissectors (e.g., McCabe, Jacobson), fine bipolar cautery, and soft cotton pledgets (may be soaked in epinephrine) can facilitate meticulous sharp dissection and gentle blunt dissection in order to maintain nerve stimulation during the microdissection. Overly aggressive blunt dissection on the nerve or use of monopolar cautery increases the risk of neuropraxia. In many cases, the encasement of the nerve is at the cricothyroid joint, such that it may be challenging to identify a non-encased distal nerve segment beyond the area of encasement. Even in cases where the nerve must be ultimately sacrificed, identification of a distal nerve stump at the joint allows either primary nerve re-anastomosis or an ansa to recurrent nerve neurorrhaphy, which has been associated with maintenance of vocal cord tone and improved long-term vocal quality (compared to no nerve reconstruction) (Fig. 13.2). If the nerve is found to be grossly involved with tumor, the extent of nerve involvement as well as the preoperative and intraoperative functioning of the nerve must be considered. If only a superficial aspect of the nerve is involved with disease, sometimes, the epineurium can be resected with tumor, leaving the perineurium and endoneurium intact (Fig. 13.3). However, the surgeon must realize the likelihood of loss of nerve signal with this approach, resulting in either temporary or permanent nerve paresis. On the other hand, if the entire nerve is thickened and discolored, no amount of microdissection will meaningfully change the ability to both grossly completely resect disease and preserve the nerve, and the surgeon must in this case make a choice between nerve sacrifice and nerve preservation (Fig. 13.4). In such a case, a number of factors come into play including preoperative and intraoperative nerve function, biology of the disease and prognosis, and preoperative patient discussion and preference.

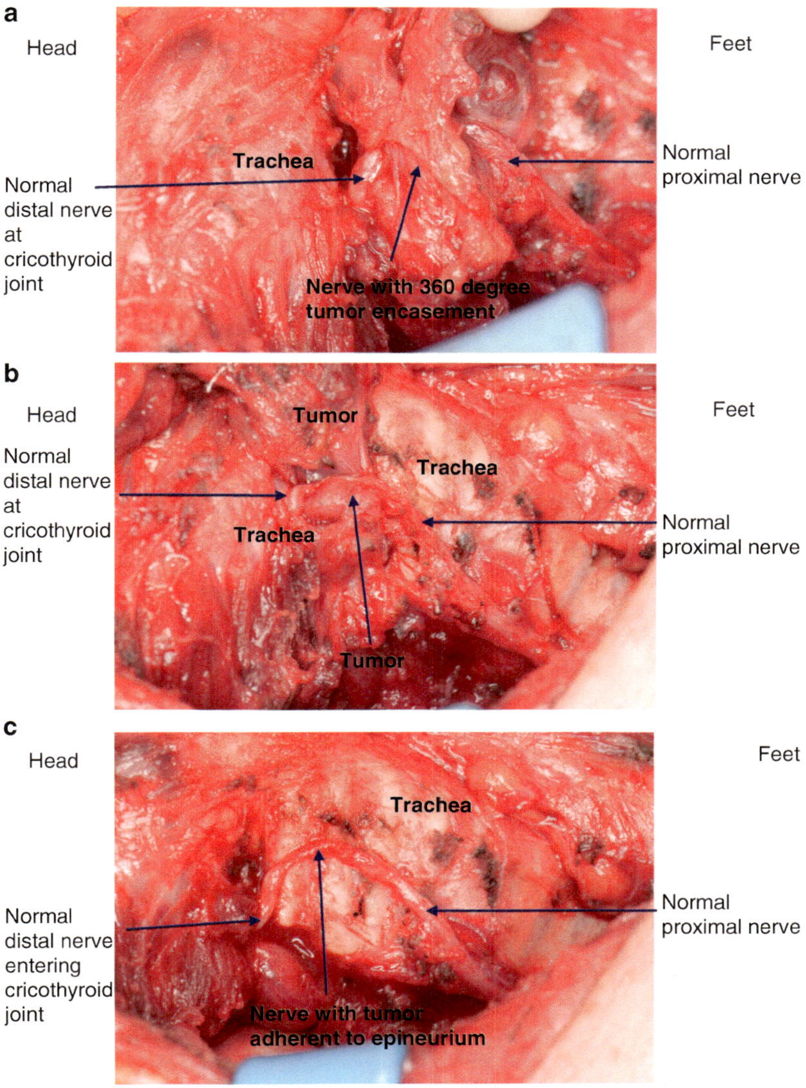

Fig. 13.1 When a recurrent laryngeal nerve is 360 degree encased in disease, every attempt should be made to microdissect the nerve free from tumor. This is best accomplished by identifying normal nerve proximal and distal to the tumor when possible (**a**) and then microdissecting between the normal nerve segments to attempt to free the nerve from the tumor (**b**). Upon completion of dissection, the nerve may be found to have tumor intimately adherent to the epineurium; in which case, an intraoperative decision must be made between leaving minimal residual disease adherent to the nerve and further microdissection of the nerve, versus nerve sacrifice (**c**). In this particular case, the nerve was preoperatively functional and maintained strong intraoperative neural signal, and the disease was not felt to be clinically rapidly progressive, culminating in a decision to accept minimal residual disease adherent to the nerve in order to maintain nerve function

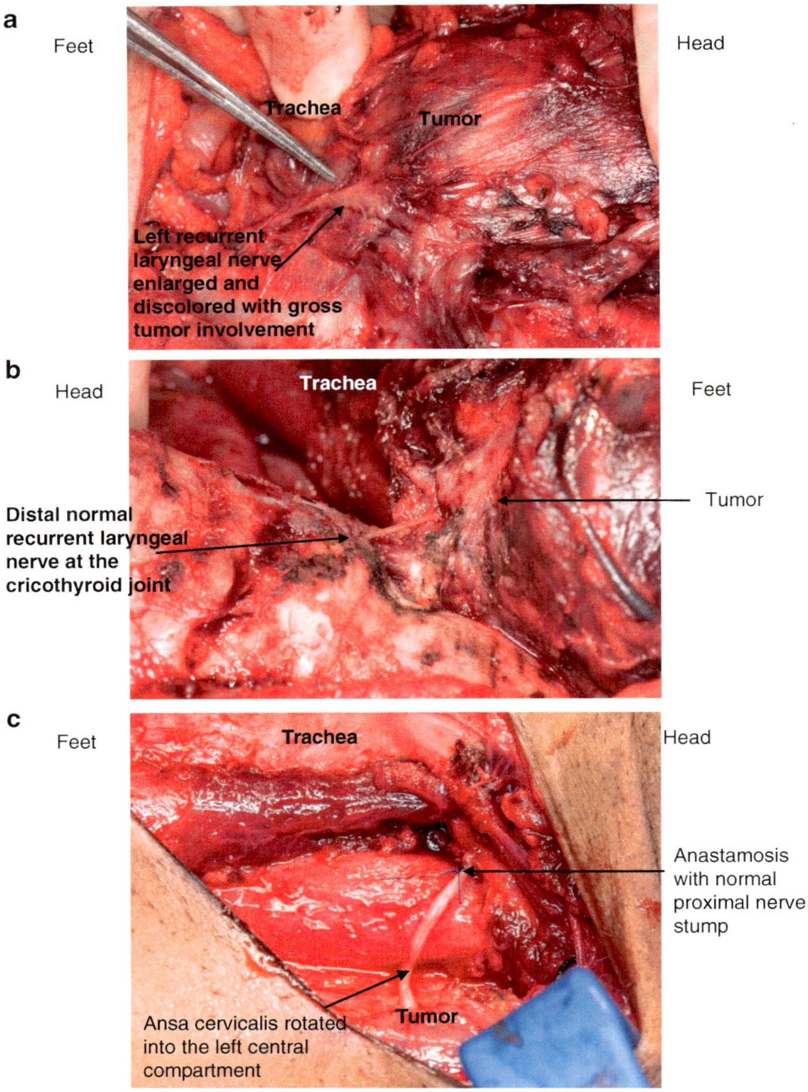

Fig. 13.2 Left recurrent laryngeal nerve encasement and gross involvement (thickened, discolored) in a patient with anaplastic thyroid cancer (**a**). While this nerve required sacrifice for tumor extirpation, the identification of the uninvolved distal nerve stump at the cricothyroid joint (**b**) enabled a left ansa cervicalis to left recurrent laryngeal nerve graft (**c**)

Conclusion

Locoregionally advanced thyroid cancer relatively more commonly affects the recurrent laryngeal nerve(s) and requires substantially heightened preoperative evaluation and multidisciplinary discussion, as well as focused intraoperative nerve monitoring with dynamic decision-making by the surgeon. Thorough preoperative evaluation, including cross-sectional imaging to evaluate any extrathyroidal extension, and dynamic evaluation of the true vocal folds, is mandatory for surgical planning. Preoperative multidisciplinary discussion regarding possible neoadjuvant and adjuvant treatments can allow the surgeon to tailor surgery within the scope of the patient's global care plan. Nerve monitoring, whether intermittent or continuous, is a necessary adjunct for intraoperative decision-making during surgical resection of invasive thyroid cancer.

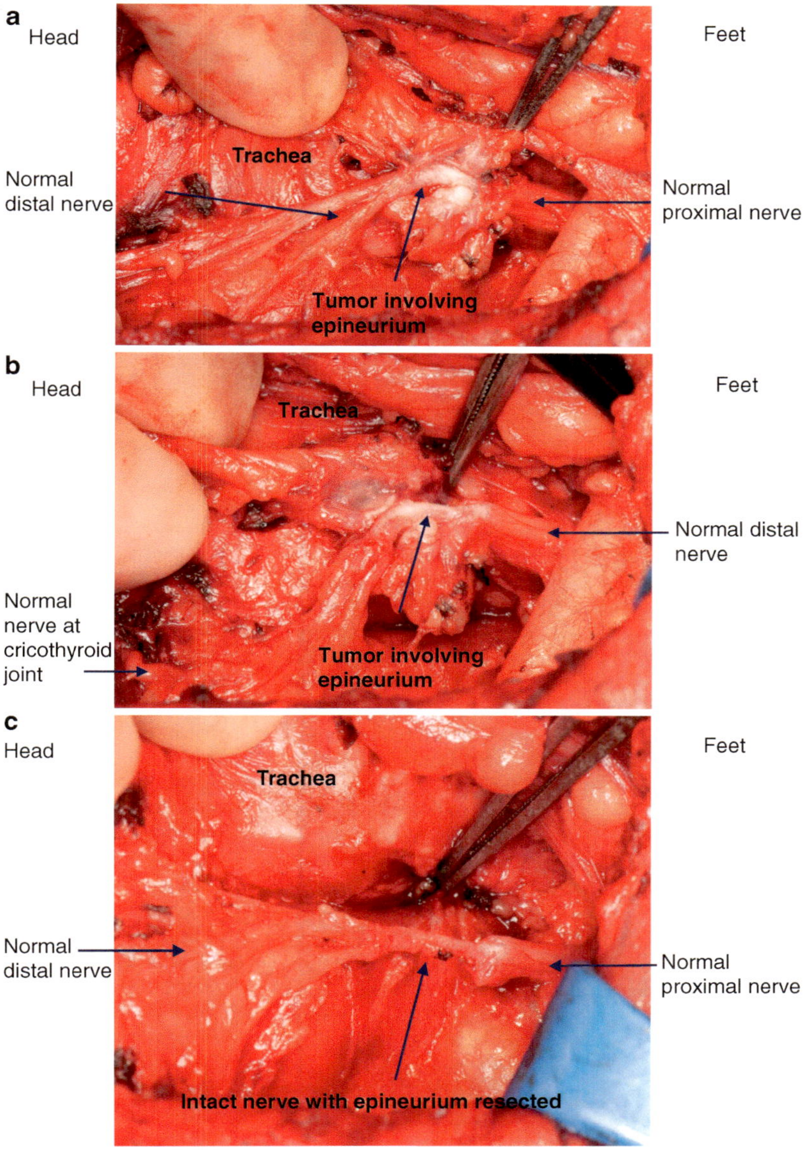

Fig. 13.3 Medullary thyroid cancer involving the epineurium of the right recurrent laryngeal nerve (**a**, **b**). With meticulous microdissection, the epineurium was resected, preserving the perineurium and endoneurium (**c**). Although this nerve maintained nerve signal, many nerves with this degree of dissection will at least temporarily lose nerve signal

Intraoperative loss of signal requires intraoperative reassessment of goals and priorities, with occasional need to abort surgery (with possibility of later staged surgery) on the contralateral side. Availability and perceived effectiveness of adjuvant therapies, as well as patient and tumor factors, must be taken into account when making an intraoperative decision to sacrifice the recurrent laryngeal nerve, or to preserve the nerve with R1/R2 disease resection.

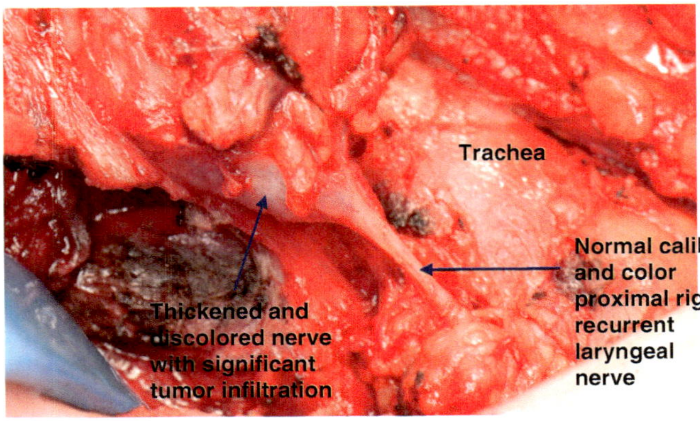

Fig. 13.4 The right recurrent laryngeal nerve is significantly enlarged and discolored (purple) in an area of infiltration with extrathyroidal medullary thyroid cancer

References

1. Falk SA, McCaffrey TV. Management of the recurrent laryngeal nerve in suspected and proven thyroid cancer. Otolaryngol Head Neck Surg. 1995;113(1):42–8.
2. Ortiz S, Rodríguez JM, Soria T, et al. Extrathyroid spread in papillary carcinoma of the thyroid: clinicopathological and prognostic study. Otolaryngol Head Neck Surg. 2001;124(3):261–5.
3. Russell MD, Kamani D, Randolph GW. Modern surgery for advanced thyroid cancer: a tailored approach. Gland Surg. 2020;9(Suppl 2):S105–19.
4. van Beek DJ, Almquist M, Bergenfelz AO, Musholt TJ, Nordenström E. Complications after medullary thyroid carcinoma surgery: multicentre study of the SQRTPA and EUROCRINE® databases. Br J Surg. 2020;
5. Hundahl SA, Cady B, Cunningham MP, et al. Initial results from a prospective cohort study of 5583 cases of thyroid carcinoma treated in the United States during 1996. U.S. and German Thyroid Cancer Study Group. An American College of Surgeons Commission on Cancer Patient Care Evaluation study. Cancer. 2000;89(1):202–17.
6. Nayyar SS, Thiagarajan S, Malik A, Chakraborthy A, Velayutham P, Chaukar D. Risk factors predisposing for recurrent laryngeal nerve palsy following thyroid malignancy surgery: experience from a tertiary oncology centre. Eur Arch Otorhinolaryngol. 2020;277(4):1199–204.
7. Haugen BR, Alexander EK, Bible KC, et al. 2015 American Thyroid Association Management Guidelines for Adult Patients with Thyroid Nodules and Differentiated Thyroid Cancer: The American Thyroid Association Guidelines Task Force on Thyroid Nodules and Differentiated Thyroid Cancer. Thyroid. 2016;26(1):1–133.
8. Scharpf J, Tuttle M, Wong R, et al. Comprehensive management of recurrent thyroid cancer: an American Head and Neck Society consensus statement: AHNS consensus statement. Head Neck. 2016;38(12):1862–9.
9. Shindo ML, Caruana SM, Kandil E, et al. Management of invasive well-differentiated thyroid cancer: an American head and neck society consensus statement. Head Neck. 2014;36(10):1379–90.
10. Sinclair CF, Bumpous JM, Haugen BR, et al. Laryngeal examination in thyroid and parathyroid surgery: an American Head and Neck Society consensus statement: AHNS Consensus Statement. Head Neck. 2016;38(6):811–9.
11. Randolph GW, Dralle H, International Intraoperative Monitoring Study G, et al. Electrophysiologic recurrent laryngeal nerve monitoring during thyroid and parathyroid surgery: international standards guideline statement. Laryngoscope. 2011;(121 Suppl 1):S1–16.
12. Schneider R, Randolph GW, Dionigi G, et al. International neural monitoring study group guideline 2018 part I: staging bilateral thyroid surgery with monitoring loss of signal. Laryngoscope. 2018;128 Suppl 3:S1–S17.
13. Wu CW, Dionigi G, Barczynski M, et al. International neuromonitoring study group guidelines 2018: part II: optimal recurrent laryngeal nerve management for invasive thyroid cancer-incorporation of surgical, laryngeal, and neural electrophysiologic data. Laryngoscope. 2018;128 Suppl 3:S18–27.
14. Randolph GW, Kamani D. The importance of preoperative laryngoscopy in patients undergoing thyroidectomy: voice, vocal cord function, and the preoperative detection of invasive thyroid malignancy. Surgery. 2006;139(3):357–62.
15. Salari B, Hammon RJ, Kamani D, Randolph GW. Staged surgery for advanced thyroid cancers: safety and oncologic outcomes of neural monitored surgery. Otolaryngol Head Neck Surg. 2017;156(5):816–21.
16. Chan WF, Lo CY, Lam KY, Wan KY. Recurrent laryngeal nerve palsy in well-differentiated thyroid carcinoma: clinicopathologic features and outcome study. World J Surg. 2004;28(11):1093–8.

17. Maniakas A, Dadu R, Busaidy NL, et al. Evaluation of overall survival in patients with anaplastic thyroid carcinoma, 2000–2019. JAMA Oncol. 2020;
18. Jozaghi Y, Zafereo M, Williams MD, et al. Neoadjuvant selpercatinib for advanced medullary thyroid cancer. Head Neck. 2021;43(1):E7–E12.
19. Ritter A, Ganly I, Wong RJ, et al. Intraoperative nerve monitoring is used routinely by a significant majority of head and neck surgeons in thyroid surgery and impacts on extent of surgery-Survey of the American Head and Neck Society. Head Neck. 2020;42(8):1757–64.
20. Cavicchi O, Burgio L, Cioccoloni E, et al. Intraoperative intermittent neuromonitoring of inferior laryngeal nerve and staged thyroidectomy: our experience. Endocrine. 2018;62(3):560–5.
21. Sinclair CF, Tellez MJ, Ulkatan S. Continuous laryngeal adductor reflex versus intermittent nerve monitoring in neck endocrine surgery. Laryngoscope. 2020;
22. Phelan E, Schneider R, Lorenz K, et al. Continuous vagal IONM prevents recurrent laryngeal nerve paralysis by revealing initial EMG changes of impending neuropraxic injury: a prospective, multicenter study. Laryngoscope. 2014;124(6):1498–505.
23. Brauckhoff K, Vik R, Sandvik L, et al. Impact of EMG changes in continuous vagal nerve monitoring in high-risk endocrine neck surgery. World J Surg. 2016;40(3):672–80.
24. Robertson ML, Steward DL, Gluckman JL, Welge J. Continuous laryngeal nerve integrity monitoring during thyroidectomy: does it reduce risk of injury? Otolaryngol Head Neck Surg. 2004;131(5):596–600.
25. Eid I, Miller FR, Rowan S, Otto RA. The role of nerve monitoring to predict postoperative recurrent laryngeal nerve function in thyroid and parathyroid surgery. Laryngoscope. 2013;123(10):2583–6.
26. Schneider R, Machens A, Lorenz K, Dralle H. Intraoperative nerve monitoring in thyroid surgery-shifting current paradigms. Gland Surg. 2020;9(Suppl 2):S120–8.
27. Calo PG, Medas F, Erdas E, et al. Role of intraoperative neuromonitoring of recurrent laryngeal nerves in the outcomes of surgery for thyroid cancer. Int J Surg. 2014;12 Suppl 1:S213–7.
28. Schneider R, Sekulla C, Machens A, Lorenz K, Thanh PN, Dralle H. Dynamics of loss and recovery of the nerve monitoring signal during thyroidectomy predict early postoperative vocal fold function. Head Neck. 2016;38 Suppl 1:E1144–51.
29. Chi SY, Lammers B, Boehner H, Pohl P, Goretzki PE. Is it meaningful to preserve a palsied recurrent laryngeal nerve? Thyroid. 2008;18(3):363–6.
30. Kamani D, Darr EA, Randolph GW. Electrophysiologic monitoring characteristics of the recurrent laryngeal nerve preoperatively paralyzed or invaded with malignancy. Otolaryngol Head Neck Surg. 2013;149(5):682–8.
31. Nishida T, Nakao K, Hamaji M, Kamiike W, Kurozumi K, Matsuda H. Preservation of recurrent laryngeal nerve invaded by differentiated thyroid cancer. Ann Surg. 1997;226(1):85–91.
32. Lang BH, Lo CY, Wong KP, Wan KY. Should an involved but functioning recurrent laryngeal nerve be shaved or resected in a locally advanced papillary thyroid carcinoma? Ann Surg Oncol. 2013;20(9):2951–7.

Nerve Monitoring in Remote Access Thyroid Surgery

14

Nicholas R. Scott-Wittenborn, Areej Shihabi, Jonathon O. Russell, Emad Kandil, and Ralph Tufano

Introduction

Over the past 30 years, there has been a movement by the surgical community to adopt minimally invasive surgical approaches. Remote access thyroid surgery is emblematic of this shift [1]. A number of different approaches have been developed, including trans-oral endoscopic thyroidectomy vestibular approach (TOETVA), trans-oral neck surgery, retro-auricular (both robotic and non-robotic), and a number of approaches through the breast and axilla (both robotic and non-robotic). All of these approaches seek to cause less disruption of tissue, reduce visible scars, and improve the visibility of the delicate structures associated with thyroid surgery.

Surgery of the thyroid gland is a challenging and delicate endeavor. The complexity of the surgery is due to the intimate relationship between the thyroid and the recurrent laryngeal nerve (RLN). The nerve can be injured in a myriad of ways: thermal injury, devascularization, and complete severance are some of the more common etiologies. The rate of injury is low, especially in high-volume centers, where it is commonly published to be less than 2% [2, 3]. However, rates of RLN injury from low-volume centers are generally higher and can approach 10%. When an injury to the RLN does occur, the sequelae can have a significant effect on the patient and include dysphagia, changes in voice, aspiration, and need for tracheostomy [4]. Such injuries are associated with a significant number of malpractice lawsuits [5–7].

Intraoperative neuromonitoring (IONM) of the recurrent laryngeal nerve (RLN) has been increasingly utilized for surgery since the creation of the electrode endotracheal tube by *Goldstone* et al. in 1991 [8]. Traditionally, visual identification of the RLN was the gold standard to prevent injury; however, IONM is now a common adjunct which surgeons use to help assess the RLN's functioning throughout the surgery and predict postoperative vocal fold function. Currently, over half of thyroid surgeons use IONM, especially younger fellowship-trained surgeons [9]. While all thyroid surgeries must emphasize protection of the RLN, the use of a trans-axillary approach to thyroid surgery poses a risk to a different neural structure: the brachial plexus. Monitoring of this crucial structure is fundamentally different from IONM of RLN but is an important part of this new surgical approach,

N. R. Scott-Wittenborn · J. O. Russell (✉) · R. Tufano
Department of Otolaryngology, Head and Neck Surgery, Johns Hopkins University, Baltimore, MD, USA
e-mail: Switten2@jhmi.edu; Jrusse41@jhmi.edu; Rtufano@jhmi.edu

A. Shihabi · E. Kandil
Department of Surgery, Tulane University School of Medicine, New Orleans, LA, USA
e-mail: ashihabi@tulane.edu; ekandil@tulane.edu

© The Author(s), under exclusive license to Springer Nature Switzerland AG 2022

J. Scharpf, G. W. Randolph (eds.), *Intraoperative Cranial Nerve Monitoring in Otolaryngology-Head and Neck Surgery*, https://doi.org/10.1007/978-3-030-84916-0_14

particularly since brachial plexus injuries are a common source of lawsuits [10].

Intraoperative Nerve Monitoring

There are two general methods of IONM for the RLN in thyroid surgery: intermittent and continuous. Intermittent nerve monitoring involves the delivery of an intermittent stimulus to complete an electrical circuit and demonstrate normal nerve function. It has become a common part of thyroid surgery, and its use has been standardized with prescribed ways of responding to signal loss [11]. Despite these advances, there is still mixed evidence whether it prevents RLN injury [2].

Continuous intraoperative nerve monitoring (C-IONM) relies on the delivery of a constant stimulus with the abrogation of this response signaling that nerve injury could be occurring. The earliest version of C-IONM used an electrode placed on the vagal nerve in order to have a continuous stimulation to the RLN [12]. While there were concerns about the safety of stimulating the vagal nerve [13], some surgeons state that vagal monitoring is safe and effective [14]. The major drawback to this monitoring method is that it requires increased dissection to reveal the vagal nerve to allow for placing of the electrode. The nerve must be dissected from the carotid sheath and have a 360-degree exposure for the electrode to be placed [15]. This can cause injury to the nerve itself [13].

The most promising type of continuous monitoring is laryngeal adductor reflex continuous intraoperative nerve monitoring (LAR-C-IONM). This new technology provides continuous monitoring of the RLN but does not require the added dissection of the vagal nerve. Instead, the electrodes on the ETT are not just the receiver but also the stimulator. They trigger the laryngeal adductor reflex, which has a reflex arc that travels from the superior laryngeal nerve, through the vagus to the RLN. Thus, it is able to monitor sensory, motor, and central components [16]. There are now studies which show (LAR-C-IONM) may have a benefit over conventional IONM as it gives the surgeon constant feedback about the vital status of the nerve; however, intermittent nerve monitoring is by far the most common [17].

RLN Monitoring in Remote Access Thyroid and Parathyroid Surgery

There are few studies which directly compare RLN monitoring in remote access thyroid surgery vs. trans-cervical. One study looked at the rates of loss of signal between retro-auricular and trans-cervical thyroidectomy with RLN monitoring and found no difference in rates [18]. Another study which looked at the feasibility in IONM of the RLN in both trans-oral and facelift incision thyroidectomy approaches showed some initial difficulty with adequate monitoring for the first 15 cases, with a failure rate of 46%; but this rate decreased to 4% subsequently [19]. However, most studies do not report any problems with RLN monitoring via remote access sites [20]. It is also clear that IONM of the RLN continues to allow for identification of the RLN even with these different approaches. Overall, there does not appear to be a significant difference in the implementation of or outcomes associated with RLN in remote access thyroid surgery.

Currently, the majority of high-volume surgeons offering remote access techniques utilize IONM of the RLN in a fashion similar to that employed with open surgery [21–23]. Some modifications are adopted by various surgeons to each system depending on the individual and local circumstances. For example, with the trans-oral endoscopic approach, our group utilizes a ball-tip thoracic or spinal nerve stimulator set to a relatively high stimulus amplitude (3 mA) given the diffuse nature of the delivered stimulus with that specific probe tip. Other centers have found that the stimulator may be connected to a laparoscopic hook, cautery probe, or other long device that allows the circuit to be completed laparoscopically or robotically. While circumstances necessitate adaptation, the general technique of nerve monitoring with intermittent stimulation remains the standard. Continuous nerve monitoring is not routinely utilized by most practitioners at this time due to the logistical challenges in accessing and placing an electrode on the vagus nerve.

Gasless Trans-Axillary Thyroidectomy and the Brachial Plexus

Trans-axillary robotic surgery is a relatively new remote access approach to the thyroid. In 2005, *Lobe* et al. reported the first trans-axillary robotic thyroidectomy [24]. This technique has become more common; *Kandil* et al. reported the largest experience in the United States with over 100 cases [25]. In addition, there have been case reports with larger numbers of procedures from Asia [26, 27]. Prior to the development of TOETVA, the trans-axillary approach was one of the few ways to avoid cervical scarring and the negative effect such scars have on quality of life [27–30]. Another benefit is that the trans-axillary approach leads to earlier return to functional activities [31]. However, one of the major drawbacks to this approach is that the positioning of the patient's arm for access during surgery can cause injury to the brachial plexus [25, 32].

The etiology of the injury to the brachial plexus comes from the stretch of and traction on the brachial plexus by having the shoulder internally rotated while the elbow is flexed [33]. Peripheral nerves are able to undergo roughly 20% stretch prior to injury. This positioning, with the arm overhead, leads to the brachial plexus being stretched unnaturally [34]. In addition, this position also leads to pressure-induced ischemia which can cause nerve injury [35]. Rates of brachial plexus nerve injury range from 2% to 5% during the trans-axillary approach [31, 36].

One of the ways to prevent injuries to the brachial plexus is through the monitoring of somatosensory evoked potentials (SSEP) of the median nerve. SSEP as a nerve monitoring technique was first developed in the 1970s [37]. Since that time, a number of other surgical subspecialties have used such monitoring for the same purpose [38–41].

Pathophysiology of Nerve Injury

The nerve injury classification introduced by Seddon and refined by Sunderland is helpful in demonstrating the principles behind the use of IONM of the brachial plexus (Table 14.1) [42, 43]. The principle is that as there is increasing damage to the axons and Schwann cells of the nerve, via stretching and compression, the nerve monitoring will detect such changes at or before Sunderland grade 1, and the positional insults may be relieved. This will prevent the injury from progression to a grade 3 or 4, in which recover is less likely.

SSEPs: Basic Principles

SSEP is the central measurement of electrical activity of a proximal site after stimulation of a distal part of the somatosensory system, and

Table 14.1 Nerve damage and recovery according to the Sunderland and Seddon classification

Sunderland	Seddon	Injury	Recovery
Grade I	Neurapraxia	Limited demyelination	Spontaneous
Grade II	Axonotmesis	Axonal damage but intact endoneurium	Spontaneous but delayed
Grade III	Axonotmesis	Axonal and endoneurial damage with perineurium intact	Possible
Grade IV	Axonotmesis	Axonal, endoneurial, and perineural damage with epineurium intact	Possible but unlikely
Grade V	Neurotmesis	Complete nerve disruption	No

Information derived from Seddon [42] and Sunderland [43]

therefore SSEP can be used to monitor for damage to a nerve. In an SSEP, the peripheral somatosensory nerve sends a signal through the dorsal root ganglion, the dorsal column, and the brainstem before finally ending in the cortex, where electrodes detect the signal [44].

SSEPs can be recorded from any of the peripheral nerves feeding into the brachial plexus, including the median, ulnar, and radial nerves, though monitoring is usually done of just the median nerve. While this is a simple system in theory, in reality, SSEP monitoring is complex, and there are a variety of nuances which must be understood by the surgeon.

First, there are basic terms that the surgeon must be familiar with. The two most important terms are latency and amplitude. Amplitude is measured in μV. Its technical definition is the height of the apex of the initial deflection of the wave form to the greatest point of deflection peak. Amplitudes are traditionally under the 10 μV's range [45]. Latency is defined as the time from stimulation until the downward defection of the initial peak of the waveform. Short latencies are the peaks and troughs within the first 40 msec after a single stimulation to the upper limb and are the type used when monitoring the brachial plexus [46].

There are several other components to an SSEP system that the surgeon must also know. The duration of stimulation provided to the nerve is a variable measured in milliseconds, and the frequency of the simulation is another variable, and the preferred rate is 3–5 Hz; up to 8 Hz is acceptable [46].

The International Federation of Clinical Neurophysiology (IFCN) guidelines are as follows: electrical stimulus: 100–300 ms duration square wave pulse with a target of a pulse width maintained at 300 ms with intensity 10% above the motor threshold; each SSEP record should be made with an average of 100–200 total pulses [47].

The signal is then monitored for either a change in latency of 10% or a decrease in amplitude of greater than 50% [48]. Once either of these thresholds is met, the patient should be repositioned by the surgeon in order to discontinue any stretch on the brachial plexus and to decrease compressive ischemia.

SSEP Electrodes

While beyond the scope this chapter, a brief mention of electrodes is needed so that the surgeon may understand SSEPs more thoroughly. The basic signals needed for monitoring the median nerve monitoring are in Table 14.2 [44]. These electrodes are then used to make a montage of the different electrical signals which can be interpreted by the electrophysiologist. The cortical electrodes should be placed in the contralateral side of the monitored nerve, Fc (contralateral frontal) and Pc (contralateral parietal). Scalp electrodes may utilize a reference frontal scalp electrode (FpZ), according to the International 10–20 system [47].

In addition to these proximal detecting electrodes, the stimulator electrodes should be placed over the nerve course. The cathode should be 2 cm proximal to the anode, and the ground lead should be placed distally as well [47].

Table 14.2 Stimulation signals needed for median nerve monitoring

Signal name	Correlation
EP	Propagated volley passing under Erb's point
N13	Stationary cervical potential recorded from the dorsal neck
P14	Subcortically generated far-field potential recorded referentially from the scalp
N18	Subcortically generated far-field potential best recorded referentially from the scalp ipsilateral to the side of stimulation
N20	Primary somatosensory cortex recorded using a bipolar derivation to subtract the widespread far-field potentials from the superimposed primary cortical activity in the centro-parietal region contralateral to the side of stimulation

Naming: The waveform peaks have polarity, which is considered negative (N) on upward deflection and positive (P) on downward one. Based on the post-stimulus latency (in ms), each one is assigned an integer
Information derived from: Leeman [44]

Utility of Nerve Monitoring

One of the main challenges in assessing the benefit of IONM is that the rate of injury to the recurrent laryngeal nerve is rare. For open surgery, the number of patients needed to power the correlation between IONM and RLN paralysis/palsy would be over nine million patients for benign pathology of the thyroid and 40,000 for thyroid malignancy [49]. Multiple large studies on open surgery have been inconclusive [49–56]. Given that there are significantly less procedures performed with remote access thyroid surgery, it is unclear to what degree IONM of the RLN provides. More well-conducted studies are needed on this subject to provide a more definitive answer.

While there is also a lack of thyroid operation-specific data on the ability of SSEP to prevent injury to the brachial plexus, other surgical specialties have shown reductions in injury rates as high as 80% when using SSEP [57]. Importantly, thyroid surgeons who use a trans-axillary approach for thyroidectomy advocate for its use as a necessary part to the procedure [58]. There are also studies which report shorter operative times with SSEP monitoring [31]. Still, well-conducted studies are needed in order to ensure that monitoring of the brachial plexus SSEPs is useful.

One of the drawbacks of this system though is that it requires a neurophysiologist to assess the stimulation and response of the nerve. This increase in personnel and material means additional cost of and complexity in the surgery. The system also requires the surgeon to pay attention to another series of inputs, which may detract from his ability to concentrate on the surgery. Despite these considerations, the use of SSEP monitoring during trans-axillary surgery is an important tool to prevent injury to the brachial plexus.

It should be noted though that SSEPS are not the only way to monitor nerve function of the brachial plexus. There is also the use of electric motor evoked potentials to evaluate impending nerve injury and may be more sensitive as they tend to predict changes 10–20 minutes earlier than SSEPS. Only one study for trans-axillary thyroidectomy has used these more sensitive monitoring techniques [59].

Another way to reduce brachial plexus injury in these patients is using proper positioning of the patients' arm in order to relieve the stretch and possible ischemic effects. In one center, this decreased the brachial plexus injury rate from 5% to 0% [31]. Other steps are to reduce total time of stretch by positioning the patient as late as possible in the surgery [25].

While other specialties have shown that certain populations are more at risk for peripheral nerve injury, specifically patients who are obese, underweight, and diabetic, the same trend has been reported in the literature of thyroid surgery [31].

Conclusion

In conclusion, IONM for the RLN monitoring with remote access follows the same principles of other IONM monitoring for thyroid and parathyroid surgery. Small modifications can be employed as needed with specific techniques, but the generalities are consistent. CIONM is a newer technology that may even improve upon the current paradigm of intermittent RLN monitoring but currently is difficult to utilize with remote access techniques. With a trans-axillary approach, the brachial plexus is at risk, and nerve monitoring of this structure with SSEP is an important tool to alert the surgeon to impending nerve injuries. Given the high rate of complications seen in some centers, the benefit of such monitoring outweighs any drawbacks associated with cost or complexity.

References

1. Russell JO, et al. Minimally invasive and remote-access thyroid surgery in the era of the 2015 American Thyroid Association guidelines. Laryngoscope Investig Otolaryngol. 2016;1(6):175–9.
2. Randolph GW, et al. Electrophysiologic recurrent laryngeal nerve monitoring during thyroid and parathyroid surgery: international standards guideline statement. Laryngoscope. 2011;121 Suppl 1:S1–16.

3. Shindo M, Chheda NN. Incidence of vocal cord paralysis with and without recurrent laryngeal nerve monitoring during thyroidectomy. Arch Otolaryngol Head Neck Surg. 2007;133(5):481–5.
4. Caragacianu D, Kamani D, Randolph GW. Intraoperative monitoring: normative range associated with normal postoperative glottic function. Laryngoscope. 2013;123(12):3026–31.
5. Lydiatt DD. Medical malpractice and the thyroid gland. Head Neck. 2003;25(6):429–31.
6. Angelos P. Ethical and medicolegal issues in neuromonitoring during thyroid and parathyroid surgery: a review of the recent literature. Curr Opin Oncol. 2012;24(1):16–21.
7. Gartland RM, et al. A long, unnerving road: malpractice claims involving the surgical management of thyroid and parathyroid disease. World J Surg. 2019;43(11):2850–5.
8. Goldstone AC, Schettino RL. Electrode endotracheal tube. 1991, Google Patents.
9. Sturgeon C, Sturgeon T, Angelos P. Neuromonitoring in thyroid surgery: attitudes, usage patterns, and predictors of use among endocrine surgeons. World J Surg. 2009;33(3):417–25.
10. Na. Practice Advisory for the Prevention of Perioperative Peripheral Neuropathies: A Report by the American Society of Anesthesiologists Task Force on Prevention of Perioperative Peripheral Neuropathies. Anesthesiology. 2000;92(4):1168–82.
11. Sinclair CF, Kamani D, Randolph GW. The evolution and progress of standard procedures for intraoperative nerve monitoring. Ann Thyr. 2019;4.
12. Marin Arteaga A, et al. Modification of the surgical strategy for the dissection of the recurrent laryngeal nerve using continuous intraoperative nerve monitoring. World J Surg. 2018;42(2):444–50.
13. Terris DJ, Chaung K, Duke WS. Continuous vagal nerve monitoring is dangerous and should not routinely be done during thyroid surgery. World J Surg. 2015;39(10):2471–6.
14. Schneider R, et al. Superiority of continuous over intermittent intraoperative nerve monitoring in preventing vocal cord palsy. Br J Surg. 2020.
15. Stankovic P, et al. Continuous intraoperative neuromonitoring (cIONM) in head and neck surgery-a review. HNO. 2020;68(Suppl 2):86–92.
16. Sinclair CF, Téllez MJ, Ulkatan S. Noninvasive, tube-based, continuous vagal nerve monitoring using the laryngeal adductor reflex: feasibility study of 134 nerves at risk. Head Neck. 2018;40(11):2498–506.
17. Sinclair CF, Téllez MJ, Ulkatan S. Continuous laryngeal adductor reflex versus intermittent nerve monitoring in neck endocrine surgery. Laryngoscope. 2020.
18. Ban MJ, et al. Analysis of neuromonitoring signal loss during retroauricular versus conventional thyroidectomy. Laryngoscope. 2019;129(9):2199–204.
19. Ji YB, et al. Feasibility and efficacy of intraoperative neural monitoring in remote access robotic and endoscopic thyroidectomy. Oral Oncol. 2020;103:104617.
20. Wang Y, et al. Implementation of intraoperative neuromonitoring for transoral endoscopic thyroid surgery: a preliminary report. J Laparoendosc Adv Surg Tech A. 2016;26(12):965–71.
21. Inabnet WB 3rd, Suh H, Fernandez-Ranvier G. Transoral endoscopic thyroidectomy vestibular approach with intraoperative nerve monitoring. Surg Endosc. 2017;31(7):3030.
22. Castellsagué X, et al. HPV involvement in head and neck cancers: comprehensive assessment of biomarkers in 3680 patients. J Natl Cancer Inst. 2016;108(6):djv403.
23. Jonas J. Total-endoscopic thyroid resection in ABBA-technique: comments on the integration of intraoperative neuromonitoring. Zentralbl Chir. 2016;141(5):565–9.
24. Lobe TE, Wright SK, Irish MS. Novel uses of surgical robotics in head and neck surgery. J Laparoendosc Adv Surg Tech. 2005;15(6):647–52.
25. Kandil E, et al. Transaxillary gasless robotic thyroidectomy: a single surgeon's experience in North America. Arch Otolaryngol Head Neck Surg. 2012;138(2):113–7.
26. Ikeda Y, et al. Endoscopic neck surgery by the axillary approach. J Am Coll Surg. 2000;191(3):336–40.
27. Ikeda Y, et al. Clinical benefits in endoscopic thyroidectomy by the axillary approach. J Am Coll Surg. 2003;196(2):189–95.
28. Juarez MC, et al. Objectively measuring social attention of thyroid neck scars and transoral surgery using eye tracking. Laryngoscope. 2019;129(12):2789–94.
29. Casserly P, Kirby R, Timon C. Outcome measures and scar aesthetics in minimally invasive video-assisted parathyroidectomy. Arch Otolaryngol Head Neck Surgry. 2010;136(3):260–4.
30. Best AR, Shipchandler TZ, Cordes SR. Midcervical scar satisfaction in thyroidectomy patients. Laryngoscope. 2017;127(5):1247–52.
31. Huang S, et al. Somatosensory evoked potential: preventing brachial plexus injury in transaxillary robotic surgery. Laryngoscope. 2019;129(11):2663–8.
32. Landry CS, et al. Robot assisted transaxillary surgery (RATS) for the removal of thyroid and parathyroid glands. Surgery. 2011;149(4):549–55.
33. Alzahrani HA, et al. Gasless trans-axillary robotic thyroidectomy: the technique and evidence. Gland Surg. 2017;6(3):236–42.
34. Grant GA, Goodkin R, Kliot M. Evaluation and surgical management of peripheral nerve problems. Neurosurgery. 1999;44(4):825–39; discussion 839–40.
35. Desai DC, Uribe A, Lachman T. Brachial plexus injury due to compression: an alternate mechanism of injury: case report and review of the literature. Am Surg. 1997;63(6):487–9.
36. Garstka ME, et al. Conventional robotic endoscopic thyroidectomy for thyroid cancer. Endocrinol Metab Clin N Am. 2019;48(1):153–63.
37. Deletis V, Sala F. Intraoperative neurophysiological monitoring of the spinal cord during spinal cord and

spine surgery: a review focus on the corticospinal tracts. Clin Neurophysiol. 2008;119(2):248–64.
38. Jellish WS, et al. Hands-up positioning during asymmetric sternal retraction for internal mammary artery harvest: a possible method to reduce brachial plexus injury. Anesth Analg. 1997;84(2):260–5.
39. Schwartz DM, et al. Neurophysiological identification of position-induced neurologic injury during anterior cervical spine surgery. J Clin Monit Comput. 2006;20(6):437–44.
40. Kamel IR, et al. The use of somatosensory evoked potentials to determine the relationship between patient positioning and impending upper extremity nerve injury during spine surgery: a retrospective analysis. Anesth Analg. 2006;102(5):1538–42.
41. Bhalodia VM, et al. Transcranial electric motor evoked potential detection of compressional peroneal nerve injury in the lateral decubitus position. J Clin Monit Comput. 2008;22(4):319–26.
42. Seddon HJ. A classification of nerve injuries. Br Med J. 1942;2(4260):237–9.
43. Sunderland S. A classification of peripheral nerve injuries producing loss of function. Brain. 1951;74(4):491–516.
44. Leeman SA. SSEPs: from limb to cortex. Am J Electroneurodiagnostic Technol. 2007;47(3):165–77.
45. Schomer DL, et al. Niedermeyer's electroencephalography basic principles, clinical applications, and related fields, in somatosensory and pain evoked potentials normal responses, abnormal waveforms, and clinical applications in neurological diseases. Oxford University Press; 2017.
46. Allison T, et al. Potentials evoked in human and monkey cerebral cortex by stimulation of the median nerve. A review of scalp and intracranial recordings. Brain. 1991;114(Pt 6):2465–503.
47. Cruccu G, et al. Recommendations for the clinical use of somatosensory-evoked potentials. Clin Neurophysiol. 2008;119(8):1705–19.
48. Nuwer MR, et al. Somatosensory evoked potential spinal cord monitoring reduces neurologic deficits after scoliosis surgery: results of a large multicenter survey. Electroencephalogr Clin Neurophysiol. 1995;96(1):6–11.
49. Dralle H, et al. Risk factors of paralysis and functional outcome after recurrent laryngeal nerve monitoring in thyroid surgery. Surgery. 2004;136(6):1310–22.
50. Pisanu A, et al. Systematic review with meta-analysis of studies comparing intraoperative neuromonitoring of recurrent laryngeal nerves versus visualization alone during thyroidectomy. J Surg Res. 2014;188(1):152–61.
51. Sanabria A, et al. Neuromonitoring in thyroidectomy: a meta-analysis of effectiveness from randomized controlled trials. Eur Arch Otorhinolaryngol. 2013;270(8):2175–89.
52. Lombardi CP, et al. "The final countdown": is intraoperative, intermittent neuromonitoring really useful in preventing permanent nerve palsy? Evidence from a meta-analysis. Surgery. 2016;160(6):1693–706.
53. Zheng S, et al. Effect of intraoperative neuromonitoring on recurrent laryngeal nerve palsy rates after thyroid surgery–a meta-analysis. J Formos Med Assoc. 2013;112(8):463–72.
54. Bai B, Chen W. Protective effects of intraoperative nerve monitoring (IONM) for recurrent laryngeal nerve injury in thyroidectomy: meta-analysis. Sci Rep. 2018;8(1):7761.
55. Wong KP, et al. Systematic review and meta-analysis on intra-operative neuro-monitoring in high-risk thyroidectomy. Int J Surg. 2017;38:21–30.
56. Yang S, et al. Systematic review with meta-analysis of intraoperative neuromonitoring during thyroidectomy. Int J Surg. 2017;39:104–13.
57. Pajewski TN, Arlet V, Phillips LH. Current approach on spinal cord monitoring: the point of view of the neurologist, the anesthesiologist and the spine surgeon. Eur Spine J. 2007;16 Suppl 2(Suppl 2):S115–29.
58. Davis SF, et al. Detection and prevention of impending brachial plexus injury secondary to arm positioning using ulnar nerve somatosensory evoked potentials during transaxillary approach for thyroid lobectomy. Am J Electroneurodiagnostic Technol. 2011;51(4):274–9.
59. Luginbuhl A, et al. Detection of evolving injury to the brachial plexus during transaxillary robotic thyroidectomy. Laryngoscope. 2012;122(1):110–5.

15 Nerve Monitoring During Parathyroid Surgery

Phillip K. Pellitteri and Nicholas C. Purdy

Introduction

Surgery for parathyroid disease has undergone an evolutionary renaissance over the past two decades. This has primarily been accomplished through the development of accurate preoperative localization techniques and the advent of biochemical confirmation of adequate removal of hyperfunctional tissue through the assessment of intraoperative parathyroid hormone levels. Consonant with these developments has been the introduction of nerve monitoring techniques implemented to track the neurophysiologic status of the recurrent laryngeal nerve during surgery. This technique has been popularized and enthusiastically embraced for use in thyroid surgery, where nerve identification and preservation are directly applicable due to the anatomic course of the recurrent laryngeal nerve and its relationship to the thyroid gland. Although the parathyroid glands may be less proximate to the recurrent nerve, they nevertheless occupy an anatomic compartment in which the recurrent nerve resides. As such, during surgical exploration for parathyroid disease, the nerve may be at risk for iatrogenic injury. It is then as a result of this relationship within the central neck compartment that nerve monitoring techniques are also being used during surgery for parathyroid disease. This chapter examines the use of nerve monitoring in parathyroid surgery and discusses the techniques employed and the clinical scenarios where monitoring may be of greatest application and benefit.

Surgical disorders of the parathyroid glands resulting in parathyroid hyperfunction include those which arise directly within the glands and those that are sponsored by metabolic influences that secondarily involve the parathyroid glands. Disorders arising directly in the gland may be categorized into single gland disease, commonly referred to as parathyroid adenoma, and multiple gland disease, referred to as parathyroid hyperplasia. Collectively they are termed primary hyperparathyroidism. Those parathyroid disorders which secondarily occur as a result of metabolic influences, primarily renal, are termed secondary hyperparathyroidism and are associated with multiple gland disease or diffuse hyperplasia. The etiologic distinction between these entities is beyond the scope of this chapter; however, each entity may involve a different level of risk to recurrent laryngeal nerve function when applied to central compartment neck exploration.

P. K. Pellitteri (✉)
Department of Otolaryngology/HNS, Geisinger Commonwealth School of Medicine, Geisinger Wyoming Valley Medical Center, Wilkes Barre, PA, USA

N. C. Purdy
Geisinger Commonwealth School of Medicine, Danville, PA, USA

© The Author(s), under exclusive license to Springer Nature Switzerland AG 2022
J. Scharpf, G. W. Randolph (eds.), *Intraoperative Cranial Nerve Monitoring in Otolaryngology-Head and Neck Surgery*, https://doi.org/10.1007/978-3-030-84916-0_15

The risk of complications in central compartment neck surgery for parathyroid disorders, as for thyroid surgery, primarily involves injury to the recurrent laryngeal nerve(s) and fellow parathyroid glands. It has been generally acknowledged that because of the less proximate relationship of parathyroid glands to the recurrent nerve, risk of injury during parathyroidectomy is less than for thyroid surgery. However, circumstances may exist whereby the parathyroid gland(s) being dissected during exploration may occupy an anatomic relationship to the nerve which places the nerve at significant risk for injury. It is in these scenarios where implementing nerve monitoring techniques could provide the greatest benefit in recurrent laryngeal nerve protection intraoperatively.

A review of the anatomic course of the recurrent laryngeal nerve, relative to parathyroid gland locations, is important for parathyroid surgery. It aids in assessing the predictive capability of localization imaging. These modalities have gained greater acceptance in the evaluation of surgical parathyroid disorders. The course of right and left recurrent nerves differ, but the embryo-anatomic relationship of the parathyroid glands in relation to each nerve is similar. The left vagus nerve courses from the carotid sheath at the left base of the neck to pass anterior to the aortic arch. The left recurrent laryngeal nerve then passes under the aortic arch to ascend in the tracheoesophageal groove just lateral to the trachea. The right vagus nerve runs from behind the internal jugular vein at the right base of the neck crossing anterior to the subclavian artery. The right recurrent nerve branches and then passes up and around the subclavian artery coursing medially along the pleura and superiorly behind the common carotid artery to enter the neck in a more lateral orientation than does the left recurrent nerve. It ascends to a paratracheal position in the last centimeter of its course as it approaches the inferior constrictor muscle. Thus, the right recurrent nerve ascends in a more oblique course than does the straighter vertical course of the left recurrent nerve. The relationship of the parathyroid glands to the nerve is crucial when identifying which parathyroid gland, superior or inferior, is being sought. Because of the embryonic relationship of the inferior parathyroid gland and thymus (third branchial pouch derivatives), the inferior parathyroid gland will reliably reside in an orientation ventral to the recurrent laryngeal nerve. The superior parathyroid gland (fourth pouch derivative) will lie in a dorsal orientation with the nerve, within proximity to the laryngeal entry point of the nerve (Fig. 15.1). Because of this superior parathyroid gland/recurrent nerve relationship, abnormal superior glands being dissected during exploration may require both identification and protection of the nerve to avoid injury.

The ability to preoperatively assess the location of putative hyperfunctional parathyroid glands, and thus potential risk to the recurrent nerve, has been augmented by more accurate and practical localization techniques. Although a thorough discussion of the various modalities utilized for parathyroid gland localization is beyond the intent of this discussion, it is important to point out that cross-sectional imaging techniques, such as sestamibi SPECT/CT and 4D CT, provide the greatest benefit in establishing gland locations which may be in close relationship to the recurrent laryngeal nerve and, thus, a situation for which nerve monitoring may be most useful during surgical exploration. Imaging which demonstrates descent of an enlarged superior parathyroid gland, located dorsal to the laryngeal nerve, a so called "pseudo-ectopic" location, may be expected to reside close to the nerve in a para-esophageal location (Fig. 15.2). The predictive value of such localization, with reference to the anatomic course of the nerve, is important in planning conduct of the exploration and utilizing the protective potential for nerve monitoring. Similarly, imaging which demonstrates true ectopic parathyroid gland locations, such as in the mediastinal compartment, may benefit from nerve monitoring to avoid surgical injury to the recurrent nerve (Fig. 15.3).

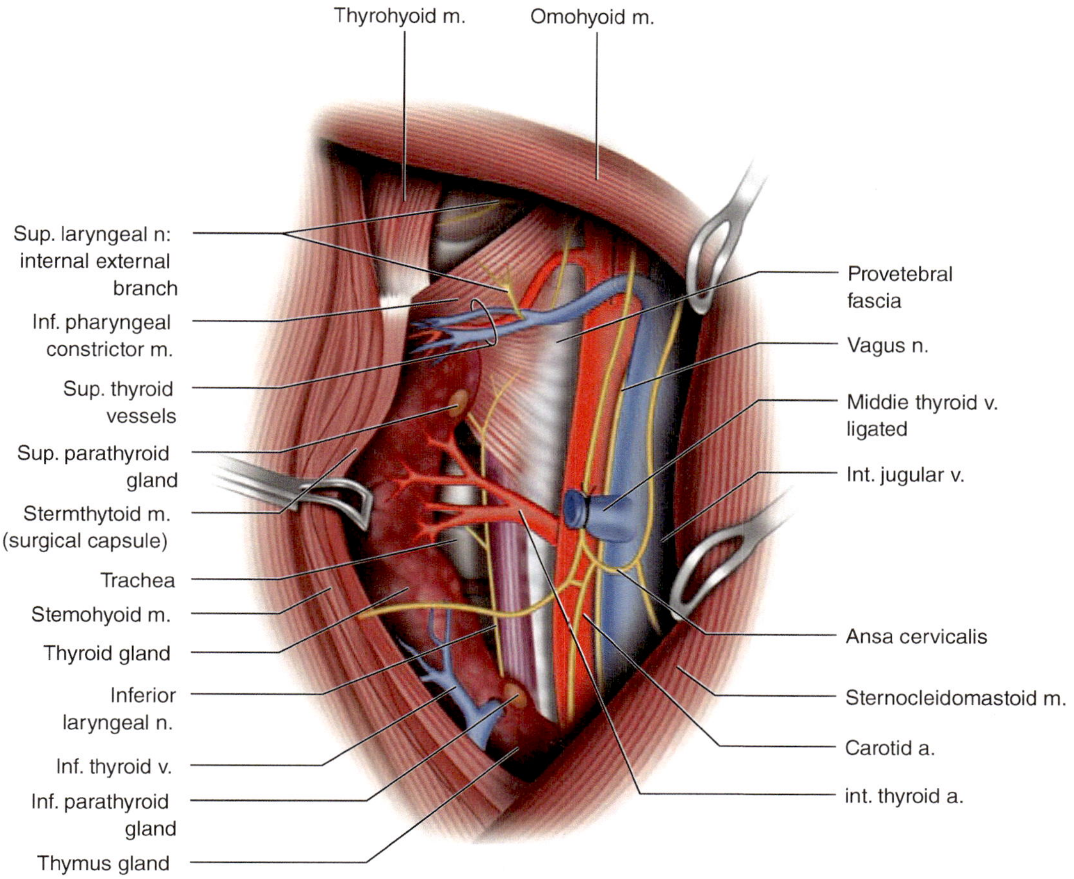

Fig. 15.1 Illustration of the normal relationship of the parathyroid glands to the recurrent laryngeal nerve and related central compartment neck structures

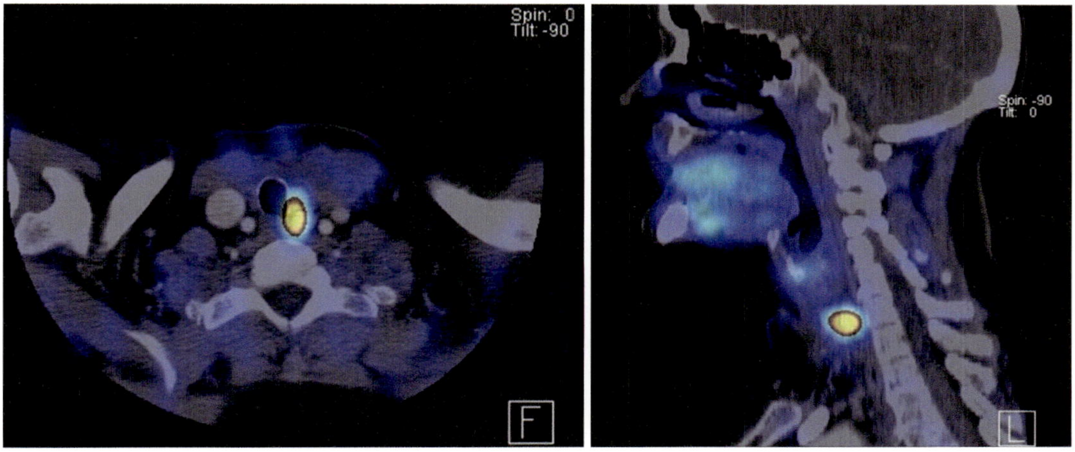

Fig. 15.2 CT sestamibi fusion (axial and sagittal) imaging demonstrating enlarged superior parathyroid gland, located dorsal to the laryngeal nerve, a so-called "pseudo-ectopic" location, may be expected to reside close to the nerve in a para-esophageal location

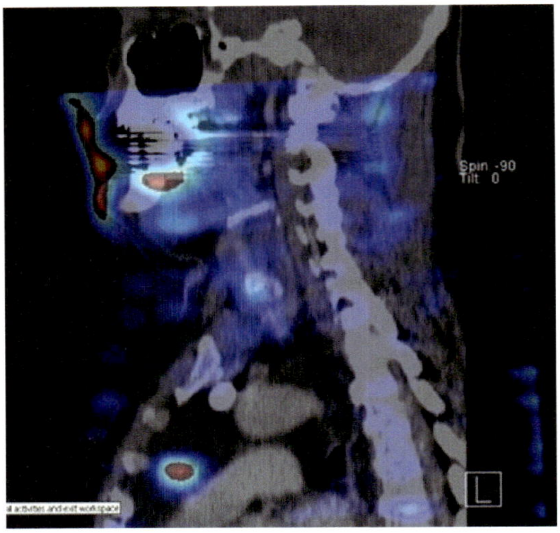

Fig. 15.3 CT sestamibi fusion imaging demonstrating a true ectopic parathyroid gland location in the mediastinal compartment

Neck Exploration

Neck exploration for parathyroid disease may be categorized into three procedural components. These include (1) disease etiology, (2) imaging results, and (3) history of previous surgical treatment. Targeted surgery involves preoperative localization whereby an abnormal hyperfunctional parathyroid gland is identified in a patient with laboratory evidence of primary hyperparathyroidism. Surgical success is predicated on identification and removal of the gland localized with a subsequent decline in serum parathyroid hormone measured intraoperatively (IOPTH), thereby biochemically confirming removal of all hyperfunctional parathyroid tissue. Bilateral comprehensive exploration, as a planned procedure, is implemented for patients with disease entities known to manifest as a multi-glandular disease, i.e., renal-induced secondary hyperparathyroidism, multiple endocrine neoplasia type I, and non-MEN-associated familial hyperparathyroidism. Patients with these disorders may be expected to have multiple glands possessing hyperfunctional capability requiring subtotal/total parathyroidectomy, depending on intraoperative findings and IOPTH results. Recalcitrant hyperparathyroidism, primary or secondary/tertiary, will often require reoperative exploration, potentially posing increased risk to the recurrent laryngeal nerve. The decision to pursue re-exploration is based on the clinical presentation and severity of recalcitrant disease and is very dependent upon accurate localization of hyperfunctional tissue. A similar clinical scenario involves parathyroid exploration after thyroidectomy, as endocrine disorders involving both the thyroid and parathyroid glands can occur in the same patient. Depending on the location of the abnormal gland, the surgeon may be faced with operating in a fibrotic field with increased risk to the nerve.

Nerve Monitoring Techniques

Preservation of recurrent laryngeal nerve function is of the utmost importance during parathyroid surgery. Visual identification of the recurrent laryngeal nerve remains the gold standard for nerve management during head and neck endocrine surgery. However, a visually intact nerve does not always indicate a physiologically functional nerve. Patients may still suffer significant functional consequences, despite the absence of visible anatomic injury. In order to address this issue, several intraoperative nerve monitoring techniques have gained greater acceptance during parathyroid surgery [1].

Despite enjoying greater popularity, the clearly defined role of intraoperative nerve monitoring in parathyroid surgery remains unclear in the literature. In the only investigation examining the use of intraoperative nerve monitoring exclusive to parathyroid surgery, the study authors concluded that nerve monitoring may not provide additional benefit in preventing recurrent laryngeal nerve injury [1]. It is our belief, however, that clinical scenarios exist which will benefit from the application of nerve monitoring during parathyroid surgery and that a knowledge of available techniques will provide potentially useful adjuncts in the surgeon's armamentarium in support of a successful endocrine surgical practice.

Perhaps the most widely practiced technique to manage the recurrent laryngeal nerve during parathyroid surgery is intermittent intraoperative nerve monitoring. This method utilizes a handheld monopolar probe to directly stimulate the vagus nerve, recurrent laryngeal, or superior laryngeal nerve. The electrophysiologic response is recorded by needle electrodes placed directly in the vocal muscles or by surface electrodes on the endotracheal tube.

Intermittent intraoperative nerve monitoring provides surgeons with several pieces of valuable information during parathyroid surgery. Notably, it can be used to confirm the identity as well as the functional integrity of the recurrent laryngeal nerve. In the event of a nerve injury, nerve monitoring will provide assistance in locating the potential site of injury. If the injury is of a reversible cause, the monitoring system can identify intraoperative recovery of nerve function.

The evolution of nerve monitoring has led to a technique known as continuous intraoperative nerve monitoring (CIONM). This form of nerve monitoring provides real-time information to aid in the surgical dissection of the RLN. It involves dissection of the desired nerve with placement of circumferential electrodes around the nerve. By actively measuring latency and amplitude changes of the nerve, the surgeon can anticipate impending neurophysiologic injury, such as thermal or traction injury, which may not be anatomically evident and which will potentially limit hazardous maneuvers in high-risk parathyroid surgery.

Continuous monitoring of the vagus nerve has gained traction in thyroid surgery over the past several years. However, it should be noted that vagal nerve monitoring requires additional dissection and has the potential for added morbidity. Some authors feel it should not be routinely used in thyroid surgery due to a narrowed risk to benefit ratio [2]. Other investigators believe this to be a safe and effective technology, when applied and utilized in the appropriate setting [3]. Ultimately, its role in routine parathyroid surgery may be limited.

A handheld device alone, such as the Checkpoint nerve stimulator (Checkpoint Surgical, Cleveland, OH) can be used for neural monitoring. This is a compact device that is grounded to the patient and does not need additional electrodes or an external EMG monitor to provide physiologic neurofeedback. The RLN is directly stimulated, and the respective posterior cricoarytenoid muscle is palpated for contraction. Important features include an adjustable amplitude switch and the generation of a biphasic waveform to allow for safe and continuous nerve stimulation without fatigue while the probe is applied (Fig. 15.4).

While not proven to decrease recurrent laryngeal nerve injury in parathyroid surgery, knowledge of, and familiarity with, these techniques can provide a valuable adjunct to aid in surgical decision-making. (We recommend familiarizing yourself with the physiology of these techniques, as discussed in previous chapters.)

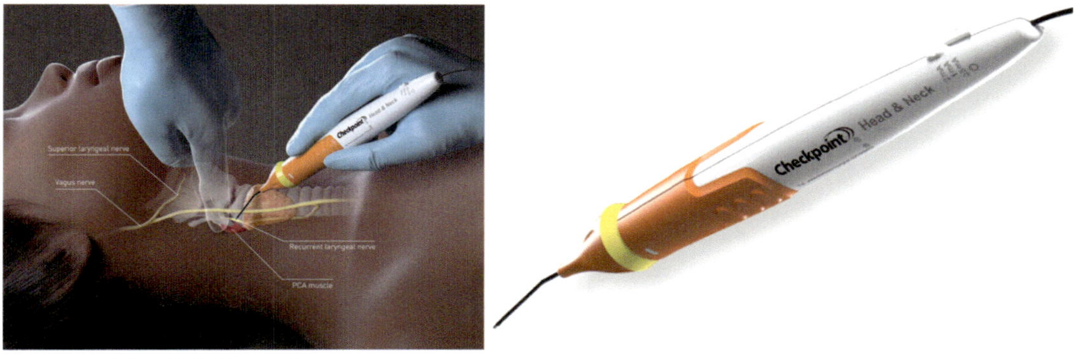

Fig. 15.4 Checkpoint nerve monitoring instrument

Neuromonitoring Applications

Recognizing that protection of the recurrent laryngeal nerve is a major goal during central neck compartment surgery, intraoperative nerve monitoring has gained wide acceptance by surgeons over the past decade [4]. This shift has occurred despite controversy involving the value of neuromonitoring in avoiding nerve injury. Moreover, the predominant reports advocating for neuromonitoring have been generated by its application in thyroid surgery. There exists little data involving the use of neuromonitoring solely in parathyroid surgery. Existing reports combine the experience of thyroid and parathyroid surgery as single study populations, or with thyroidectomy alone [4]. One study which described an investigation dedicated to the use of nerve monitoring in parathyroid surgery was reported by Mourad in 2016. This investigation endeavored to describe differences in nerve injury in patients undergoing parathyroid surgery with and without nerve monitoring using a historical cohort as control. The authors noted no statistical difference in nerve injury between the two groups. Of interest was that, in the nine total patients incurring vocal paralysis, four had undergone re-exploration procedures [1]. Advocates of neuromonitoring in central neck surgery remain consistent in mandating visualization of the recurrent nerve during dissection as the gold standard for prevention of nerve injury [5]. Neuromonitoring, especially when implementing the continuous mode, will provide feedback to the surgeon during dissection of and around the nerve during thyroidectomy, alerting the surgeon to potential injurious maneuvers. The same experience has not been described for parathyroid surgery, where nerve dissection and manipulation are not usually required in most instances. There are circumstances, however, whereby the recurrent laryngeal nerve may be at greater risk during parathyroid surgery and thus where nerve monitoring may be of benefit.

In most instances, image-directed parathyroid surgery for focal enlarged abnormal glands is straightforward and relatively risk-free. In these instances, the recurrent nerve is not uniformly identified, and even larger glands have no dense attachments to the gland requiring nerve manipulation. This is especially true for abnormal inferior glands, which reside ventral and further from the nerve. The superior glands are located closer to the nerve and are usually lateral to the laryngeal nerve entry point. However, larger superior glands which descend in the neck due to gravity do so in a space which may allow them to reside posterior or dorsal to the nerve in a para-esophageal orientation. These so-called "pseudo-ectopic" glands can be visualized by imaging techniques, alerting the surgeon that nerve dissection and manipulation may be required in order to remove the parathyroid gland (Fig. 15.5). Planned bilateral neck exploration, requiring 4-gland identification and subtotal/total parathyroidectomy for multiple gland disease, does not usually require mandatory identification and/or manipulation of the recurrent laryngeal nerve. For disease entities manifested by multi-gland disease, standard localization techniques are rarely employed, owing to the need to identify all four parathyroid glands intraoperatively. There are instances however, most notably in renal failure-induced secondary hyperparathyroidism, where excessively large parathyroid glands will be encountered and where these glands may be located very closely to the recurrent laryngeal nerve. Although distinctly uncommon, situations like this will potentially benefit from neuromonitoring if identified preoperatively. As previously mentioned, a visually intact nerve does not always indicate a functional nerve. Thus, similar to staged thyroid surgery, IONM can be used to confirm the functional status of the ipsilateral nerve prior to proceeding with contralateral neck exploration [6]. It is not unreasonable to obtain imaging in these patients preoperatively to determine if excessively large glands are present.

Neuromonitoring of the recurrent laryngeal nerve will provide the greatest benefit in patients requiring re-exploration for hyperparathyroidism. This may occur in the clinical setting of recalcitrant primary hyperparathyroidism or, less commonly, tertiary hyperparathyroidism

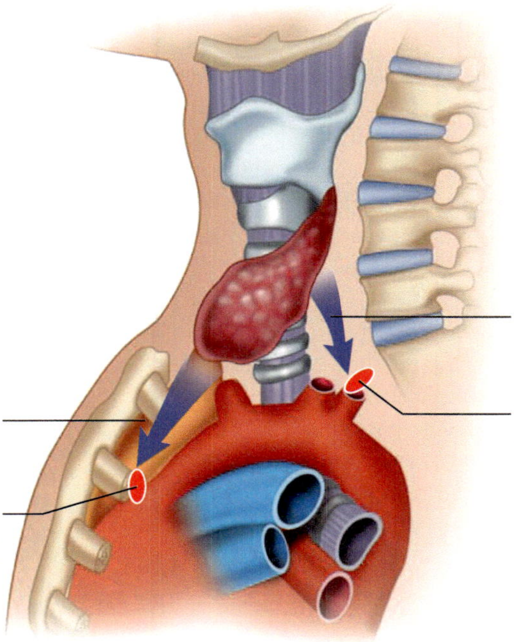

Fig. 15.5 Illustration depicting the pattern of ectopic gland migration relative to gland origin, superior and inferior

following renal transplantation after initial subtotal parathyroidectomy. Depending on the degree of exploration initially conducted and the neck side to be explored, the re-operating surgeon may encounter significant surgical fibrosis making dissection a formidable exercise. This has the potential to place the recurrent nerve at substantial risk of injury. In such circumstances, nerve monitoring will provide for both nerve identification and protection during dissection. The same may be true in the setting of parathyroid exploration following thyroidectomy, where it should be anticipated that surgical fibrosis around the recurrent laryngeal nerve(s) will hinder dissection and pose a heightened risk for nerve injury.

The authors find the Checkpoint nerve stimulator particularly useful in situations whereby altered anatomy and significant tissue fibrosis is found [7]. This technology can be used for both localization and intermittent nerve monitoring. By decreasing the stimulus on the selective amplitude switch, the location of the nerve can be narrowed to increasingly smaller areas of the surgical field. The adjustable stimulus can also be used to assess for changes in nerve function throughout the procedure.

Although rarely encountered, more extensive surgical dissection may be required in patients with parathyroid cancer. Hemithyroidectomy is usually performed in conjunction with parathyroid cancer resection. There will usually be surrounding desmoplastic tissue changes and inflammation resulting in a more difficult nerve identification process. Use of IONM can assist in nerve identification, integrity, and functionality both pre- and post-gland excision.

At the conclusion of parathyroidectomy, the nerve can be confirmed to be physiologically intact, thus reassuring the surgeon of functionally intact vocal cords. Conversely, if an anatomically intact nerve does not stimulate, the surgeon can investigate further into the presence of reversible causes of nerve paralysis, such as an improperly placed surgical clip or ligature, which can then be removed.

Intraoperative Recurrent Laryngeal Nerve Injury

In the unfortunate situation of a recurrent nerve injury identified intraoperatively, IONM can provide information on the approximate location of the injury and potentially guide treatment. By stimulating the nerve in a distal to proximal fashion starting at the point of laryngeal nerve entry, the point at which the nerve loses the electrical response can be identified as the site of injury. If the nerve is intact, the surgeon should begin an investigation into a potentially reversible cause. If the nerve is found to be transected, a primary nerve repair should be performed, using microsurgical techniques. If a tension-free repair is not possible, consideration should be given to ansa cervicalis nerve anastomosis or, potentially, urgent thyroplasty.

Summary

The use of intraoperative nerve monitoring for parathyroid surgery provides a powerful tool for endocrine surgeons of all skill sets. Its value extends beyond simple confirmation of the nerve after visual identification. Methods exist to assist in nerve identification when tissue fibrosis is encountered, warn of impending injury through continuous physiologic monitoring, and potentially guide decision-making, if a nerve injury should occur. Parathyroid surgeons must have a thorough understanding of the pathophysiology of hyperparathyroidism in order to select appropriate surgical candidates, together with identifying situations in which nerve monitoring provides benefit. While nerve monitoring does not guarantee absolute nerve safety, the authors feel that it represents a beneficial tool for head and neck endocrine surgeons when applied appropriately.

References

1. Mourad M, Kadakia S, Jategaonkar A, et al. Intraoperative nerve monitoring during parathyroid surgery: the fort worth experience. Head and Neck. 2017;39(8):1662–4.
2. Terris DJ, Chaung K, Duke WS. Continuous vagal nerve monitoring is dangerous and should not routinely be done during thyroid surgery. World J Surg. 2015;39(10):2471–6.
3. Bacuzzi A, Dralle H, Randolph GW, et al. Safety of continuous intraoperative neuromonitoring (C-IONM) in thyroid surgery. World J Surg. 2016;40:768–9.
4. Randolph GW, Kamani D. Intraoperative electrophysiologic monitoring of the recurrent laryngeal nerve during thyroid and parathyroid surgery: Experience with 1,381 nerves at risk. Laryngoscope. 2017;127(1):280–6.
5. Steurer M, Passler C, Denk DM, Schneider B, Niederle B, Bigenzahn W. Advantages of recurrent laryngeal nerve identification in thyroidectomy and parathyroidectomy and the importance of preoperative and postoperative laryngoscopic examination in more than 1000 nerves at risk. Laryngoscope. 2002;112(1):124–33.
6. Fontenot TE, Randolph GW, Setton TE, et al. Does intraoperative nerve monitoring reliably aid in staging of total thyroidectomies? Laryngoscope. 2015;125(9):2232–5.
7. Lawson BR, Kamani D, Shama M, et al. Safety and reliability of a handheld stimulator for neural monitoring during thyroid surgery. Laryngoscope. 2020;130(2):561–5.

Part III

Facial Nerve, Glossopharyngeal Nerve, Hypoglossal Nerve, Brachial Plexus and Spine Monitoring

Lisa Orloff

Facial Nerve Monitoring: Extratemporal Facial Nerve

16

Julia E. Noel and Lisa A. Orloff

Introduction

The extratemporal facial nerve, or seventh cranial nerve, innervates the muscles of facial expression via the frontal, zygomatic, buccal, and marginal mandibular branches. Injury to this nerve is the most feared complication of parotid surgery and can cause both cosmetic and functional morbidity. While permanent dysfunction is uncommon, up to 40% of patients undergoing parotid surgery may experience temporary facial nerve impairment [1–3]. Ocular and oral deficits are the most devastating, contributing to unwanted side effects and diminished quality of life [4–6].

Nerve injury may occur as a result of stretch, compression, entrapment, thermal injury, ischemia, or division, whether intentional or inadvertent. The likelihood of postoperative dysfunction is influenced by the size, type, and location of a tumor within the gland. An inflamed, scarred, or re-operative field also increases the potential for a nerve-related complication.

Intraoperative nerve monitoring is a tool now used by the majority of otolaryngologists-head and neck surgeons to optimize motor nerve preservation during parotidectomy [7]. The goals of monitoring are to facilitate early nerve identification and mapping, warn of stimulation and reduce unintended trauma, as well as evaluate and prognosticate function at the end of surgery [8]. This chapter will review the types, technique, interpretation, and benefits of intraoperative electrophysiologic monitoring of the extratemporal facial nerve.

Monitoring Methods and Systems

Facial nerve monitoring can be accomplished visually or electrophysiologically. In visual monitoring, an assistant informs the surgeon of facial movements that are evoked mechanically during dissection or electrically with a nerve stimulator. While a simple approach, this information is often used in combination with electrophysiologic monitoring to ensure properly functional equipment and confirm expected responses.

Electrophysiologic monitoring of facial muscle electromyographic (EMG) activity is the more sensitive and quantifiable method. Several electrophysiologic nerve monitoring systems are available commercially. The selection varies geographically as well as based on the preferences and familiarity of the monitoring physician. These systems have between two and eight channels, though two to four are most commonly used in parotid surgery. Recent updates aim to reduce artifact and improve the user interface, but the

J. E. Noel · L. A. Orloff (✉)
Department of Otolaryngology Head & Neck Surgery, Stanford University School of Medicine, Stanford, CA, USA
e-mail: jnoel@stanford.edu; Lorloff@stanford.edu

© The Author(s), under exclusive license to Springer Nature Switzerland AG 2022
J. Scharpf, G. W. Randolph (eds.), *Intraoperative Cranial Nerve Monitoring in Otolaryngology-Head and Neck Surgery*, https://doi.org/10.1007/978-3-030-84916-0_16

fundamental technology remains consistent. Multichannel systems continuously track facial muscle activity and provide immediate feedback regarding mechanically evoked response during dissection. An adjustable pulsed-current stimulation probe is also built in to allow the surgeon the ability to actively stimulate nerve branches. Stimulation results in an audible and visible response that can then be interpreted by the surgeon or electrophysiologist.

Technique

Electrodes are placed transcutaneously into the facial muscles innervated by any or all of the four aforementioned dominant branches (frontal, zygomatic, buccal, marginal mandibular), as depicted in Fig. 16.1. For parotidectomy, two to four channels can be monitored. In two-channel monitoring, electrodes are inserted into the orbicularis oculi and oris muscles. This is sufficient for monitoring the main trunk, though the surgeon should be aware that responses will only be evoked with stimulation of these muscles. If a broader field is desired, four channels can be employed to monitor all main facial nerve branches. Ground and stimulator electrodes are also placed in a separate location. All electrodes are then inserted into a circuit box.

A sterile stimulator probe is also included in the field, with parameters for intensity, duration, rate, and event threshold as determined by the operator. There is no consensus regarding appropriate stimulation values specific to extratemporal facial nerve monitoring. Typical starting parameters include intensity of 0.5 mA, duration of 100 microseconds, rate of 4 bursts/second, and threshold of 100 microvolts. Setup for four-channel monitoring is shown in Fig. 16.2. Stimulating current may be set higher for nerve "seeking" or stimulation through more soft tissue, and threshold may be increased to reduce noise. As the desired output is determined by EMG, it is important to communicate to the anesthesiologist that long-term neuromuscular blockade should be avoided [9].

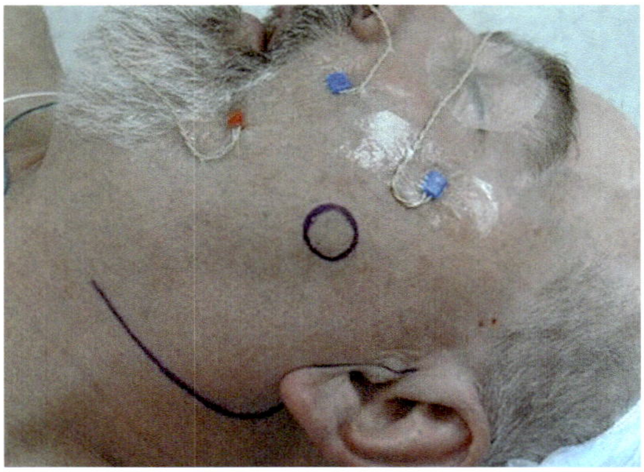

Fig. 16.1 Intraoperative facial nerve monitoring during parotidectomy demonstrating electrode positioning for three-channel monitoring of the zygomatic, marginal mandibular, and cervical branches. The electrodes are placed in the corresponding orbicularis oculi, orbicularis oris, and mentalis muscles

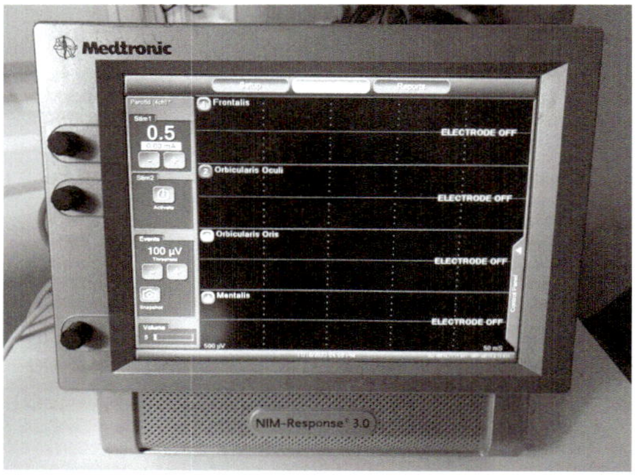

Fig. 16.2 Typical setup for a four-channel EMG monitoring device recording output from the frontalis, orbicularis oculi, orbicularis oris, and mentalis muscles

Interpretation

Accurate interpretation of evoked responses during nerve monitoring is critical to achieve the previously described goals of facial nerve monitoring. Nerve excitability is derived from a change in ion permeability across axonal cell membranes that generates an action potential. A single, synchronous burst of motor unit action potentials is generally associated with direct mechanical nerve stimulation. Virtually, all patients will demonstrate some degree of facial EMG activity related to head turning, tissue retraction, tumor dissection, irrigation, electrocautery, or other surgical maneuvers. While this is most often due to force or heat transmitted from the working area, it is often the first indicator that a facial nerve trunk or branch may be approaching. Maintenance of this burst signal with manipulation throughout the case is indicative of preserved facial nerve function [10].

Multiple asynchronous motor unit discharges that result in tonic or train EMG activity might occur during prolonged tumor dissection or retraction. Train potentials, especially when high in amplitude (>500microvolts), indicate significant compression or stretch of the facial nerve that can be associated with decreased postoperative function. Release of retraction and temporary cessation of dissection are recommended in this scenario.

Electrically evoked stimulation with the handheld stimulation probe is used to help locate, confirm, and map the facial nerve branches. The resolution of electrical mapping is directly related to the stimulus intensity and may be adjusted for the given scenario. When determining the precise location of a nerve trunk or branch, the stimulus is maintained at a minimum level to evoke an EMG response. This allows distinction from the immediately adjacent fascia, sensory nerves, or gland parenchyma. Higher amplitudes might be used to rule out the presence of the nerve within tissue targeted for division. Though this maneuver reduces the likelihood of false-negative results, the absence of an electrically evoked response does not exclude the possibility of facial nerve within the stimulated tissue. Ultimately, information obtained from nerve monitoring is adjunctive, and surgical judgement and knowledge of anatomic relationships must supersede.

Spontaneous EMG activity of the facial muscles will also be evident with lightening of anesthesia. This response is important to recognize as it will interfere with the ability to evoke stimulated responses. In addition, it often precedes patient movement by several seconds and can help guide depth of anesthesia.

At the conclusion of dissection, electrical stimulus is applied proximal to the site of dissection to assess neural integrity and function and aid in predicting postoperative function. Normal response thresholds typically indicate preserved postoperative function, and a recent retrospective study has suggested a post-dissection threshold of 0.25 mA to predict normal movement [2]. Elevated thresholds correlate with some degree of paresis, and absent thresholds indicate at least temporary loss of integrity. This should prompt the surgeon to ensure the nerve is physically intact and attempt repair if a transection is encountered [11]. Alternatively, decreased post-dissection to pre-dissection maximum response amplitudes have also been suggested to indicate nerve conduction abnormalities [12].

Benefits

A growing body of literature has come to support the routine use of facial nerve monitoring during parotidectomy, and its potential benefits are numerous [3, 8, 13–16]. A survey of US physicians in 2005 found the majority (60%) of otolaryngologists-head and neck surgeons employed facial nerve monitoring during parotid surgery. Among those performing greater than ten parotidectomies per year, 79% reported use. Intuitively, surgeons who used nerve monitoring in training are more likely to continue to do so in practice [7]. International literature reflects similar patterns, with 75% of otolaryngologist-head and neck surgeons in Germany and up to 90% in the United Kingdom using intraoperative nerve monitoring during parotidectomy [17, 18].

The ability to actively stimulate is especially useful in cases where nerve localization and preservation might otherwise be difficult. Anatomic landmarks may be distorted by large or deep lobe tumors. Scarring from prior infection, operation, or radiation therapy also renders identification and subsequent dissection challenging. Surgeons pursuing a retrograde approach to the facial nerve also benefit from early confirmation of small, peripheral branches leading back to the main trunk. Particularly with these more superficial branches, differentiation of motor from sensory nerves is aided by electrically evoked stimulation.

The literature addressing the use of facial nerve monitoring and correlation with post-parotidectomy functional outcomes is limited and suffers from a lack of randomized data. A retrospective study of 267 German patients reported a reduced rate of transient palsy with monitoring, but no impact on final function [15]. Conversely, a prospective cohort of patients with benign parotid tumors found no relationship between EMG monitoring and temporary or long-term postoperative facial paralysis [19]. Most recently, the only prospective randomized trial reported more severe immediate facial nerve dysfunction in non-monitored patients, with no difference in overall incidence or final functional status [20]. Overall, the aggregate data supports the effectiveness of facial nerve monitoring in mitigating the incidence and severity of at least immediate weakness [1].

Another potential benefit of nerve monitoring is reduction in operative time. An analysis of 58 cases for recurrent pleomorphic adenoma reported longer surgery duration when monitoring was not used [21]. Similarly, prospective study demonstrated reduced case length for superficial parotidectomy when monitoring was used, regardless of ultimate tumor histology [19].

Nerve monitoring is particularly useful in the teaching setting. In this context, intraoperative monitoring has been shown to correlate with preserved nerve function and significantly lower operative times [22]. Furthermore, feedback to the surgeon in training hones skills of structure recognition and surgical finesse. The trainee learns to differentiate nerve branches from adjacent and similar appearing tissue, to reduce mechanical trauma from dissection and retraction, and to be alerted to facial nerve proximity when not anticipated.

Finally, it is reassuring to the patient to know that all measures are being taken to preserve facial nerve function. Indeed, 14% of US otolaryngologists-head and neck surgeons cite medicolegal protection as a primary motivation to employ electrophysiologic monitoring [7]. Though review of salivary gland litigation did not identify cases filed specifically on the grounds of failure to use monitoring, surgeons using this technology were less likely to have undergone malpractice litigation for nerve injury than their non-monitoring counterparts [23].

Limitations and Potential Complications

A primary criticism of nerve monitoring technology is the potential for unreliable feedback [7]. The surgeon must be familiar with and able to interpret EMG waveform and amplitude in the context of what is transpiring in the operative field. False-positive errors most often occur with stimulus evoked EMG, typically when stimulation of a structure adjacent the facial nerve results in a positive signal through conduction of current. This may lead to incorrect identification of a nerve branch. The error can be minimized by reducing the amplitude to the threshold stimulus level. Bipolar stimulators, which have a narrower field of current conduction, may alternatively be used. Other sources of artifact signal include cautery use, bimetallic instrument contact, lightening of anesthesia, cold saline irrigation, or inadvertent pressure on the electrode or facial muscle by an assistant.

False-negative errors can also occur and are generally more dangerous as they provide a false sense of security. Reliance on this feedback can lead to subsequent nerve division. As mentioned previously, anatomic knowledge and judgement are paramount and primary. Current shunted away by overlying fluid or soft tissue may result in inadequate depolarizing current, despite having directly stimulated the facial nerve. Neuromuscular blockade induces paralysis unrelated to the surgical field or dissection. Improper setup of the monitoring system or inadvertent movement of electrodes or circuit box during the case may also generate false negatives.

There have been prior case reports of nerve fatigue and temporary paresis with overstimulation [24]. It is worth noting, however, that these have resulted from continuous stimulation. The pulsed stimulation of the more current monitoring systems is unlikely to cause weakness.

Rarely, the monitoring device or electrodes can result in superficial injury. With sterile technique and thoughtful placement as well as removal, infection and prolonged bleeding or bruising can be avoided. Needle electrodes must be handled carefully, especially once removed from the patient, and disposed of appropriately. Facial burns have been reported at the sites of electrode insertion, though not with updated and approved technology [25].

Conclusions

Facial nerve monitoring is an important adjunctive tool in surgery of the parotid gland. Along with understanding of expected anatomic relationships, information obtained during monitoring assists in identification and preservation of the facial nerve. A sufficiently powered randomized clinical trial to assess the benefit of facial nerve monitoring in reducing the immediate or long-term frequency of facial nerve paralysis is unlikely to be completed, given the already widespread adoption of and surgeon preference for monitoring and its low risk to perceived high benefit. Intraoperative facial nerve monitoring is safe and simple and has many objective advantages, including mapping of the facial nerve branches, ability to differentiate facial nerve from other tissue, recognition of potentially injurious mechanical manipulation, and acquisition of prognostic information about postoperative function.

References

1. Sood AJ, Houlton JJ, Nguyen SA, Gillespie MB. Facial nerve monitoring during parotidectomy: a systematic review and meta-analysis. In: Otolaryngology – head and neck surgery (United States), vol. 152. SAGE Publications Inc.; 2015. p. 631–7. https://doi.org/10.1177/0194599814568779.
2. Haring CT, Ellsperman SE, Edwards BM, et al. Assessment of intraoperative nerve monitoring parameters associated with facial nerve outcome in parotidectomy for benign disease. JAMA Otolaryngol Head Neck Surg. 2019;145(12):1137–43. https://doi.org/10.1001/jamaoto.2019.1041.
3. Eisele DW, Wang SJ, Orloff LA. Electrophysiologic facial nerve monitoring during parotidectomy. Head Neck. 2009;32(3):399–405. https://doi.org/10.1002/hed.21190.
4. Saadi R, Shokri T, Schaefer E, Hollenbeak C, Lighthall JG. Depression rates after facial paralysis. Ann Plast Surg. 2019;83(2):190–4. https://doi.org/10.1097/SAP.0000000000001908.
5. Ryzenman JM, Pensak ML, Tew JM. Facial paralysis and surgical rehabilitation: a quality of life analysis in a cohort of 1,595 patients after acoustic neuroma surgery. Otol Neurotol. 2005;26(3):516–21. https://doi.org/10.1097/01.mao.0000169786.22707.12.
6. Lydiatt DD. Medical malpractice and facial nerve paralysis. Arch Otolaryngol Head Neck Surg. 2003;129(1):50–3. https://doi.org/10.1001/archotol.129.1.50.
7. Lowry TR, Gal TJ, Brennan JA. Patterns of use of facial nerve monitoring during parotid gland surgery. Otolaryngol Head Neck Surg. 2005;133(3):313–8. https://doi.org/10.1016/j.otohns.2005.03.010.
8. Guntinas-Lichius O, Eisele DW. Facial nerve monitoring. Adv Otorhinolaryngol. 2016;78:46–52. https://doi.org/10.1159/000442124.
9. Naguib M, Brull SJ, Kopman AF, et al. Consensus statement on perioperative use of neuromuscular monitoring. Anesth Analg. 2018;127(1):71–80. https://doi.org/10.1213/ANE.0000000000002670.
10. Kircher ML, Kartush JM. Pitfalls in intraoperative nerve monitoring during vestibular schwannoma surgery. Neurosurg Focus. 2012;33(3):E5. https://doi.org/10.3171/2012.7.FOCUS12196.
11. Guntinas-Lichius O, Silver CE, Thielker J, et al. Management of the facial nerve in parotid cancer: preservation or resection and reconstruction. Eur Arch Oto Rhino Laryngol. 2018; https://doi.org/10.1007/s00405-018-5154-6.
12. Mamelle E, Bernat I, Pichon S, et al. Supramaximal stimulation during intraoperative facial nerve monitoring as a simple parameter to predict early functional outcome after parotidectomy. Acta Otolaryngol. 2013; https://doi.org/10.3109/00016489.2013.771283.
13. Witt RL. Facial nerve monitoring in parotid surgery: the standard of care? Otolaryngol Head Neck Surg. 1998; https://doi.org/10.1016/S0194-5998(98)70103-2.
14. Petrides GA, Subramaniam N, Pham M, Clark JR. Reducing the morbidity of parotidectomy for benign pathology. ANZ J Surg. 2020; https://doi.org/10.1111/ans.16008.
15. Savvas E, Hillmann S, Weiss D, Koopmann M, Rudack C, Alberty J. Association between facial nerve monitoring with postoperative facial paralysis in parotidectomy. JAMA Otolaryngol Head Neck Surg. 2016;142(9):828–33. https://doi.org/10.1001/jamaoto.2016.1192.
16. Chiesa-Estomba CM, Larruscain-Sarasola E, Lechien JR, et al. Facial nerve monitoring during parotid gland surgery: a systematic review and meta-analysis.

Eur Arch Oto Rhino Laryngol. 2020; https://doi.org/10.1007/s00405-020-06188-0.

17. Hopkins C, Khemani S, Terry RM, Golding-Wood D. How we do it: nerve monitoring in ENT surgery: current UK practice. Clin Otolaryngol. 2005;30(2):195–8. https://doi.org/10.1111/j.1365-2273.2004.00933.x.
18. Preuss SF, Guntinas-Lichius O. On the diagnosis and treatment of parotid gland tumors. Results of a nationwide survey of ENT hospitals in Germany. HNO. 2006; https://doi.org/10.1007/s00106-006-1394-7.
19. Grosheva M, Klussmann JP, Grimminger C, et al. Electromyographic facial nerve monitoring during parotidectomy for benign lesions does not improve the outcome of postoperative facial nerve function: a prospective two-center trial. Laryngoscope. 2009;119(12):2299–305. https://doi.org/10.1002/lary.20637.
20. Graciano AJ, Fischer CA, Coelho GV, Steck JH, Paschoal JR, Chone CT. Facial nerve dysfunction after superficial parotidectomy with or without continuous intraoperative electromyographic neuromonitoring: a prospective randomized pilot study. Eur Arch Oto Rhino Laryngol. 2018;275(11):2861–8. https://doi.org/10.1007/s00405-018-5130-1.
21. Liu H, Wen W, Huang H, et al. Recurrent pleomorphic adenoma of the parotid gland: intraoperative facial nerve monitoring during parotidectomy. Otolaryngol Head Neck Surg (United States). 2014;151(1):87–91. https://doi.org/10.1177/0194599814528098.
22. Deneuve S, Quesnel S, Depondt J, et al. Management of parotid gland surgery in a university teaching hospital. Eur Arch Oto Rhino Laryngol. 2010;267(4):601–5. https://doi.org/10.1007/s00405-009-1088-3.
23. Hong SS, Yheulon CG, Sniezek JC. Salivary gland surgery and medical malpractice. Otolaryngol Head Neck Surg (United States). 2013;148(4):589–94. https://doi.org/10.1177/0194599813475566.
24. Love JT, Marchbanks JR. Injury to the facial nerve associated with the use of a disposable nerve stimulator. Otolaryngology. 1978;86(1) https://doi.org/10.1177/019459987808600112.
25. Russell MJ, Gaetz M. Intraoperative electrode burns. J Clin Monit Comput. 2004;18(1):25–32. https://doi.org/10.1023/B:JOCM.0000025254.73456.db.

Spinal Accessory Nerve Monitoring in Head and Neck Surgery

17

Nicole Molin and Jeffrey C. Liu

Introduction

The spinal accessory nerve (SAN) is a vital structure encountered in many surgeries of the head and neck. The anatomy is complex, and identification intraoperatively is key to preventing injury and subsequent postoperative shoulder syndrome. Intraoperative nerve monitoring is widely used in various head and neck surgeries; however, it has more recently been applied to the SAN, although literature to support the use is variable and relatively limited. This chapter will detail the anatomy of the SAN, review the presentation and prevalence of postoperative shoulder syndrome, summarize surgeries that put the SAN at risk, and finally review the literature on SAN monitoring in head and neck surgery.

N. Molin (✉)
Department of Otolaryngology Head and Neck Surgery, Lewis Katz School of Medicine at Temple University, Philadelphia, PA, USA
e-mail: Nicole.molin@tuhs.temple.edu

J. C. Liu
Department of Otolaryngology Head and Neck Surgery, Lewis Katz School of Medicine at Temple University, Philadelphia, PA, USA

Department of Surgical Oncology, Fox Chase Cancer Center, Philadelphia, PA, USA
e-mail: Jeffrey.Liu@temple.edu

Anatomy

The SAN or cranial nerve 11 (CN XI) has both a spinal and cranial root joined together only briefly as they course through the jugular foramen. The cranial root originates in the dorsolateral surface of the medulla oblongata and eventually joins with the superior ganglion of the vagus nerve [1]. The spinal root, which provides somatic motor function to the sternocleidomastoid (SCM) and trapezius muscles, arises from the cervical spinal nerves of vertebral levels C1 to C5 within the accessory nucleus of the dorsolateral part of the ventral horn. The nerves course between the dorsal and ventral spinal roots to form a trunk that ascends to enter the posterior cranial fossa through the foramen magnum, exiting through the jugular foramen [2, 3]. Though the spinal portion arises from cervical rootlets, the fibers join briefly with the cranial fibers in the jugular foramen, prior to exiting the cranial cavity. The nerve then courses in proximity to the internal jugular vein (IJV). At the level of the superior border of the posterior belly of the digastric, the SAN most commonly courses lateral to the IJV, but can less commonly course medially and rarely directly through the IJV [4]. The nerve continues its complex course through the neck traversing anterior to the transverse process of the atlas and descending medial to the styloid process and stylohyoid and digastric muscles. It subse-

© The Author(s), under exclusive license to Springer Nature Switzerland AG 2022
J. Scharpf, G. W. Randolph (eds.), *Intraoperative Cranial Nerve Monitoring in Otolaryngology-Head and Neck Surgery*, https://doi.org/10.1007/978-3-030-84916-0_17

quently enters the deep surface of the SCM, where it may anastomose with fibers of C2–C5 and rarely with C1 [5]. The contribution of these cervical fibers to motor function is not fully understood [6]. This segment of the SAN also serves as an important landmark for subdividing level II of the neck, marking the boundary between levels IIa and IIb [7]. The proximal IJV is used as a landmark to identify the proximal SAN in the anterior triangle and Erb's point in the posterior triangle. If an imaginary line is drawn from this point to the thyroid notch, the SAN will enter the posterior triangle within 2 cm above this level and exit within 2 cm below it [8]. The SAN begins its course through the posterior triangle of the neck as it emerges from the posterior border of the SCM, approximately 7–9 cm above the clavicle, passing about 1–2 cm superiorly to Erb's point [1]. Within the posterior triangle of the neck, the nerve crosses superficial to the levator scapulae and enters the trapezius muscle approximately 5 cm above the clavicle [2, 3].

Postoperative Shoulder Syndrome

Any surgery that injures the SAN can result in postoperative shoulder syndrome, which is caused by trapezius muscle denervation. When first described in the 1950s, the findings of postoperative shoulder syndrome were viewed as minor and acceptable side effects following radical neck dissection (RND) [9]. Most neck dissections now are function sparing, which include preservation of the SCM and SAN making postoperative shoulder syndrome less common [10]. Patients with postoperative shoulder syndrome present with pain, weakness, and deformity of the shoulder girdle. They can have destabilization of the scapula with progressive flaring, drooping, lateral and anterior rotation, as well as decreased ability to abduct the shoulder above 90 degrees. Secondary glenohumeral stiffness from scapulohumeral girdle muscle weakness and postoperative immobility can also contribute to shoulder disability [11]. For those with SAN preservation, improvement in symptoms from postoperative shoulder syndrome can be seen 6 months to a year postoperatively as the nerve fibers recover and regenerate [12].

The prevalence of shoulder dysfunction varies by the type of surgery. Following posterior triangle lymph node biopsy, the prevalence is between 3% and 8% [8] [13]. The prevalence of findings following neck dissection is variable and is highest after RND when the SAN is sacrificed. The presence of shoulder droop following RND ranges from 44% to 100%, modified radical neck dissection with SAN preservation (MRND) 0% to 30%, selective neck dissection (SND) levels II–V 56%, and SND levels I–III 13%. Reduction in shoulder active abduction range of motion following unilateral RND ranges between 92% and 94%, bilateral RND 100%, and MRND 23%. The prevalence of reduced neck range of motion following RND is as high as 45% and 13% following MRND [14].

Postoperative shoulder syndrome may have a significant impact on patient's quality of life (QOL) and is a significant source of malpractice litigations [15]. The impact on QOL after neck dissection has been evaluated using a variety of validated questionnaires – SF-36 [16], SF-12 [17], or HNQOL [18] . Validated patient-reported outcomes have been reported in the literature that specifically evaluate shoulder function such as the Shoulder and Pain Disability Index (SPADI) and Constant Shoulder Score [19]. While the impact on quality of life is multifactorial, in general, those with the highest decline in QOL tend to be those patients who had SAN resection [12].

Surgeries that Risk the SAN

Compromise of the SAN is a known complication of many head and neck surgeries, in particular those closer in proximity to the posterior triangle and lateral skull base.

Neck Dissection

Neck dissection, also referred to as cervical lymphadenectomy, is a commonly performed procedure for head and neck cancer and widely known to risk the SAN. SAN injury can occur even when the nerve is macroscopically intact.

Injuries can be on a spectrum of neural dysfunction, from neuropraxia and axonotmesis to neurotmesis [20]. The observed morbidity and disability of postoperative shoulder syndrome motivated a trend from RND toward MRND. Demonstration of similar survival and regional control with MRND over RND further supported this transition [21, 22]. SND is also becoming more accepted for appropriate patients [23]. As alluded to above QOL seems to be less affected in those patients who undergo SND involving levels I–III, although care should be taken to protect the proximal segment of the SAN as it courses along the IJV toward the SCM in level II of the neck. Neck dissections involving level V tend to be associated with higher risk to the distal portion of the SAN as it emerges from the posterior border of the SCM and courses through the posterior triangle.

Surgery in the Posterior Triangle

Surgery in the area of the posterior triangle, such as lymph node biopsy, puts the SAN at risk and makes up a majority of malpractice claims related to SAN iatrogenic injury [15]. SAN injury is estimated to occur after 3–8% of posterior triangle lymph node biopsies [8, 13]. As the nerve courses through the posterior triangle, it is surrounded by fibrofatty tissue and associated with a chain of five to ten lymph nodes; however, the nerve may also course superficially to these nodes [8].

Lateral Skull Base Surgery

The SAN is at particular risk in lateral skull base surgery that involves the jugular foramen. Here, the SAN exits the skull base with cranial nerves IX and X, and all these nerves are at risk. The jugular foramen is divided into three compartments, CN IX exits through the anterior compartment and CN X and XI through the middle compartment [24]. Care must be taken to preserve the SAN in this complex space. The most common tumors of this area are glomus jugulare, schwannomas, and meningiomas [25].

SAN Monitoring

SAN injury has a significant impact on patients, and despite the trend toward nerve-sparing surgeries, SAN injury still remains a worrisome complication. The SAN function can be preserved in a variety of ways intraoperatively. Visible and palpable muscle response of the SCM and trapezius can signal proximity of the nerve without the use of electrodes. Given the size of these muscles, this response is most often noticeable. Electromyography (EMG) measures action potentials of a muscle via electrodes placed into the muscle of interest. The SAN can be monitored by placement of electrodes into the trapezius muscle. EMG can be further divided into evoked, passive, and continuous monitoring, the former two methods can be utilized for SAN monitoring. Evoked nerve monitoring involves the surgeon stimulating the nerve to create a measured response. In contrast, passive nerve monitoring relies on analysis of various discharge patterns that occur throughout the operation and does not involve active stimulation of the nerve. Continuous monitoring involves continuously stimulating the nerve of interest for the entire procedure while measuring response; this method is available only for select nerves, not including the SAN [26].

EMG SAN monitoring is set up in a similar manner to that of facial nerve monitoring, with electrodes placed into the trapezius muscle [27]. Typically, bursts and trains of motor unit potential activity during surgery are continuously monitored in addition to deliberate electrical stimulation of the nerve while recording compound muscle action potential of the innervated muscle [20]. SAN monitoring can aid in identification of the nerve and alert the surgeon of proximity even prior to identification. The surgeon can stimulate the nerve directly at the end of the case to assess function, with the goal of preventing postoperative shoulder syndrome [27].

Currently, there is no standard of care when it comes to intraoperative SAN monitoring in head and neck surgery, leaving the decision at the discretion of the surgeon. As SAN monitoring is a relatively newer innovation, literature on the topic is limited [20] [28]. Data supporting SAN monitoring to prevent postoperative shoulder syndrome is variable. Intraoperative SAN monitoring during MRND has been shown to improve postoperative EMG scores; however, clinical scores related to postoperative shoulder syndrome were similar, whether nerve monitoring was used or not [29]. Lee and colleagues also studied 25 consecutive patients undergoing selective neck dissection with spinal accessory nerve monitoring and had no patient with postoperative shoulder syndrome sequelae other than mild pain; however, there was no comparative control group [28].

If the decision is made to use SAN monitoring, certain parameters can aid in predicting which patients may suffer from shoulder function decline postoperatively. These include threshold increment of greater than 0.25–0.5 mA [20, 30] and amplitude decrement of greater than 72% during surgery [30]. These findings may not always correlate with clinical outcomes and seem to have more specificity than sensitivity in predicting shoulder dysfunction [20, 31]. While these parameters are not completely predictive, the information can help in counseling patients in the postoperative period and may help in setting expectations for recovery. We were not able to identify any literature documenting the frequency of SAN monitoring use during neck dissection among surgeons.

Conclusion/Summary

The spinal accessory nerve (SAN) is a vital structure encountered in many surgeries of the head and neck. The anatomy of the SAN is complex, and identification intraoperatively is key in preventing injury. Postoperative shoulder syndrome resulting from SAN compromise has a significant impact on patient's QOL. Intraoperative SAN monitoring can be used to identify the SAN, as well as assess nerve integrity during and at the end of surgery. Literature to support the use of SAN monitoring is variable and relatively limited, and decision for use is based on surgeon preference and discretion.

References

1. Overland J, Hodge JC, Breik O, Krishnan S. Surgical anatomy of the spinal accessory nerve: review of the literature and case report of a rare anatomical variant. J Laryngol Otol. 2016;130(10):969.
2. Wilkinson JL. Neuroanatomy for medical students [Internet]. Butterworth-Heinemann; 1992. Available from: https://books.google.com/books?id=wbp8yQEACAAJ.
3. Rea P. Chapter 11 – Spinal accessory nerve. In: Rea PBT-CA of the CN, editor. San Diego: Academic Press; 2014. p. 117–25. Available from: http://www.sciencedirect.com/science/article/pii/B9780128008980000117.
4. Hinsley ML, Hartig GK. Anatomic relationship between the spinal accessory nerve and internal jugular vein in the upper neck. Otolaryngol Neck Surg. 2010;143(2):239–41.
5. Standring S. Gray's anatomy E-book: the anatomical basis of clinical practice. Elsevier Health Sciences; 2016.
6. Weisberger EC. The efferent supply of the trapezius muscle: a neuroanatomic basis for the preservation of shoulder function during neck dissection. Laryngoscope. 1987;97(4):435–45.
7. Robbins KT, Clayman G, Levine PA, Medina J, Sessions R, Shaha A, et al. Neck dissection classification update: revisions proposed by the American Head and Neck Society and the American Academy of Otolaryngology–Head and Neck Surgery. Arch Otolaryngol Neck Surg [Internet]. 2002;128(7):751–8. Available from: https://doi.org/10.1001/archotol.128.7.751.
8. Nason RW, Abdulrauf BM, Stranc MF. The anatomy of the accessory nerve and cervical lymph node biopsy. Am J Surg. 2000;180(3):241–3.
9. Ewing MR, Martin H. Disability following "radical neck dissection". An assessment based on the postoperative evaluation of 100 patients. Cancer. 1952;5(5):873–83.
10. Goldstein DP, Ringash J, Bissada E, Jaquet Y, Irish J, Chepeha D, et al. Scoping review of the literature on shoulder impairments and disability after neck dissection. Head Neck. 2014;36(2):299–308.

11. Johnson JT, Rosen CA. Bailey's head & neck surgery otolaryngology. Lippincott; 2014.
12. Terrell JE, Welsh DE, Bradford CR, Chepeha DB, Esclamado RM, Hogikyan ND, et al. Pain, quality of life, and spinal accessory nerve status after neck dissection. Laryngoscope [Internet]. 2000;110(4):620–6. Available from: https://doi.org/10.1097/00005537-200004000-00016.
13. Valtonen EJ, Lilius HG. Late sequelae of iatrogenic spinal accessory nerve injury. Acta Chir Scand. 1974;140(6):453–5.
14. Gane EM, Michaleff ZA, Cottrell MA, McPhail SM, Hatton AL, Panizza BJ, et al. Prevalence, incidence, and risk factors for shoulder and neck dysfunction after neck dissection: a systematic review. Eur J Surg Oncol [Internet]. 2017;43(7):1199–218. Available from: http://www.sciencedirect.com/science/article/pii/S0748798316309660.
15. Morris LGT, Ziff DJS, DeLacure MD. Malpractice litigation after surgical injury of the spinal accessory nerve: an evidence-based analysis. Arch Otolaryngol Neck Surg [Internet]. 2008;134(1):102–7. Available from: https://doi.org/10.1001/archotol.134.1.102.
16. Ware Jr JE. SF-36 health survey. 1999;
17. Ware JE, Keller SD, Kosinski M. SF-12: how to score the SF-12 physical and mental health summary scales. Health Institute, New England Medical Center; 1995.
18. Terrell JE, Nanavati KA, Esclamado RM, Bishop JK, Bradford CR, Wolf GT. Head and neck cancer—specific quality of life: instrument validation. Arch Otolaryngol Neck Surg. 1997;123(10):1125–32.
19. Constant CR, Murley AG. A clinical method of functional assessment of the shoulder. Clin Orthop Relat Res. 1987;214:160–4.
20. McGarvey AC, Hoffman GR, Osmotherly PG, Chiarelli PE. Intra-operative monitoring of the spinal accessory nerve: a systematic review. J Laryngol Otol. 2014;128(9):746.
21. Chu W, Strawitz JG. Results in suprahyoid, modified radical, and standard radical neck dissections for metastatic squamous cell carcinoma: recurrence and survival. Am J Surg [Internet]. 1978;136(4):512–5. Available from: http://www.sciencedirect.com/science/article/pii/0002961078902726.
22. Jesse RH, Ballantyne AJ, Larson D. Radical or modified neck dissection: a therapeutic dilemma. Am J Surg [Internet]. 1978;136(4):516–9. Available from: http://www.sciencedirect.com/science/article/pii/0002961078902738.
23. Muzaffar K. Therapeutic selective neck dissection: a 25-year review. Laryngoscope [Internet]. 2003;113(9):1460–5. Available from: https://doi.org/10.1097/00005537-200309000-00005.
24. Lloyd S. Accessory nerve: anatomy and surgical identification. J Laryngol Otol [Internet]. 2007;121(12):1118–25. Available from: http://libproxy.temple.edu/login?url=https://search.proquest.com/docview/274820196?accountid=14270.
25. Griessenauer CJ, McGrew B, Matusz P, De Caro R, Loukas M, Tubbs RS. Surgical approaches to the Jugular Foramen: a comprehensive review. J Neurol Surg B Skull Base [Internet]. 2015/11/16. 2016;77(3):260–4. Available from: https://pubmed.ncbi.nlm.nih.gov/27175322.
26. Stankovic P, Wittlinger J, Georgiew R, Dominas N, Hoch S, Wilhelm T. Continuous intraoperative neuromonitoring (cIONM) in head and neck surgery—a review. HNO. 2020:1–7.
27. Midwinter K, Willatt D. Accessory nerve monitoring and stimulation during neck surgery. J Laryngol Otol. 2002;116(4):272–4.
28. Lee C-H, Huang N-C, Chen H-C, Chen M-K. Minimizing shoulder syndrome with intra-operative spinal accessory nerve monitoring for neck dissection. Acta Otorhinolaryngol Ital. 2013;33(2):93.
29. Lanišnik B, Žitnik L, Levart P, Žargi M, Rodi Z. The impact on post-operative shoulder function of intra-operative nerve monitoring of cranial nerve XI during modified radical neck dissection. Eur Arch Oto Rhino Laryngol. 2016;273(12):4445–51.
30. Birinci Y, Genc A, Ecevit MC, Erdag TK, Guneri EA, Oztura I, et al. Spinal accessory nerve monitoring and clinical outcome results of nerve-sparing neck dissections. Otolaryngol Neck Surg. 2014;151(2):253–9.
31. Witt RL, Rejto L. Spinal accessory nerve monitoring in selective and modified neck dissection. Laryngoscope. 2007;117(5):776–80.

Glossopharyngeal (CN IX) and Hypoglossal (CN XII) Nerve Stimulation and Monitoring

18

Maria V. Suurna and David L. Steward

Glossopharyngeal Nerve (CN IX)

The glossopharyngeal nerve has primarily a sensory function but does have a motor component that innervates the stylopharyngeus muscle, which is involved in elevating the larynx and dilating the pharynx during swallowing. The glossopharyngeal nerve exits the jugular foramen posterior-medial to the styloid process before innervating the stylopharyngeus muscle [1] and is vulnerable to injury during surgery for tumors of the jugular foramen [2, 3]. Because branches of the vagus (CN X) also innervate muscles involved in deglutition, monitoring both simultaneously is necessary to differentiate the glossopharyngeal component during surgery [4, 5]. Reduction in the ratio of glossopharyngeal to vagal amplitude is associated with soft palate dysfunction, dysphagia, and loss of gag reflex [6]. Combined glossopharyngeal and vagal nerve monitoring has also been used to perform selective rhizotomy in treatment of glossopharyngeal neuralgia with a reported 88% success rate [7]. Techniques for simultaneous CN IX and X monitoring include a modified endotracheal tube to include surface electrodes abutting the soft palate (IX) in addition to those abutting the vocal folds (X) [5], or with electromyography (EMG) needle electrodes placed within the soft palate (IX) and cricothyroid (X) muscles [7]. Either way, a 50% difference in the IX/X signal ratio appears significant.

Hypoglossal Nerve (CN XII)

Overview

The hypoglossal nerve provides primary motor innervation to the tongue, the function of which is critical for speaking, swallowing, and maintaining the oropharyngeal airway. The hypoglossal nerve exits the skull through the hypoglossal canal near the jugular foramen and descends between the carotid bifurcation traversing horizontally along the hyoid deep to the digastric muscle and tendon and then ascends superiorly and medially innervating the extrinsic and intrinsic tongue muscles along the way [8–13]. A cervical contributing branch of C1 tags along with the hypoglossal nerve in its horizontal segment to provide innervation to the geniohyoid muscle. Other cervical contributing branches of C1–C2 descend below the hyoid where the hypoglossal

M. V. Suurna (✉)
Department of Otolaryngology-Head and Neck Surgery, Weill Cornell Medicine, New York, NY, USA
e-mail: mas9390@med.cornell.edu

D. L. Steward
Department of Otolaryngology-Head and Neck Surgery, University of Cincinnati, College of Medicine, Cincinnati, OH, USA
e-mail: David.Steward@uc.edu

© The Author(s), under exclusive license to Springer Nature Switzerland AG 2022
J. Scharpf, G. W. Randolph (eds.), *Intraoperative Cranial Nerve Monitoring in Otolaryngology-Head and Neck Surgery*, https://doi.org/10.1007/978-3-030-84916-0_18

turns horizontally to innervate the infra-hyoid strap musculature along with ascending branches of C2–C3 as part of the ansa hypoglossal/ansa cervicalis nerve loop [14, 15]. The hypoglossal nerve has traditionally been vulnerable to injury during surgery of the tongue and upper neck including head and neck cancers, hypoglossal to facial nerve anastomosis, tumors of the jugular foramen, and carotid endarterectomy [13]. Hypoglossal nerve stimulation and monitoring have successfully been used selectively for some of these cases [16–20]. More recently, hypoglossal nerve stimulation with monitoring has become critical to distal nerve branch identification to facilitate accurate cuff electrode placement for hypoglossal nerve stimulator implantation to treat obstructive sleep apnea (OSA), in both adults and children [21–25]. This has resulted in renewed interest in distal hypoglossal neuroanatomy and its clinical relevance to selective hypoglossal cranial nerve stimulator implants for OSA [10, 26] (Fig. 18.1). Perhaps in no other surgery involving the lower cranial motor nerves are direct surgeon stimulation and EMG monitoring of the various branches of the nerve more critical to the successful outcome of surgery [27–29]. Commercially available, FDA-approved hypoglossal nerve stimulation (HNS) implants manufactured by Inspire Medical Systems (Minneapolis, MN), when activated, deliver neurostimulation from a pulse generator via a wire and electrode cuff placed precisely on the hypoglossal nerve to result in tongue advancement to open the pharyngeal airway. HNS therapy for OSA is based on the concept that selective stimulation of the nerve fibers that protrude and stiffen the tongue muscles will prevent the upper airway collapse and resolve airway obstruction during sleep. Failure to include the branches to the genioglossus (GG) muscle (which protrudes the tongue) and/or failure to exclude the branches to the styloglossus (SG) and hyoglossus (HG) muscles (which retract the tongue) within the cuff electrode (Fig. 18.2) will result in failure to improve OSA with hypoglossal nerve stimulation therapy [30–32] Current surgical technique also encourages identification and inclusion of the C1 branch which innervates geniohyoid muscle, resulting in anterior hyoid bone movement to further increase hypopharyngeal airway opening. However, inclusion of the C1 branch to the geniohyoid muscle appears less critical to surgical implant success than inclusion of the GG and exclusion of the SG/HG muscles [33].

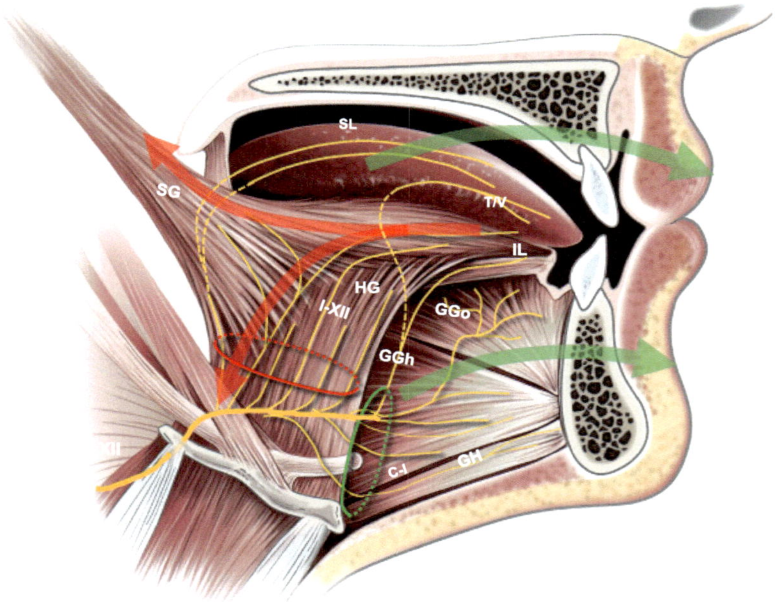

Fig. 18.1 Hypoglossal nerve (XII) anatomy. Styloglossus muscle (SG), hyoglossus (HG), genioglossus horizontal (GGh), genioglossus oblique (GGo), transverse/vertical muscles (T/V), superior longitudinal (SL), inferior longitudinal (IL), geniohyoid (GH), cervical nerve 1 (C1); red, direction of action lateral division; green, direction of action of the medial division (Reprinted with permission)

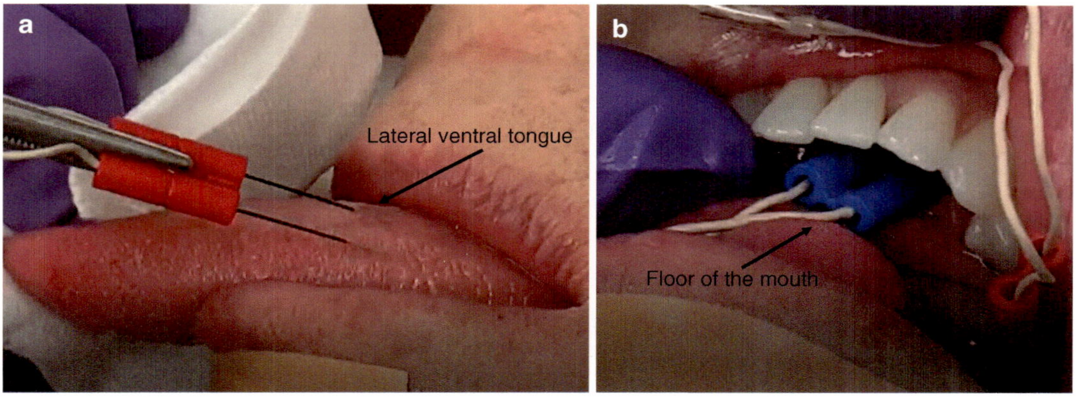

Fig. 18.2 Images taken from the head of the patient. (**a**) Insertion of EMG needle electrodes into styloglossus/hyoglossus muscle. (**b**) Insertion of EMG needles into genioglossus muscle

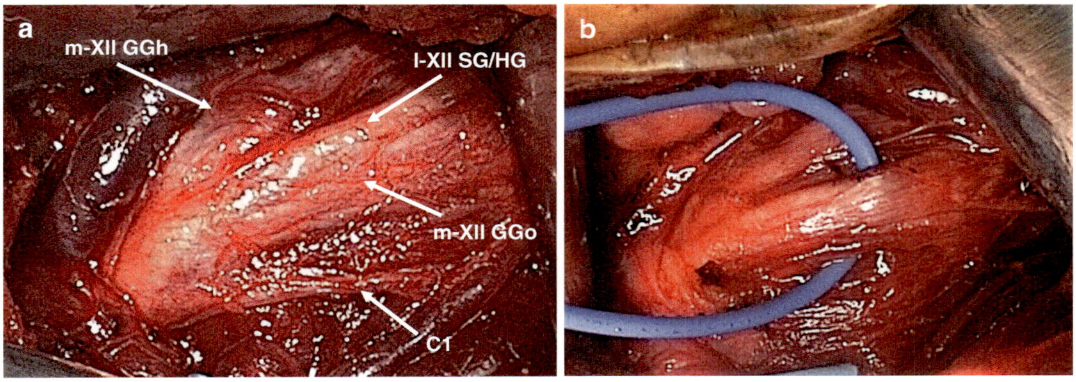

Fig. 18.3 (**a**) Intraoperative hypoglossal (HG) (XII) nerve anatomy. Lateral division styloglossus/hyoglossus (l-XII SG/HG), medial division genioglossus horizontal (m-XII GGh), and genioglossus oblique (m-XII GGo); cervical nerve 1 (C1). (**b**) Separation of the lateral and medial nerve divisions using a vessel loop

Hypoglossal Nerve Branch Identification with Stimulation and Monitoring: Technical Aspects

Accurate intraoperative identification of inferior/medial and superior/lateral fibers of the hypoglossal nerve is essential for precise neurostimulator cuff placement. Nerve activity is monitored by analyzing EMG responses to selective bipolar stimulation of the distal branches of the nerve. It is imperative that no muscle relaxant or paralytic agents are used as part of general anesthesia during the procedure to allow monitoring during nerve stimulation for accurate branch identification as well as to permit monitoring during cuff placement to minimize trauma from excessive traction. Typically, single-use Prass Paired EMG 18 mm needle electrodes (Medtronic Xomed, Ref 8,227,304) are used to measure GG and SG/HG responses to nerve branch stimulation. Blue-color-coded EMG needles are inserted into the GG muscle through the floor of the mouth just off the midline on the side of the implant, avoiding Wharton's duct (Fig. 18.3a). The red-color-coded EMG needles are placed submucosally into HG/SG muscles along the ventral side of the lateral tongue about 5 cm from the tip of the tongue (Fig. 18.3b). The electrodes are connected to a nerve integrity monitoring (NIM) system.

During dissection, the hypoglossal nerve is identified deep to the anterior portion of the submandibular gland as it is retracted posteriorly,

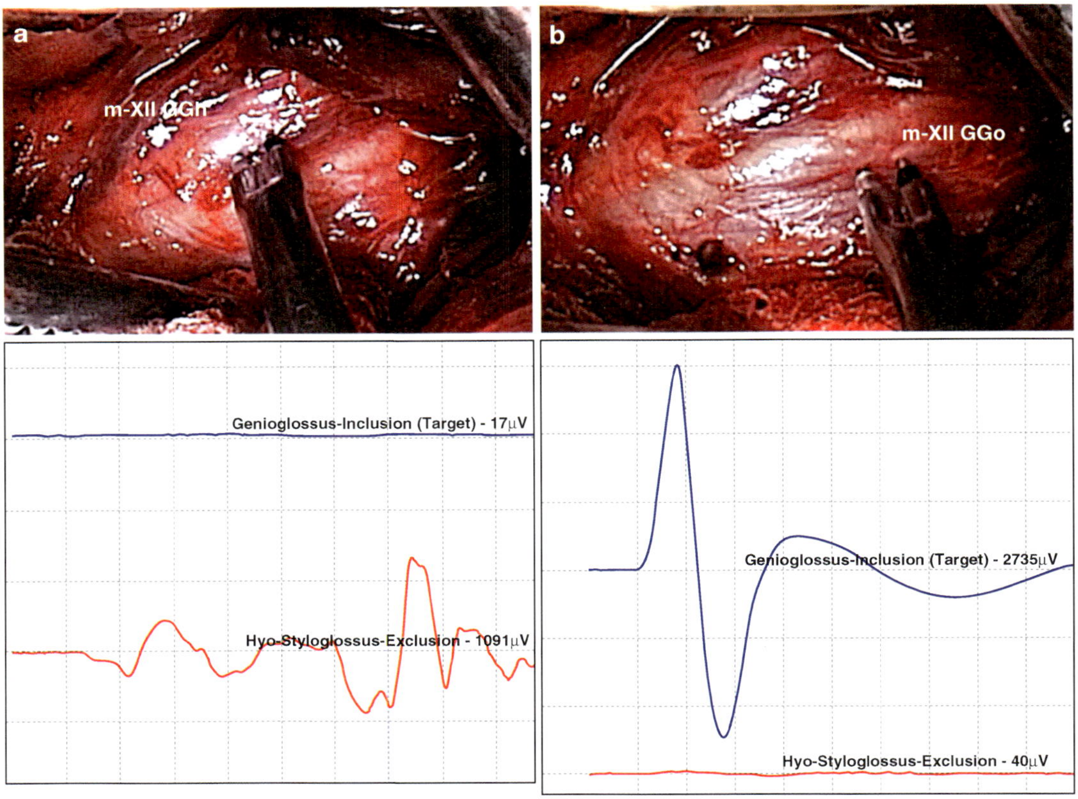

Fig. 18.4 (**a**) EMG response on the hyoglossus/styloglossus channel to stimulation of the lateral division. (**b**) EMG response on the genioglossus channel to stimulation of the medial division

digastric tendon as it is retracted inferiorly, and mylohyoid muscle as it is retracted anterior and superiorly. Distal dissection of the nerve is performed, separating it from the ranine vein. Once the branching point of inferior/medial and superior/lateral fibers is visually identified, a Bipolar Stimulating Probe (Medtronic Xomed, Ref 8,225,401) is used to stimulate the nerve using 0.1 to 0.3 mA to confirm the function of the fibers based on EMG responses recorded by the NIM system [34]. Figure 18.4 demonstrates an EMG response seen when SG/HG nerve fibers from the superior/lateral branches of the hypoglossal nerve are stimulated. Polyphasic EMG response is seen in the red SG/HG channel, and no response is present in blue GG channel (Fig. 18.4a). When GG nerve fibers from the inferior/medial branches of the hypoglossal nerve are stimulated, monophasic response is seen in GG channel and no response in SG/HG channel (Fig. 18.4b). In cases when nerve fibers innervating intrinsic muscles of the tongue are adherent to the inferior/medial division of the hypoglossal nerve, EMG activity can be observed in the SG/HG channel with a synchronous wave pattern with the GG channel (Fig. 18.5a). Distinction should be made between the EMG response when intrinsic muscle nerve fibers are present within the dissected inferior/medial branch and when late takeoff superior/lateral retractor fibers supplying SG/HG have not been adequately separated from the inferior/medial division. In case of a retained retractor branch, stimulation will produce a monophasic response in the GG channel and erratic, polyphasic response in the SG/HG channel (Fig. 18.5b). When this is observed, further dissection to identify the retractor nerve fibers should be performed to avoid their inclusion in the stimulation cuff; otherwise, mixed activation and poor outcomes will result.

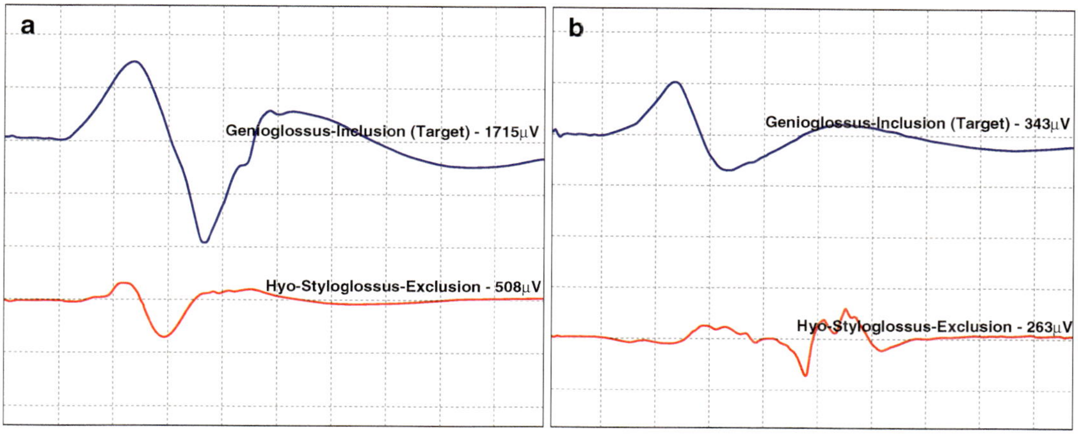

Fig. 18.5 (**a**) Synchronous activity of SG/HG channel mimicking the wave in GG channel indicating presence of fibers to intrinsic muscles. (**b**) Monophasic response in the GG channel and erratic, polyphasic response in the SG/HG channel indicating presence of retained late retractor fibers

Additional testing to confirm selective inclusion of the medial branches of the hypoglossal nerve should be performed at the completion of device implantation, prior to closing, to confirm implant function. The nerve stimulation is performed using the implanted pulse generator connected to the nerve stimulation cuff using standard manufacturer settings. For the FDA-approved and commercially available Inspire device (Minneapolis, MN), the device function and tongue response are commonly tested by using standard bipolar [+ − +] setting at 1.0 V. Unrestricted forward protrusion of the tongue should be visualized through a transparent sterile drape. If mixed activation is observed, which manifests by ipsilateral retraction and twisting of the tongue, further nerve dissection is required to identify the late takeoff retractor branch with cuff repositioning on the more distal nerve segment and subsequent improvement in tongue protrusion.

In some cases, the tongue may have unrestricted forward protrusion at the standard bipolar setting but mixed activation when tested with unipolar settings. Postoperative device programming, particularly advanced programming for patients who do not have optimal response to or compliance with therapy, includes setting optimization and testing of the airway response at both bipolar and unipolar electrode configurations. Failure to identify mixed activation intraoperatively will result in presence of mixed activation postoperatively and will limit programming options due to unfavorable airway response with the change in electrode configuration. In order to reduce the incidence of mixed activation, EMG response can be thoroughly tested to identify activation of the SG/HG muscles using implantable pulse generator at various electrode configurations and intensities [32]. The Inspire device cuff has three electrodes, and each electrode can be programmed as a cathode (−), anode (+), or off (o). Additionally, the pulse generator can be programmed to be off, or as an anode (+). Inspire-recommended default electrode cuff setting is bipolar [+ − +]. Programming of the cuff electrodes from this default bipolar [+ − +] setting to an anode unipolar [− o −], [o − o], or [− − −] setting, where the pulse generator serves as an anode (+), can change the field of electric stimulation of the nerve leading to different patterns of muscle activation [31]. If mixed activation occurs with unipolar stimulation, further dissection and cuff repositioning may be necessary to optimize programming options postoperatively.

Summary

Intraoperative nerve stimulation and monitoring of the glossopharyngeal and hypoglossal nerves are both feasible and safe. Recently, hypoglossal nerve monitoring with selective neurostimulation of distal branches has become critical to successful hypoglossal cranial nerve stimulator implant therapy for OSA. In addition to monitoring the nerve to avoid injury from excess traction during dissection and cuff placement, precise mapping of the nerve using NIM technology allows for accurate, selective placement of the electrode cuff on the inferior/medical branches of the nerve to allow for optimization of the upper airway opening and therapy outcomes. In no other surgery involving the lower cranial nerves is direct surgeon involvement in nerve stimulation and interpretation of various signal waveforms as critical for success as with this procedure.

References

1. Ozveren MF, Türe U, Ozek MM, Pamir MN. Anatomic landmarks of the glossopharyngeal nerve: a microsurgical anatomic study. Neurosurgery. 2003;52(6):1400–10.
2. Ozveren MF, Türe U. The microsurgical anatomy of the glossopharyngeal nerve with respect to the jugular foramen lesions. Neurosurg Focus. 2004;17(2):E3.
3. Lai PF, Wu X, Lan SH, Tang B, Huang HY, Hong T. Anatomical study of a surgical approach through the neck to the jugular foramen under endoscopy. Surg Radiol Anat. 2020; https://doi.org/10.1007/s00276-020-02574-9.
4. Singh R, Husain AM. Neurophysiologic intraoperative monitoring of the glossopharyngeal and vagus nerves. J Clin Neurophysiol. 2011;28(6):582–6.
5. Fukuda M, Takao T, Hiraishi T, Yajima N, Saito A, Fujii Y. Novel devices for intraoperative monitoring of glossopharyngeal and vagus nerves during skull base surgery. Surg Neurol Int. 2013;4:97.
6. Kullmann M, Tatagiba M, Liebsch M, Feigl GC. Evaluation of the predictive value of intraoperative changes in motor-evoked potentials of caudal cranial nerves for the postoperative functional outcome. World Neurosurg. 2016;95:329–34.
7. Zhang W, Chen M, Zhang W, Chai Y. Use of electrophysiological monitoring in selective rhizotomy treating glossopharyngeal neuralgia. J Craniomaxillofac Surg. 2014;42(5):e182–5.
8. Mu L, Sanders I. Human tongue neuroanatomy: nerve supply and motor endplates. Clin Anat. 2010;23:777–91.
9. Iaconetta G, Solari D, Villa A, Castaldo C, Gerardi RM, Califano G, Montagnani S, Cappabianca P. The hypoglossal nerve: anatomical study of its entire course. World Neurosurg. 2018;109:e486–92.
10. Delaey P, Duisit J, Behets C, Duprez T, Gianello P, Lengelé B. Specific branches of hypoglossal nerve to genioglossus muscle as a potential target of selective neurostimulation in obstructive sleep apnea: anatomical and morphometric study. Surg Radiol Anat. 2017;39(5):507–15.
11. Bassiri Gharb B, Tadisina KK, Rampazzo A, Hashem AM, Elbey H, Kwiecien GJ, Doumit G, Drake RL, Papay F. Microsurgical anatomy of the terminal hypoglossal nerve relevant for neurostimulation in obstructive sleep apnea. Neuromodulation. 2015;18(8):721–8.
12. Yigit E, Dursun E, Omeroglu E, Sunter AV, Edizer DT, Terzi S, Coskun ZO, Demirci M. The course of lower cranial nerves within the neck: a cadaveric dissection study. Eur Arch Otorhinolaryngol. 2018;275(10):2541–8.
13. Kikuta S, Jenkins S, Kusukawa J, Iwanaga J, Loukas M, Tubbs RS. Ansa cervicalis: a comprehensive review of its anatomy, variations, pathology, and surgical applications. Anat Cell Biol. 2019;52(3):221–5.
14. Vacher C, Caix P. Anatomie du couple nerf hypoglosse, anse cervicale [Anatomy of the hypoglossal nerve and the hypoglossal ansa cervicalis]. Rev Stomatol Chir Maxillofac. 2004;105(3):160–4.
15. Manoli A, Ploumidou K, Georgopapadakos N, Stratzias P, Skandalakis PN, Angelis S, Apostolopoulos AP, Filippou DK. Hypoglossal nerve: anatomy, anatomical variations comorbidities and clinical significance. J Long-Term Eff Med Implants. 2019;29(3):197–203.
16. Kim SY, Im HW, Choi YD, Kim K, Kim JW, Kim YH, Seo HG. Intraoperative monitoring of hypoglossal nerve using hypoglossal motor evoked potential in infratentorial tumor surgery: a report of two cases. Ann Rehabil Med. 2018;42(2):352–7.
17. Walshe P, Shandilya M, Rowley H, Zahirovich A, Walsh RM, Walsh M, Timon C. Use of an intraoperative nerve stimulator in identifying the hypoglossal nerve. J Laryngol Otol. 2006;120(3):185–7.
18. Kojima A, Saga I, Ishikawa M. Intraoperative hypoglossal nerve mapping during carotid endarterectomy: technical note. World Neurosurg. 2018;113:249–53.
19. Skinner SA. Neurophysiologic monitoring of the spinal accessory nerve, hypoglossal nerve, and the spinomedullary region. J Clin Neurophysiol. 2011;28(6):587–98.
20. Duque CS, Londoño AF, Penagos AM, Urquijo DP, Dueñas JP. Hypoglossal nerve monitoring, a potential application of intraoperative nerve monitoring in head and neck surgery. World J Surg Oncol. 2013;11:225. https://doi.org/10.1186/1477-7819-11-225.
21. Strollo PJ Jr, Soose RJ, Maurer JT, de Vries N, Cornelius J, Froymovich O, Hanson RD, Padhya TA, Steward DL, Gillespie MB, Woodson BT, Van de Heyning PH, Goetting MG, Vanderveken OM, Feldman N, Knaack L, Strohl KP, STAR Trial Group. Upper-airway stimulation for obstructive sleep apnea. N Engl J Med. 2014;370(2):139–49.

22. Woodson BT, Gillespie MB, Soose RJ, Maurer JT, de Vries N, Steward DL, Baskin JZ, Padhya TA, Lin HS, Mickelson S, Badr SM, Strohl KP, Strollo PJ Jr, STAR Trial Investigators. Randomized controlled withdrawal study of upper airway stimulation on OSA: short- and long-term effect. Otolaryngol Head Neck Surg. 2014;151(5):880–7.
23. Woodson BT, Strohl KP, Soose RJ, Gillespie MB, Maurer JT, de Vries N, Padhya TA, Badr MS, Lin HS, Vanderveken OM, Mickelson S, Strollo PJ Jr. Upper airway stimulation for obstructive sleep apnea: 5-year outcomes. Otolaryngol Head Neck Surg. 2018;159(1):194–202.
24. Caloway CL, Diercks GR, Keamy D, de Guzman V, Soose R, Raol N, Shott SR, Ishman SL, Hartnick CJ. Update on hypoglossal nerve stimulation in children with Down syndrome and obstructive sleep apnea. Laryngoscope. 2020;130(4):E263–7.
25. Diercks GR, Wentland C, Keamy D, Kinane TB, Skotko B, de Guzman V, Grealish E, Dobrowski J, Soose R, Hartnick CJ. Hypoglossal nerve stimulation in adolescents with down syndrome and obstructive sleep apnea. JAMA Otolaryngol Head Neck Surg. 2018;144(1):37–42.
26. Heiser C, Knopf A, Hofauer B. Surgical anatomy of the hypoglossal nerve: a new classification system for selective upper airway stimulation. Head Neck. 2017;39(12):2371–80.
27. Heiser C, Maurer JT, Steffen A. Functional outcome of tongue motions with selective hypoglossal nerve stimulation in patients with obstructive sleep apnea. Sleep Breath. 2016;20(2):553–60.
28. Zhu Z, Hofauer B, Heiser C. Improving surgical results in complex nerve anatomy during implantation of selective upper airway stimulation. Auris Nasus Larynx. 2018;45(3):653–6.
29. Steffen A, Kilic A, König IR, Suurna MV, Hofauer B, Heiser C. Tongue motion variability with changes of upper airway stimulation electrode configuration and effects on treatment outcomes. Laryngoscope. 2018;128(8):1970–6.
30. Heiser C, Hofauer B, Lozier L, Woodson BT, Stark T. Nerve monitoring-guided selective hypoglossal nerve stimulation in obstructive sleep apnea patients. Laryngoscope. 2016;126(12):2852–8.
31. Sturm JJ, Modik O, Suurna MV. Neurophysiological monitoring of tongue muscle activation during hypoglossal nerve stimulation. Laryngoscope. 2020;130(7):1836–43.
32. Sturm JJ, Lee CH, Modik O, Suurna MV. Intraoperative identification of mixed activation profiles during hypoglossal nerve stimulation. J Clin Sleep Med. 2020;16(10):1769–74.
33. Kumar AT, Vasconcellos A, Boon M, Huntley C. Inclusion of the first cervical nerve does not influence outcomes in upper airway stimulation for treatment of obstructive sleep apnea. Laryngoscope. 2020;130(5):E382–5.
34. Heiser C, Thaler E, Boon M, Soose RJ, Woodson BT. Updates of operative techniques for upper airway stimulation. Laryngoscope. 2016;126 Suppl 7:S12–6.

Brachial Plexus and Spinal Nerve Monitoring

19

Arbaz A. Momin, Maxwell Y. Lee, Navkiranjot Kaur, and Michael P. Steinmetz

Introduction

Operating around the spine and brachial plexus entails risk to neural structures. When neural structures are at risk during an operation, a surgeon may elect to include intraoperative neuromonitoring (IOM) in order to minimize postoperative complications. IOM allows the surgeon to assess, in real time, the integrity of neural structures while a patient is under general anesthesia and cannot participate in a face-to-face neurological examination. IOM may provide real-time assessments; however, interpretation of the results of the neuromonitoring modality can pose a significant challenge to even a highly skilled surgeon.

IOM is only beneficial if it provides an early enough warning for an intervention to be completed or altered in order to reverse or minimize neurological injury. Additionally, the IOM modality needs to have low false positives, low false negatives, and predefined alarm criteria, be easily interpretable, and be cost-effective. IOM modalities need to have a low false positive rate to prevent spending time unnecessarily performing interventions repeatedly due to warnings that are not correlated with a true injury. For example, when a warning is issued during a case, the surgical, anesthesia, and monitoring teams spend valuable time double-checking blood pressure, medications, level of anesthesia, etc. False negatives can lead to a false sense of confidence when an intervention should have been performed. Validated alarm criteria need to be determined prior to surgical operation, and IOM output needs to be easily interpretable in order to inform the surgeon which signals correspond to the onset of impairment.

The overarching goal of IOM is to allow changes in intraoperative strategies based on real-time assessment of neural structures to potentially avoid, minimize, or reverse neurological deficits. IOM allows surgeons to be more aggressive with maneuvers during spinal deformity correction or tumor resection procedures that otherwise may not have been possible without IOM. However, IOM is not beneficial or cost-effective to be used in every surgical case. Operative cases which have significantly low incidence and magnitude of postoperative neurological deficits should not utilize IOM. IOM should be applied to cases in which incidence of deficit and injury are substantial and in cases where intervention, change in approach, or

A. A. Momin (✉) · M. Y. Lee · N. Kaur
Cleveland Clinic Lerner College of Medicine of Case Western Reserve University, Education Institute, Cleveland Clinic, Cleveland, OH, USA
e-mail: momina@ccf.org; LEEM10@ccf.org; KAURN2@ccf.org

M. P. Steinmetz
Center for Spine Health, Department of Neurosurgery, Neurological Institute, Cleveland Clinic Foundation, Cleveland, OH, USA
e-mail: STEINMM@ccf.org

© The Author(s), under exclusive license to Springer Nature Switzerland AG 2022
J. Scharpf, G. W. Randolph (eds.), *Intraoperative Cranial Nerve Monitoring in Otolaryngology-Head and Neck Surgery*, https://doi.org/10.1007/978-3-030-84916-0_19

strategy is possible when a warning is triggered. Most importantly, the surgeon must recognize that each IOM modality has its own limitations, and even if the most perfect IOM strategy is deployed and executed, the risk of neurological deterioration from an adverse neurological event still remains.

This chapter will review the commonly used IOM modalities, the anatomical/physiological focus of each modality, advantages/disadvantages of each modality, and the impact of anesthesia on the specific modalities in spine and brachial plexus surgeries. Additionally, we will discuss the use of multimodal IOM, the importance of team-based communication, and developing a plan prior to surgical intervention.

Intraoperative Neuromonitoring (IOM) in Spine Surgery

Stagnara Wake-Up Test

One of the first intraoperative neuromonitoring test developed was the Stagnara wake-up test [1]. This test, as the name suggests, involves gradually waking the patient by decreasing anesthesia until voluntary movement of the lower extremities is achieved. This test assesses the functional integrity of the spinal cord by detecting gross motor movements. This test provides a gross approximation of the function of the primary motor cortex, nerve roots, and peripheral nerves; however, it fails to measure the sensory system and fine motor changes or provide information on nerve root injury. Since this test requires the patient to be adequately awake to follow commands, results of the test are highly dependent on patients' willingness to participate.

The administration of this test is highly dependent upon the anesthesia used during the procedure. The anesthetic used must be short acting and reversible in order to generate a wakeful state. Some have suggested that the value of this test may be indirect since the reduction of anesthesia required to perform this test inevitably leads to an increase in blood pressure and improved spinal cord perfusion [2].

The advantages of the Stagnara wake-up test include straightforward interpretation and high accuracy in detecting gross motor changes, if properly administered. Since the test is not reliant on electrophysiological recordings and is primarily focused on gross movement from the patient, the results are easy to interpret. For instance, if a patient is unable to move both upper and lower extremities, then the patient may not be adequately awake to follow commands. Global ischemic injury or cervical spine injury should be considered in cases where the patient is responsive and able to move facial muscles, but unable to move upper and lower extremities.

One major limitation of this test is that it does not provide continuous monitoring but instead provides a snapshot of spinal cord function at a single point in time, usually toward the end of a procedure. Administering this test increases operative time and the risk of air embolisms, self-extubation, and neural compression due to positional changes. It requires a surgical and anesthesia team trained and prepared to perform such a maneuver. The necessity of the patient to be awake in order to effectively administer this test poses a major limitation of this IOM modality. Many challenges and risks are encountered when repeatedly waking up a patient from anesthesia and re-anaesthetizing them after the test is complete; therefore, this test is rarely performed multiple times. Due to the risks associated with waking up a patient from anesthesia and the lack of continuous monitoring, this test is rarely performed as an IOM technique. Today, it is most commonly used as a final confirmatory test for a potential true positive. Specifically, a wake-up test may be performed before making a decision to abort a surgical procedure.

Somatosensory Evoked Potentials (SSEP)

SSEPs were first incorporated into clinical practice in the 1980s and became reliable and reproducible by 1986 [3–5]. This was the first effective continuous monitoring modality that could assess the function of the spinal cord intraoperatively.

The anatomical focus of SSEPs is to assess the posterior columns of the spinal cord. The dorsal column-medial lemniscus pathway (DCML) (also known as the posterior column-medial lemniscus pathway, PCML) is the sensory pathway of the central nervous system that communicates sensation of fine touch, vibration, and proprioception.

Intraoperative monitoring with this modality consists of electrodes placed on a distal limb and scalp. An electrical stimulus is delivered to the distal limb, and recordings are made along the spinal pathway up to the scalp. The most common distal region that is stimulated in the lower extremity is the posterior tibial nerve at the medial malleolus. This is performed in a transcutaneous fashion. In the upper extremity, the median or ulnar nerve is stimulated. Comparisons between upper extremity median nerve monitoring and lower extremity monitoring can help signal the surgeon to brachial plexus injury during preoperative positioning [6]. In the lower extremity, a somatosensory impulse travels through the posterior tibial nerve and generates a popliteal potential as the impulse traverses the popliteal fossa. The impulse then reaches the lumbosacral plexus and moves into the cauda equina generating a N21 lumbar potential. The electrical impulse then moves into the dorsal root and enters the spinal cord and travels through the dorsal column and arrives at the cortex. At the cortical level, a P37/P40 potential is generated. SSEPs do not monitor the slower conducting fibers of the spinothalamic pathway, the sensory pathway to the thalamus that conveys sensations of crude touch, pain, and temperature. Upper extremity SSEP pathway will be discussed in the brachial plexus section.

The SSEP output is low in amplitude and requires averaging of responses over a prolonged period of time; therefore, detecting a change in SSEPs from baseline may take 5 minutes or longer depending on the ambient level of artifact [7]. Initial baselines of SSEPs are determined immediately before or after incision. Additionally, baseline recording can be performed before or after positioning. There is no clear consensus on what defines a significant change from baseline. This is largely due to interobserver variability, and what constitutes a significant change is highly dependent on the type of procedure being performed. Some argue that SSEP latency changes of 7–14% and amplitude changes of 45–50% from baseline are tolerable without causing postoperative neurological deficits [8–10]. Most spine surgeons would agree that decrease in amplitude of 50% or greater or latency increases of 10% or greater signals injury to the dorsal column pathways [11–13]. When an SSEP change is triggered, alternative causes such as technical faults, alterations in blood pressure, and body temperature need to be ruled out.

Hypothermia, hypotension, and anesthesia can all influence SSEP recordings. SSEPs are influenced by all anesthetics to some degree. Propofol increases latency and decreases the amplitude of cortical SSEPs. However, opioids have minimal effects on SSEP waveforms. During SSEP monitoring, infusion of opioids is recommended. Muscle relaxants act primarily at the neuromuscular junction and have little influence on electrophysiological recordings of SSEPs. Volatile anesthetics depress the amplitude of SSEPs and prolong the latency in a dose-dependent manner. IV agents tend to have negligible effects on cortical SSEPs. Therefore, when cortical SSEPs are being recorded, intravenous anesthetics should be incorporated since volatile anesthetics at high concentrations can eliminate cortical SSEPs [14].

SSEPs are considered to have high specificity for injury but low sensitivity. In a large survey of Scoliosis Research Society surgeons by Nuwer et al. (1995), 80% of spine surgeons reported using SSEP monitoring. In 51,263 spine surgeries, the true-negative rate was 97.94%, and the true-positive rate 0.42%. This large study demonstrated a sensitivity of 77% and specificity of 98.5% for SSEPs [15]. SSEPs are more sensitive to motor changes as a result of mechanical injuries that effect the entire cord rather than vascular injuries. Most commonly, postoperative paraparesis with normal SSEPs is the result of anterior spinal artery syndrome. This phenomenon is seen because the anterior spinal artery selectively provides blood flow to the anterolateral columns and spares the posterior column of the spinal cord [16]. In cases where false negatives are present, this can also be due to purely motor deficits or nerve root-related injuries that are not directly monitored by SSEPs [17–19].

The advantage of using SSEPs is that this modality provides continuous monitoring unlike the single time point snapshot provided by the wake-up test. One limitation of using SSEPs is that it does not monitor motor function directly. In cases where the entire cord is expected to be affected (i.e., spinal correction surgery for scoliosis) due to stretching of all neural and vascular structures, monitoring of the dorsal column can serve as an adequate proxy for motor pathway monitoring. The primary disadvantage of this modality is that SSEPs need to be summed up over a period of time (3–5 minutes), delaying the results of this modality. Additionally, SSEPs monitoring capabilities are limited to the dorsal column and do not provide direct information about motor pathway or nerve root injuries; therefore, SSEPs should be utilized as an adjunct modality alongside other IOM modalities, i.e., multimodal monitoring.

Motor Evoked Potentials (MEPs)

Since SSEPs are limited to monitoring only the dorsal column and do not have the capability to directly monitor the motor tracts, MEPs were developed to monitor the motor pathways of the anterior and anterolateral spinal cord. Intraoperative monitoring via transcranial motor evoked potentials (TC-MEPs) has been performed for over 20 years [20, 21]. TC-MEPs have become widely used after a device designed to produce them was approved by the FDA in 2002. The anatomical focus of this IOM modality is to assess the motor pathways.

Subdermal electrodes on the head produce trains of high-voltage stimuli to activate the motor cortex and subsequently the corticospinal tract which leads to either a muscle contraction (muscle MEP or CMAPs) or a nerve action potential (D-wave). Compound muscle action potentials (CMAPs), an all-or-nothing response as a result of synchronized activation of a group of motor neurons, are commonly recorded at the abductor pollicus brevis (hand) or adductor hallucis brevis (foot). These areas are rich in corticospinal tract innervation. Nerve action potentials (D-wave), which reflect direct conduction of corticospinal neurons, can be directly recorded with an epidural electrode that is placed over the upper thoracic spinal cord [22]. In an awake patient, single pulse electrical stimulation of the cortical white matter will produce a D-wave followed by multiple succeeding I-waves that can be recorded. The D-wave is the result of nerve action potential generated by stimulating the white matter directly and is independent of synapses. However, the I-waves are produced by internuncial neurons and are highly dependent on synaptic activity for their production. In an awake patient, a single train of stimulus can produce muscle MEP because sufficient D-wave and I-waves can reach the anterior horn cells and summate to bring the anterior horn cells to threshold and produce a peripheral nerve action potential. However, I-waves are strongly diminished with general anesthesia, and a partial synaptic blockage is induced by the anesthetic at the anterior horn cells. This combined effect of anesthesia makes it more difficult for the anterior horn cells to reach threshold and fire a peripheral nerve action potential to generate a muscle MEP. Under general anesthesia, anterior horn cells will fire more easily when trains of stimuli are delivered as compared to a single stimulus. Because the D-wave is resistant to anesthetic depression, trains of stimuli produce multiple D-waves that can summate at the anterior horn cells to generate a peripheral nerve action potential and a subsequent muscle response. Because a single stimulus will not be able to produce a muscle MEP, IOM studies need to utilize trains of stimuli to overcome the effects of general anesthesia.

One alarm criteria proposed by Calancie et al. for muscle MEPs is the threshold criterion [23]. This criterion is based upon the premise that the threshold required to generate a muscle MEP increases when the corticospinal tract is damaged. Generally, increases in threshold of more than 100 V are an early indication of injury to the corticospinal tract. The issue with using this criterion is that the threshold increases gradually during surgery and thresholds are highly influenced by anesthesia. Another criterion is the disappearance of muscle MEPs; however, this does not always indicate an irreversible injury. For example, in a study of intramedullary spinal cord tumor resection surgeries, loss of muscle MEP without more than a 50% change in D-wave was associated with only transient neurological deficits [24]. Similar to SSEPs, some researchers have proposed the alarm criterion to be greater than 50% reduction in amplitude; however, high natural variability in muscle MEPs leads to increased false positives and false negatives [25]. The exact alarm criteria for MEPs have not been established within the literature.

IOM responses that are highly dependent on synaptic function will have marked reductions in amplitude and increased latency with the use of inhaled anesthetic agents. Muscle MEPs are highly depressed with the use of halogenated anesthetics; these agents should be avoided when recording muscle MEPs. The effect of inhaled anesthetics is likely due to depression of synaptic transmission either at the level of the anterior horn cells on lower motor neurons leading to diminished myogenic response or in the cortex on internuncial synapses leading to the loss of I-waves. Muscle relaxants have a profound blockade effect at the neuromuscular junction, which prevents recording of muscle MEPs. Similar to SSEPs, opioid analgesics have less of an effect on MEPs than inhaled anesthetics. As a component of total intravenous anesthetic, infusions of propofol combined with ketamine and dexmedetomidine have produced acceptable monitoring conditions of MEPs [26].

In a retrospective study of 235 C4–C5 spine procedures, TC-MEP had a sensitivity of 100% and specificity of 99% for acute C5 radiculopathy [27]. In a prospective series of 103 spine procedures, D-wave monitoring correctly predicted motor outcomes in all 97 recordable cases [28]. In a study of 1121 idiopathic scoliosis patients, a 65% decrease in MEP amplitude predicted postoperative motor deficit 100% of the time, whereas SSEPs picked up a change 43% of the time [7].

The advantage of using MEP monitoring is that they provide repeatable snapshots of spinal cord function. This modality is superior to the wake-up test because it can be performed multiple times throughout the operation. Contrary to SSEPs, which require up to 5 minutes for summation before results can be presented, MEP monitoring can provide immediate assessment of motor pathways after high-risk maneuvers are performed and are more sensitive than SSEPs in detecting spinal cord ischemia [29, 30]. However, MEP can only be helpful if they are performed at consistent intervals. If MEPs are performed at a varying rate during surgery, the exact timing of an injury may not be known, and mitigation is not possible. The surgeon determines a plan with the monitoring technician at the beginning of the case and typically performs MEPs at 30-minute intervals throughout the entire case. Additionally, MEPs need to be performed frequently because MEPs tend to fade with length of surgery, anesthesia, and blood loss. A sudden change indicates a problem, but slow decline over time, a consistent trend, may not be worrisome, especially toward the end of the case. The disadvantage of using muscle MEPs is that the waveform produced is complex to interpret and MEPs do not have a standardized metric of what defines a significant change. Additionally, muscle MEPs cannot provide enough information about intraoperative injury to nerve roots. Overall, MEP monitoring has advantages over SSEPs; however, MEPs still require other monitoring modalities as adjuncts in order to provide a comprehensive multimodal monitoring plan for spine procedures [31].

Spontaneous Electromyography

Spontaneous electromyography (sEMG) or free-running EMG was first introduced in the 1990s [32]. Prior to the introduction of sEMGs, dermatomal SSEPs were used to evaluate nerve root function. Dermatomal SSEPs involve recording cerebral-evoked responses to stimulation of specific sensory dermatomes. When this modality was used in the OR, individual dermatomal fields were stimulated; however, the recordings of dermatomal SSEPs were not specific enough to isolate individual nerve roots and were highly influenced by anesthesia. As mentioned in the SSEP section, dermatomal SSEPs also require approximately 3–5 minutes of signal summation time to produce results. Within this summation window, it is very likely that an irreversible nerve root injury would go undetected [33]. Therefore, the need for continuous, real-time nerve root monitoring was paramount.

sEMG monitors the activity of a muscle and provides the surgeon with information about the peripheral nerve that innervates that muscle. Hypothermia, ischemia, compression, or stretching of a nerve will lead to depolarization of axons and will produce a spontaneous action potential which will lead to a muscle contraction. Cold irrigation, cauterization, and use of high-speed drills can lead to neurotonic discharges even when the nerve is normal (false positives) because this modality is sensitive to temperature changes. Muscle contractions are detected by the EMG electrodes placed in the muscle. These electrodes are commonly paired intramuscular needles or wire electrodes that are placed after anesthesia. The preselected sEMG myotome is dependent upon the operative level.

Clearly defining which EMG pattern is most associated with damage to the nerve root is important for the surgeon to understand prior to operating. The traditional alarm criterion is defined as high-frequency (more than five spikes per second) EMG discharge lasting longer than 5 seconds [34]. Spontaneous EMG spikes and bursts indicate proximity of the nerve root. Alternatively, spontaneous EMG activity was classified by Romstock et al. into three different types of trains (A, B, and C). Trains were classified as seconds of sustained periodic EMG activity. According to Romstock et al., A trains were sinusoidal, symmetrical sequence of high-frequency and low-amplitude EMG waveforms and were most likely associated with significant injury to the nerve. B and C trains were not significantly associated with postoperative outcomes [35].

Compared to SSEPs and MEPs, EMG recordings are less influenced by inhaled anesthetics. However, EMG recordings are highly influenced by muscle relaxants because of their ability to inhibit electrical activity across the neuromuscular junction. Due to their inhibitory effects on neural activity and muscle contractions, manipulation or injury to nerve roots will not result in the production of EMG signal recordings. A cautious dose of short-acting muscle relaxants before laryngoscopy may be administered; however, its effects must wear off prior to starting sEMG recordings. Reversal agents may also be given prior to recordings, if necessary [36].

Spontaneous EMG monitoring is sensitive for nerve root injury and helps prevent postoperative radiculopathy [37]. In a retrospective review of 213 thoracolumbar procedures, sensitivity of sEMG was 100%, and specificity was 23.7% [38]. Jin et al. (2015) retrospectively reviewed 25 patients who underwent intramedullary spinal cord tumor resection with multimodal IOM. In their study, sEMG alerts preceded TcMEP alerts in 72% of cases, and the authors suggested that sEMG alerts may predict a detrimental MEP alert [39].

The advantage of using sEMG monitoring is that it is instantaneous and continuous. When performing instrumentation surgery, postoperative radiculopathy is much more common than postoperative myelopathy; therefore, the development of selective nerve root monitoring (i.e., sEMG) has helped detect nerve root irritation due to retraction of the spinal cord or nerve root [40, 41]. The other advantage of using sEMG is that it can be combined with SSEPs to improve specificity [42]. The limitations of sEMG include sensitivity to temperature changes which may account for the high rate of false-positive alarms, and sEMG prevents the use of neuromuscular blocking agents during recordings [42]. Another limitation of sEMG monitoring is that injury to a nerve root does not cause spontaneous synchronization in the different axons; therefore, there is no large-scale muscle movement, rather contraction of a few muscle fibers occur at a time. Because spontaneous activity may be detected in one location but not in another, even within the same muscle, placement and type of recording electrode are important [43, 44]. Chronic injury to axons can lead to fibrillations or fasciculation on sEMG recordings due to chronic denervation of muscle fibers. These signals can be distinguished from acute nerve injury by observing the time at which these signals are detected. Fibrillations and fasciculations generally occur over weeks; therefore, these signals will be present at the beginning of the operation. Overall, the real-time monitoring of nerve roots provided by sEMG provides another adjunct IOM modality that can be combined with SSEPs and MEPs to create a comprehensive monitoring plan.

Triggered Electromyography

Triggered electromyography (tEMG) was first introduced into an animal model in 1992 and was rapidly translated into humans [45]. Pedicle screw fixation has become a widely accepted technique in spine fusion surgeries, largely due to the rigidity provided for fixation. However, significant postoperative radiculopathy can be experienced when a screw is incorrectly placed due to the close proximity of neural structures to the pedicle wall. Unfortunately, screw insertion techniques are largely "blind" with some intraoperative radiography or fluoroscopy methods to assist in correct placement. In one retrospective study of 57 patients undergoing pedicle screw fixation, 11% experienced postoperative neurological complications, majority of which were related directly to nerve root impingement by a pedicle screw [46]. In order to prevent postoperative neurological complications, intraoperative SSEPs were used to monitor nerve root function. However, multiple nerve roots contribute to cortical SSEPs; therefore, damage to a single nerve root would still lead to normal cortical SSEP potentials. Dermatomal SSEPs were then used to increase the sensitivity and specificity of detecting a single nerve root injury. This technique fell out of favor because a breached pedicle screw could sit next to a nerve root without compressing the nerve root and triggering an alert signal on dermatomal SSEP monitoring. However, this screw could lead to nerve root irritation and postoperative radiculopathy. To increase the sensitivity and specificity for detecting a pedicle screw breach, triggered EMG was developed [36].

Triggered EMG evaluates the accuracy of pedicle screw placement. With this technique, a surgeon can evaluate the integrity of the pedicle wall by determining whether or not the pedicle screw has breached the cortical bone. The main premise behind this recording modality is the impedance of cortical bone. The bone has a high impedance and therefore serves as a good electrical insulator. A well-placed pedicle screw is surrounded by intact, high-impedance, cortical bone, and if the screw or pedicle hole was stimulated with current, a high stimulation threshold would have to be generated in order to overcome the impedance of the bone and stimulate the adjacent nerve root. However, when tEMG requires a low stimulation to activate an adjacent nerve root, it demonstrates lack of pedicle cortex integrity and possible perforation. Direct stimulation of an errant pedicle screw that has breached the cortical bone will evoke a muscle contraction (CMAP) in the corresponding myotome at lower stimulation intensities compared to a screw placed in an intact pedicle cortex.

A handheld mono- or bipolar stimulator is used to gradually increase the stimulating current in order to determine the threshold at which stimulating current causes a CMAP in the corresponding myotome. When testing pedicle screw placement, thresholds less than 10 mA and duration of 0.2 msec should be inspected, and screws with stimulation threshold of less than 5 mA have likely perforated the bony cortex. Well-placed screws typically have stimulation thresholds of greater than 10 mA [47, 48]. These stimulation thresholds generally hold true when the adjacent nerve root is healthy. However, when the adjacent nerve root has a preexisting injury, stimulation intensities required to generate a CMAP are higher even if the screw has perforated the bony cortex and is near the nerve. If there is uncertainty about the health of the adjacent nerve root under observation, it is possible to stimulate the nerve root directly and compare it to the screw stimulation [49]. When stimulating the nerve root directly, threshold for stimulation is approximately 2 mA of current. As a secondary check metric, all screw thresholds should be compared with each other, and any screw with a threshold significantly higher or lower than the others should be reevaluated by the surgeon and monitoring team.

Triggered EMG has a reported sensitivity of 93% for detecting misplaced hardware, whereas radiography has a reported sensitivity of 63% [50]. In a study of 36 patients, screw placement was checked with tEMG, and 13 of 239 hardware insertion were detected as malpositioned; however, radiography was normal, but incorrect positioning was confirmed by visual inspection of the pedicle wall [50]. In 2007, Raynor et al. conducted a study evaluating tEMG in the placement of 4857 screws in 1078 patients. Raynor et al. found that the specificity increased as the stimulation threshold decreased; however, as the stimulation threshold decreased, the sensitivity dropped significantly. Raynor et al. reported a specificity of 94%, 99%, and 100% at stimulation thresholds of less than 8, 4, and 2 mA, respectively [51].

The advantages of using tEMG are as follows: high sensitivity for pedicle wall breach, relatively easy technique to perform and interpret, and can still obtain reliable information during partial (<80%) neuromuscular blockade. The limitations of tEMG include false negatives due to scar tissue from prior surgeries falsely elevating stimulation thresholds and stimulating screws in irrigation fluid may lead to current shunting and falsely elevate the stimulation threshold [52, 53]. Another limitation of this technique is that stimulation thresholds are dependent upon the state and health of the nerve root. Therefore, an individual patient approach needs to be taken, and any threshold outliers should be reevaluated and investigated further. Additionally, tEMG is less sensitive for thoracic pedicle screws as compared to lumbar pedicle screws [42]. As with the majority of these IOM modalities, there is no clearly defined or accepted alarm criteria for tEMG. Despite these limitations, its quick response and easily interpretable results make this an effective adjunct modality in combination with SSEPs and MEPs.

Intraoperative Neuromonitoring (IOM) in Brachial Plexus Surgery

Due to the intricate and variable neuroanatomy present within the brachial plexus, surgical procedures in this region can be challenging and may require complex decision-making. Intraoperative electrophysiological techniques can be employed to assess nerve function, severity of injury, potential for intervention to limit injury, and potential for neural recovery. As with all neuromonitoring techniques, they are labor intensive, time-consuming, and expensive; however, IOM can provide critical information that cannot be obtained by other methods or studies. Therefore, the benefits provided by IOM must be weighed against the time investment and cost associated with IOM in brachial plexus surgery.

Somatosensory Evoked Potentials (SSEP) and Motor Evoked Potentials (MEP)

While SSEPs and MEPs have primarily been used to evaluate integrity of dorsomedial sensory and corticospinal motor tracts of the spinal cord, respectively, they can also be used to evaluate peripheral nerve function. In brachial plexus surgery, upper extremity SSEPs and MEPs are helpful in assessing spinal nerve continuity with the spinal cord and integrity of the intraforaminal and intraspinal sensory and motor pathways. These techniques, especially when combined with nerve action potentials (NAPs), yield a comprehensive assessment of anterior and posterior root function [54].

SSEPs in the upper extremity are most commonly elicited with stimulation of the median nerve and occasionally the ulnar nerve. Stimulation of these peripheral sensory nerves containing first-order neurons of the medial-lemniscus pathway results in impulse conduction through the brachial plexus and generation of an N9 potential at Erb's point. The impulse continues to travel through the dorsal column and cuneate fasciculus, generating an N13 potential over the cervical spinal cord. First-order neurons synapse at the cuneate nucleus in the medulla with second-order neurons, which decussate and project to the posterolateral thalamus. P14 and N18 potentials represent activity through these subcortical regions of the brain. Impulse conduction through third-degree neurons to the somatosensory cortex corresponds to generation of the cortical N20 potential. Prolonged or absent N9 potential over Erb's point may indicate injury at or distal to the brachial plexus, whereas prolonged N9–P14 interval with normal P14–N20 interval may indicate injury between the brachial plexus and lower medulla [55].

Intraoperatively, surgeons can directly stimulate spinal nerves close to their foramina and obtain recordings from the spine or scalp over the sensory cortex to assess sensory nerve root continuity with the spinal cord [56]. On their own, SSEPs are not useful in differentiating preganglionic from postganglionic lesions, an important distinction that impacts surgical management. As preganglionic lesions represent involvement of the central nervous system, there is little potential for recovery of motor function. However, this distinction can be made with use of additional techniques such as NAP [57]. Purely preganglionic lesions with a negative SSEP will have a positive NAP response as the cell body and peripheral sensory axons are still intact. On the other hand, postganglionic lesions result in negative SSEP and NAP. Absence of NAP may also represent a mixed process with both preganglionic and postganglionic involvement [58].

In contrast to SSEPs, MEPs assess function of the corticospinal tract but may also be used to evaluate peripheral nerve motor function. To review, transcranial magnetic or electrical stimulation of the motor cortex results in signal transmission and generation of MEP at distal muscles or motor nerves. Intraoperatively, MEPs are recorded from one or more spinal nerves. The absence of a response suggests discontinuity of the ventral root due to root avulsion or nonfunctioning axons [54, 59].

Use of SSEPs and MEPs during brachial plexus surgery is most beneficial in identification of proximal root lesions such as posterior and anterior root avulsion [54, 59, 60]. It is important to note that SSEPs and MEPs are ideally used in combination as continuity of either the dorsal or anterior root does not guarantee continuity of the other. In fact, this type of mismatch was found in 11% of roots studied via laminectomy; most of these were intact dorsal roots with avulsion of anterior [61]. In a study of 13 patients undergoing surgical brachial plexus repair for traumatic injuries, absence of SSEP was shown to have 100% sensitivity for dorsal root lesions compared to intradural exploration [62]. Absence of MEP from neck muscles was shown to have 100% sensitivity for anterior root lesions [63]. On the other hand, a positive SSEP does not always correlate with clinical function or outcome as only a few hundred fibers are required for impulse transmission and generation of SSEP [63–65]. In a study of 23 patients, examining the utility of MEPs in predicting neurological deficits following surgical enucleation of peripheral nerve schwannomas showed postoperative neurological deficits in 22% of the patients [66]. They demonstrated that even if the nerve is not transected, MEP monitoring can detect ischemia to the nerve due to compression or traction. However, they conclude that MEP alone is not enough to predict postoperative sensory or motor deficits. MEPs should be combined with other neurological monitoring modalities to improve accuracy [66].

Triggered Electromyography (tEMG)

In peripheral nerve surgeries such as brachial plexus surgery, EMG studies are the most reliable indicator of motor nerve injury [67]. Triggered or stimulated EMG is particularly helpful for identifying normal or functional motor nerves when multiple nerves lie close together or when evaluating functional continuity through a lesion. This intraoperative technique involves direct stimulation of a nerve and recording the presence or absence of compound muscle action potentials (CMAPs) at target muscles using intramuscular needle electrodes [32]. CMAPs are all-or-nothing responses; however, the stimulus threshold is a quantitative measure used in spine surgeries to assess nerve function, as described previously in this chapter.

In brachial plexus surgeries, tEMG can be used to assess lesions involving motor nerves. In an illustrative case study of a patient undergoing resection of a benign brachial plexus nerve sheath tumor, the authors identified triggered EMG to be an indispensable tool [68]. The peripheral nerve tumor is directly stimulated with fine-tipped bipolar electrodes using small current intensities. Subsequent detection of CMAPs from target muscle can allow surgeons to identify areas of the tumor or lesion that are or are not associated with functional motor fascicles. Effort can then be made to preserve fascicles that produce CMAPs. Triggered EMG is thus an excellent modality for localizing or mapping and avoiding injury to motor axons during dissection and resection of benign nerve tumors. Triggered EMG was first adapted for stimulation and resection of a desmoid tumor of the lateral cord of the brachial plexus based on CMAP generation by Press et al. [69].

Use of tEMG in brachial plexus surgery may be limited by nerve injury or discontinuity of the nerve with the muscle. In these cases, triggered nerve action potentials (NAPs) may be used to directly assess nerve function. When using tEMG, it is also important to account for false positives or false negatives. In cases where multiple nerves are in proximity, use of a monopolar device may lead to current spread to an adjacent nerve and false-positive result. Thus, bipolar stimulation may be used to provide a localized current and avoid unwanted spread. On the other hand, a false negative may result due to current shunting if both electrodes lie within a pool of fluids in the surgical field. Hook electrodes may be used to lift the neural tissue out of pooled fluids to avoid this problem [32].

Nerve Action Potentials (NAPs)

In adults, the use of NAP recordings can help differentiate from axonometic (positive NAP) and neurotmetic injuries (negative NAP) when combined with surgeon experience and CT myelography findings [70]. This is often a difficult distinction to make, even for the most experienced of surgeons. Therefore, objective intraoperative tools are welcomed to assess the severity of injury. In a nerve, stimulation of a nerve fiber membrane can produce a nerve action potential (NAP) if the intensity of the stimulation is higher than the fiber's threshold. Various axonal properties including fiber size and membrane properties alter each individual axon's threshold [71]. When a stimulus is much higher than the threshold, the NAP amplitude and area under the curve are maximal. To achieve such a stimulus, both the duration and magnitude of the applied current must be modulated. For example, high current stimulation may not be able to produce a NAP in some fibers without a long enough stimulus duration [72].

A lesion requires around 3000–4000 nerve fibers with a diameter greater than 5um in order to conduct a positive NAP. Therefore, a positive NAP indicates that a spontaneous functional recovery will likely take place, and more drastic surgical action is not indicated [73–75]. Importantly, the presence of a NAP can be detected several months earlier than clinical recovery [73]. Several studies have indicated the usefulness of intraoperative NAP (INAP) recordings in the management of brachial plexus lesions in continuity [71, 76, 77]. In fact, a review of 1019 brachial plexus injuries found that only 7% exhibited sharp laceration and transection [78]. The mechanism of injury for the majority of lesions was stretch or contusion in 49%, thoracic outlet syndrome (16%), tumors (16%), or gunshot wound (12%) [78].

Electrodes for NAP recording are often made from medical-grade stainless steel inserted into a Teflon rod and soldered to leads [76]. A loop or hook is made out of the tip of the electrode that contacts the nerve. Typically, recording electrodes contain two prongs, and stimulating electrodes contain three. The distance between the prongs on the stimulating electrode should be no less than 3–7 mm. At lower distances, very high voltages may be required [76]. The only other equipment required is a simple EMG machine.

For a simple positive control, recording of an uninjured nerve or recordings proximal to the injury should be performed. To record a NAP, turn on the trace and stimulus, making sure to observe a stimulus artifact. Next, using a stimulus duration of 0.05–0.1 ms, gradually increase the voltage intensity until a NAP is seen. After a NAP is seen on a proximal segment, the recording electrode should be moved in a stepwise fashion toward and eventually past the lesion. In lesions that do not allow measurement of proximal sections, both electrodes may have to be placed distal to the lesion [76].

There are several reasons one might fail to record a NAP. Often this is because of the placement of the electrodes – electrodes that are too close together or touching other tissues or fluid are a common problem. Additionally, the use of local anesthetics is not recommended in the area of study because this may cause false-negative signals [76, 79].

Robert et al. reported that in the treatment of 481 brachial plexus stretch injuries, a positive NAP result followed by either neurolysis or split repair resulted in a Louisiana State University Health Science Center grading system grade 3 or better result in approximately 94% of cases. In cases where the NAP result was negative and treatment was suture or graft, the grade 3 or better result occurred in about half of the cases [76]. Additionally, intraoperative NAP recordings have been useful in assessing neuromas in continuity. NAPs help assess the potential of spontaneous useful regeneration of the nerve and provides guidance on whether to proceed with neurolysis or resection of the neuroma and nerve grafting [71]. Large series have demonstrated that 92% of neuromas in continuity with the presence of a NAP, treated with neurolysis, result in positive functional outcomes [80]. NAPs have shown to be useful in confirming brachial plexus involvement close to the spine in thoracic outlet syndrome surgery. NAPs can help assess the severity of compression and functional deficits based on reductions in NAP amplitude and conduction velocity [80].

Interestingly, in a study of infants with obstetric brachial plexus lesions, NAP recordings were found to be highly specific for predicting an unfavorable lesion (neurotmesis or avulsion), but not sensitive, with specificity of 98.5% but sensitivity of 19.5%. The conclusions from this study, however, may not be generalizable in adults [73].

Lastly, reports have shown that NAP recordings provide valuable insights when combined with other intraoperative monitoring methods. Burkholder et al. presented a case report where the use of INAPs in combination with SSEPs and MEPs was important to gain an accurate picture of brachial plexus function in a patient with brachial plexus injury following a traumatic fall. While the primary function of NAPs was to assess peripheral nerve function distal to the dorsal root ganglion to help distinguish pre- and postganglionic lesions, when they found that NAP was present and there was an absence of neurogenic MEP and SSEP findings in the middle trunk of the brachial plexus, they used this information to comment on the functional continuity of the motor and sensory fibers to the spinal cord [54].

Intraoperative Neuromonitoring in Practice

Multimodal Intraoperative Monitoring (MIOM)

Every intraoperative modality has its own advantages, disadvantages, sensitivities, and specificities. No single modality is sufficient to monitor all spinal cord pathways. The overall goal of these intraoperative modalities is to detect motor and sensory deficits early enough and intervene to prevent irreversible postoperative neurological deficits from occurring. Due to the limitations of each IOM modality, combining these recording methods may provide a robust and comprehensive multimodal monitoring plan for patients. Using a multimodal IOM approach does leads to some redundancy in the monitoring of ascending and descending pathways. However, this level of redundancy is beneficial because by combining multiple modalities together, the anesthetic or electrical limitations posed by one modality may be overcome by the advantages of another modality.

An example of when multimodal IOM can be beneficial is in intramedullary spinal cord tumor (IMSCT) resection surgeries. SSEP monitoring is known to have high rates of false positives, if this was the only modality used for tumor resection; it may lead to incomplete resection and prevent total resection. Another potential issue of using only SSEPs is that it may be too slow due to the summation time required for data acquisition, and this may lead to aggressive resection and consequently irreversible neurological injury. Combination of SSEPs and MEPs in midline myelotomy during tumor resection can be beneficial. SSEPs can help determine location of midline myelotomy, and MEPs can assist in delineating tumor edges for safe maximal resection. Transcranial MEP D-wave monitoring during intramedullary tumor resections has also allowed for safer resection. Loss of less than 50% D-waves results in transient paresis and recovery within hours to weeks [81]. However, if D-waves are lost completely, then permanent paraplegia is generally seen [82].

In studies assessing IOM in resection of IMSCTs, studies have demonstrated improved outcomes and safer maximal resections of tumors when neuromonitoring is used [81, 83]. In retrospective review of 354 scoliosis cases, Bhagat et al. has reported superiority of multimodal monitoring (SSEPs/MEPs) compared to either modality alone. Bhagat et al. reported sensitivity and specificity of 100% and 99.3%, respectively, using multimodal IOM in scoliosis cases [84]. By combining multiple IOM modalities, the false-negative rate can be significantly reduced. Raynor et al. retrospectively reviewed 12,375 spine surgeries using MIOM and reported 45 (0.36%) false-negative cases with postoperative neurological injury [85]. Overall, the multimodal approach helps increase sensitivity and provides the surgeon with more information when a warning is triggered.

Team-Based Approach for IOM

Utilization of intraoperative monitoring requires a team-based approach in the operating room. There is a technical level to this team, which includes personnel trained in placing electrodes, setting up the monitoring equipment, and conducting the actual tests discussed above. The other side of this team is the interpretational level, which includes personnel trained to help decide which test is most appropriate, the meaning of different waveforms reported from the recording modalities, and how to best intervene in order to prevent permanent neurological injury. Because alarm signals generated from IOM modalities require quick interventions in order to prevent permanent injury, it is critical that the team be highly trained and each member performs their specific role effectively. Open and effective communication between surgeon, anesthesiologist, and monitoring team is paramount. Prior to surgery, surgeon and monitoring team should share objectives, expectations, and surgical plans in case alarm criteria are triggered.

Practical Considerations of IOM

There is robust class I evidence that supports the use of SSEPs and MEP recording during spinal cord surgery as a diagnostic adjust to assess cord integrity. Utilization of SSEPs and MEPs in the perioperative setting is valid and sensitive to detect neurological injury. In procedures where there is a high risk of neurological injury, the value of IOM is becoming more clear. However, the use of IOM as a therapeutic tool during spine surgery has not been shown to reduce the rate of postoperative neurological deficits or improve neurological outcomes after surgery. There is little to no class I or II evidence to support the association between IOM use and improved neurological outcomes after spine surgery. In other words, IOM can diagnostically assess and detect neurological injury to the spinal cord during surgery; however, it remains unclear whether the use of IOM actually leads to a meaningful improvement in neurological outcomes [86].

Another practical consideration of using IOM is the cost associated with conducting intraoperative monitoring. There is the cost of the additional personnel; each time a warning is issued, there is a cost associated with the response by the surgeon and anesthesiologist (i.e., increased OR time and changes in medication/anesthesia), the cost of purchasing, and maintaining the recording instrumentation. When all of these costs are summed, the overall cost of IOM during spine surgery is substantial. Currently, there is insufficient evidence to support the use of IOM during spine surgery from a purely cost-effective standpoint. This is due to the fact that while IOM can accurately detect neurological injury during a case, the use of IOM has not been shown to therapeutically improve neurological outcomes even when IOM correctly signals neurological injury. Therefore, due to the lack of evidence to demonstrate a correlation between the use of IOM and improved neurological outcomes, the high cost associated with the use of IOM is not to be adequately justified for all procedures [86].

Conclusion

When considering whether to incorporate intraoperative neuromonitoring in spine or brachial plexus surgeries, the critical information collected from monitoring should be weighed against the potential disadvantages of each IOM modality, the cost associated with the modality, and the time expenditure required to conduct IOM. If a surgeon decides that the benefits of neuromonitoring outweighs the disadvantages of IOM, then a careful team-based approach should be employed. Prior to surgery, surgeon and monitoring team should share objectives, expectations, and surgical plans in case alarm criteria are triggered. To conclude, IOM should be strongly considered in cases in which incidence of deficit and injury are substantial and in cases where intervention, change in approach, or strategy is possible when a warning signal is triggered.

References

1. Vauzelle C, Stagnara P, Jouvinroux P. Functional monitoring of spinal cord activity during spinal surgery. Clin Orthop Relat Res. 1973;93:173–8.
2. Mendiratta A, Emerson RG. Neurophysiologic intraoperative monitoring of scoliosis surgery. J Clin Neurophysiol. 2009;26:62–9.
3. Tamaki T, Noguchi T, Takano T, et al. Spinal cord monitoring as a clinical utilization of the spinal evoked potential. Clin Orthop Relat Res. 1984;184:58–64.
4. Nash CL, Brown RH. Spinal cord monitoring. J Bone Joint Surg Am. 1989;71:627–30.
5. Dinner DS, Luders H, et al. Intraoperative spinal somatosensory evoked potential monitoring. J Neurosurg. 1986;65:807–14.
6. Labrom RD, Hoskins M, Reilly CW, et al. Clinical usefulness of somatosensory evoked potentials for detection of brachial plexopathy secondary to malpositioning in scoliosis surgery. Spine (Phila Pa 1976). 2005;30:2089–93.
7. Schwartz DM, Auerbach JD, Dormans JP, et al. Neurophysiological detection of impending spinal cord injury during scoliosis surgery. J Bone Joint Surg Am. 2007;89:2440–9.
8. York DH, Chabot RJ, Gaines RW. Response variability of somatosensory evoked potentials during scoliosis surgery. Spine (Phila Pa 1976). 1987;12:864–76.
9. LaMont RL, Wasson SL, Green MA. Spinal cord monitoring during spinal surgery using somatosensory spinal evoked potentials. J Pediatr Orthop. 1983;3:31–6.
10. Lubicky JP, Spadaro JA, Yuan HA, et al. Variability of somatosensory cortical evoked potential monitoring during spinal surgery. Spine (Phila Pa 1976). 1989;14:790–8.
11. Nuwer MR, Dawson EG, Carlson LG, et al. Somatosensory evoked potential spinal cord monitoring reduces neurologic deficits after scoliosis surgery: results of a large multicenter survey. Electroencephalogr Clin Neurophysiol. 1995;96:6–11.
12. Dawson DS, Sherman JE, Kanim LE, et al. Spinal cord monitoring. Results of the Scoliosis Research Society and the European Spinal Deformity Society survey. Spine (Phila Pa 1976). 1991;16(suppl 8):S361–4.
13. York DH. A critical evaluation of the 50% criterion for SEP monitoring; 1995.
14. Banoub M, Tetzlaff J, Schubert A. Pharmacologic and physiologic influences affecting sensory evoked potentials: implications for perioperative monitoring. Anesthesiology. 2003;99:716–37.
15. Nuwer MR, Dawson EG, Carlson LG, Kanim LE, Sherman JE. Somatosensory evoked potential spinal cord monitoring reduces neurologic deficits after scoliosis surgery: results of a large multicenter survey. Electroencephalogr Clin Neurophysiol. 1995;96:6–11.
16. Deletis V, Sala F. Intraoperative neurophysiological monitoring of the spinal cord during spinal cord and spine surgery: a review focus on the corticospinal tracts. Clin Neurophysiol. 2008;119:248–64.
17. Aminoff MJ. Intraoperative monitoring by evoked potentials for spinal cord surgery: the cons. Electroencephalogr Clin Neurophysiol. 1989;73:378–80.
18. Ginsburg HH, Shetter AG, Raudezens PA. Postoperative paraplegia with preserved intraoperative somatosensory evoked potentials: case report. J Neurosur. 1985;63:296–300.
19. Loughnan BA, Hall GM. Spinal cord monitoring. Br J Anaesth. 1989;63:587–94.

20. Burke D, Hicks R, Stephen J, Woodforth I, Crawford M. Assessment of corticospinal and somatosensory conduction simultaneously during scoliosis surgery. Electroencephalogr Clin Neurophysiol. 1992;85:388–96.
21. Kalkman CJ, Drummond JC, Kennelly NA, Patel PM, Partridge BL. Intraoperative monitoring of tibialis anterior muscle motor evoked responses to transcranial electrical stimulation during partial neuromuscular blockade. Anesth Analg. 1992;75:584–9.
22. Slimp JC. Electrophysiologic intraoperative monitoring for spine procedures. Phys Med Rehabil Clin N Am. 2004;15:85–105.
23. Calancie B, Harris W, Brindle GF, Green BA, Landy HJ. Threshold-level repetitive transcranial electrical stimulation for intraoperative monitoring of central motor conduction. J Neurosurg. 2001;95:161–8.
24. Sala F, Palandri G, Basso E, Lanteri P, Deletis V, Faccioli F, et al. Motor evoked potential monitoring improves outcome after surgery for intramedullary spinal cord tumors: a historical control study. Neurosurgery. 2006;58:1129–43.
25. Krammer MJ, Wolf S, Schul DB, Gerstner W, Lumenta CB. Significance of intraoperative motor function monitoring using transcranial electrical motor evoked potentials (MEP) in patients with spinal and cranial lesions near the motor pathway. Br J Neurosurg. 2009;23:48–55.
26. Sloan TB, Heyer EJ. Anesthesia for intraoperative neurophysiologic monitoring of the spinal cord. J Clin Neurophysiol. 2002;19:430–43.
27. Bhalodia VM, Schwartz DM, Sestokas AK, et al. Efficacy of intraoperative monitoring of transcranial electrical stimulation-induced motor evoked potentials and spontaneous electromyography activity to identify acute-versus delayed-onset C-5 nerve root palsy during cervical spine surgery: clinical arti. J Neurosurg Spine. 2013;19:395–402.
28. Costa P, Peretta P, Faccani G. Relevance of intraoperative D wave in spine and spinal cord surgeries. Eur Spine J. 2013;22:8408.
29. Sloan TB, Jameson LC. Electrophysiologic monitoring during surgery to repair the thoraco-abdominal aorta. J Clin Neurophysiol. 2007;24:316–27.
30. Costa P, Bruno A, Bonzanino M, et al. Somatosensory- and motor-evoked potential monitoring during spine and spinal cord surgery. Spinal Cord. 2007;45:86–91.
31. Sloan TB, Janik D, Jameson L. Multimodality monitoring of the central nervous system using motor-evoked potentials. Curr Opin Anaesthesiol. 2008;21:560–4.
32. Holland NR. Intraoperative electromyography. J Clin Neurophysiol. 2002;19(5):444–53.
33. Toleikis JR, Carlvin AO, Shapiro DE, et al. The use of dermatomal evoked responses during surgical procedures that use intrapedicular fixation of the lumbosacral spine. Spine (Phila Pa 1976). 1993;18:2401–7.
34. Bose B, Wierzbowski LR, Sestokas AK. Neurophysiologic monitoring of spinal nerve root function during instrumented posterior lumbar spine surgery. Spine (Phila Pa 1976). 2002;27:1444–50.
35. Romstock J, Strauss C, Fahlbusch R. Continuous electromyography monitoring of motor cranial nerves during cerebellopontine angle surgery. J Neurosurg. 2000;93:586–93.
36. Leppanen RE. Intraoperative monitoring of segmental spinal nerve root function with free-run and electrically-triggered. J Clin Monitor Comput. 2005;19:437–61.
37. Padberg AM, Thuet ED. Intraoperative electrophysiologic monitoring: considerations for complex spinal surgery. Neurosurg Clin N Am. 2006;17:205–26.
38. Gunnarsson T, Krassioukov AV, Sarjeant R, Fehlings MG. Real-time continuous intraoperative electromyographic and somatosensory evoked potential recordings in spinal surgery: correlation of clinical and electrophysiologic findings in a prospective, consecutive series of 213 cases. Spine (Phila Pa 1976). 2004;2004:677–84.
39. Jin SH, Chung CK, Kim CH, Choi YD, Kwak G, Kim BE. Multimodal intraoperative monitoring during intramedullary spinal cord tumor surgery. Acta Neurochir. 2015;157(12):2149–55.
40. Dunne JW, Silbert PL, Wren M. A prospective study of acute radiculopathy after scoliosis surgery. Clin Exp Neurol. 1991;28:180–90.
41. Harper CM, Daube JR, Litchy WJ, et al. Lumbar radiculopathy after spinal fusion for scoliosis. Muscle Nerve. 1988;11:386–91.
42. Charalampidis A, Jiang F, Wilson J, Badhiwala J, Brodke D, Fehlings MG. The use of intraoperative neurophysiological monitoring in spine surgery. Global Spine J. 2020;10:104S–14S.
43. Bigelow DC, Patterson T, Weber R, Stecker MM, Judy K. Comparison of endotracheal tube and hookwire electrodes for monitoring the vagus nerve. J Clin Monit Comput. 2002;17:217–20.
44. Khan A, Pearlman RC, Bianchi DA, Hauck KW. Experience with two types of electromyography monitoring electrodes during thyroid surgery. Am J Otolaryngol. 1997;18:99–102.
45. Calancie B, Lebwohl N, Madsen P, Klose KJ. Intraoperative evoked EMG monitoring in an animal model. A new technique for evaluating pedicle screw placement. Spine (Phila Pa 1976). 1992;17:1229–35.
46. Matsuzaki H, Toiyama Y, Matsumoto F, Hoshino M, Kiuchi T, Toriyama S. Problems and solutions of pedicle screw plate fixation of lumbar spine. Spine. 1990;15:1159–65.
47. Toleikis RJ. Neurophysiological monitoring during pedicle screw placement. In: Deletis V, Shils JL, editors. Neurophysiology in neurosurgery. San Diego: Academic Press; 2002.
48. Toleikis JR, Skelly JP, Carlvin AO, Toleikis SC, Bernard TN, Burkus JK, et al. The usefulness of electrical stimulation for assessing pedicle screw placements. J Spinal Disord. 2000;13:283–9.
49. Holland NR, Kostuik JP. Continuous electromyographic monitoring to detect nerve root injury during thoracolumbar scoliosis surgery. Spine (Phila Pa 1976). 1997;22:2547–50.

50. Maguire J, Wallace S, Madigan R, Leppanen RE, Draper V. Intraoperative long-latency reflex activity in idiopathic scoliosis. Spine. 1993;18(12):1621–6.
51. Raynor BL, Lenke LG, Bridwell KH, et al. Correlation between low triggered electromyographic thresholds and lumbar pedicle screw malposition: analysis of 4857 screws. Spine (Phila Pa 1976). 2007;32:2673–8.
52. Maguire J, Wallace S, Madigan R, Leppanen R, Draper V. Evaluation of intrapedicular screw position using intraoperative evoked electromyography. Spine. 1995;20(9):1068–74.
53. Skelly JP, Toleikis JR, Carlvin AO. Pedicle screw stimulation in a fluid environment. In: The Tenth Annual Meeting of the American Society of Neurophysiological Monitoring. Denver; 1999.
54. Burkholder LM, Houlden DA, Midha R, Weiss E, Vennettilli M. Neurogenic motor evoked potentials: role in brachial plexus surgery: case report. J Neurosurg. 2003;98(3):607–10.
55. Berger JR, Blum AS. Somatosensory evoked potentials. In: Blum AS, Rutkove SB, editors. The clinical neurophysiology primer. Humana Press; 2007.
56. Oberle J, Antoniadis G, Roth SA, et al. Intraoperative electrophysiological diagnosis of spinal root avulsion during surgical repair of brachial plexus stretch injuries (Wien). Acta Neurochir. 1997;139:238–9.
57. Jones SJ, Parry CW, Landi A. Diagnosis of brachial plexus traction lesions by sensory nerve action potentials and somatosensory evoked potentials. Injury. 1981;12(5):376–82.
58. Crum BA, Strommen JA, Stucky SC. Peripheral nerve stimulation and monitoring during operative procedures. Muscle Nerve. 2007;35(2):159–70.
59. Turkof E, Millesi H, Turkof R, et al. Intraoperative electroneurodiagnostics (transcranial electrical motor evoked potentials) to evaluate the functional status of anterior spinal roots and spinal nerves during brachial plexus surgery. Plast Reconstr Surg. 1997;99:1632–41.
60. Sugioka H, Tsuyama N, Hara T, et al. Investigation of brachial plexus injuries by intraoperative cortical somatosensory evoked potentials. Arch Orthop Trauma Surg. 1982;99:143–51.
61. Carvalho GA, Nikkhah G, Matthies C, Penkert G, Samii M. Diagnosis of root avulsions in traumatic brachial plexus injuries: value of computerized tomography myelography and magnetic resonance imaging. J Neurosurg. 1997;86(1):69–76.
62. Oberle J, Antoniadis G, Kast E, Richter HP. Evaluation of traumatic cervical nerve root injuries by intraoperative evoked potentials. Neurosurgery. 2002;51(5):1182–90.
63. Kline DG, Hudson AR. Diagnosis of root avulsion (Letter). J Neurosurg. 1997;87:483.
64. Zimmerman NB, Weiland AJ. Assessment and monitoring of brachial plexus injury in the adult. In: Gelberman RH, editor. Operative nerve repair and reconstruction. Philadelphia: Lipincott; 1991. p. 1273–83.
65. Zhao S, Kim DH, Kline DG, et al. Somatosensory evoked potentials evoked by stimulating a variable number of nerve fibers in rat. Muscle Nerve. 1993;16:1220–7.
66. Sasaki H, Nagano S, Yokouchi M, et al. Utility of intraoperative monitoring with motor-evoked potential during the surgical enucleation of peripheral nerve schwannoma. Oncol Lett. 2018;15(6):9327–32.
67. O'shea K, Feinberg JH, Wolfe SW. Imaging and electrodiagnostic work-up of acute adult brachial plexus injuries. J Hand Surg (Eur Vol). 2011;36(9):747–59.
68. Kwok K, Davis B, Kliot M. Resection of a benign brachial plexus nerve sheath tumor using intraoperative electrophysiological monitoring. Oper Neurosurg. 2007;60(suppl_4):ONS-316.
69. Press JM, Rayner SL, Philip M, Monga TN, Katz RT. Intraoperative monitoring of an unusual brachial plexus tumor. Arch Phys Med Rehabil. 1992;73(3):297–9.
70. Kline DG. Nerve surgery as it is now and as it may be. Neurosurgery. 2000;46:1285–93.
71. Kline DG, Happel LT. A quarter century's experience with intraoperative nerve action potential recording. Can J Neurol Sci. 1993;20:3–10.
72. Gilliatt RW, Sears TA. Sensory nerve action potentials in patients with peripheral nerve lesions. J Neurol Neurosurg Psychiatry. 1958;21:109–18.
73. Pondaag W, Veken LP, et al. Intraoperative nerve action and compound motor action potential recordings in patients with obstetric brachial plexus lesions: clinical article. J Neurosurg. 2008;109:946–54.
74. Dg K, Br D. Evoked potentials to evaluate peripheral nerve injuries. Surg Gynecol Obstet. 1968;127:1239–48.
75. Kline DG, Hackett ER, May PR. Evaluation of nerve injuries by evoked potentials and electromyography. J Neurosurg. 1969;31:128–36.
76. Robert EG, Happel LT, Kline DG. Intraoperative nerve action potential recordings technical considerations, problems, and pitfalls. Neurosurgery. 2009;65:A97–104.
77. Haninec P, Šámal F, Tomáš R, Houstava L, Dubový P. Direct repair (nerve grafting), neurotization, and end-to-side neurorrhaphy in the treatment of brachial plexus injury. J Neurosurg. 2007;106:391–9.
78. Kim DH, Murovic JA, Tiel RL, Kline DG. Mechanisms of injury in operative brachial plexus lesions. Neurosurg Focus. 2004;16:E2.
79. Happel L, Kline D. Intraoperative neurophysiology of the peripheral nervous system. In: Deletis V, Shils JL, editors. Neurophysiology in neurosurgery. Academic Press; 2002. p. 169–95.
80. Kline DG, Hudson AR. Nerve injuries: operative results for major nerve injuries, entrapments, and tumors. Philadelphia: W.B. Saunders; 1995.
81. Sala F, Palandri G, Basso E, et al. Motor evoked potential monitoring improves outcome after surgery for intramedullary spinal cord tumors: a historical control study. Neurosurgery. 2006;58:1129–43.
82. DiCindio S, Theroux M, Shah S, et al. Multimodality monitoring of transcranial electric motor and somatosensory-evoked potentials during surgical correction of spinal deformity in patients with cerebral palsy and other neuromuscular disorders. Spine (Phila Pa 1976). 2003;28:1851–5.

83. Morota N, Deletis V, Constantini S, et al. The role of motor evoked potentials during surgery for intramedullary spinal cord tumors. Neurosurgery. 1997;41:1327–36.
84. Bhagat S, Durst A, Grover H, et al. An evaluation of multimodal spinal cord monitoring in scoliosis surgery: a single centre experience of 354 operations. Eur Spine J. 2015;24(7):1399–407.
85. Raynor BL, Padberg AM, Lenke LG, et al. Failure of intraoperative monitoring to detect postoperative neurologic deficits: a 25-year experience in 12,375 spinal surgeries. Spine. 2016;41(17):1387–93.
86. Hadley MN, Shank CD, Rozzelle CJ, Walters BC. Guidelines for the use of electrophysiological monitoring for surgery of the human spinal column and spinal cord. Neurosurgery. 2017;81(5):713–32.

Part IV

Miscellaneous Nerve Monitoring Considerations

Whitney Liddy

20 Documentation and Reimbursement

Whitney Liddy

Introduction

Intraoperative nerve monitoring (IONM) allows for real-time functional neural assessment that reaches beyond the limitations of simple visualization alone and has become a widely accepted procedure among surgeons. The benefits and cost-effectiveness of IONM have been shown in many otolaryngologic procedures from otologic/neurotologic and skull base surgery [1–3] to thyroid and parathyroid surgery [4, 5] and neck dissection [6–8]. The widespread prevalence of IONM is not only seen with experienced high-volume surgeons but with less experienced surgeons as well. IONM has been shown to improve the learning curve for more inexperienced thyroid surgeons, for example, allowing them to reach nerve outcome levels similar to more experienced surgeons [4]. Position statements have been endorsed by the American Academy of Otolaryngology – Head and Neck Surgery (AAO-HNS) for intraoperative cranial nerve monitoring and for intraoperative facial nerve monitoring (IOFNM) in otologic surgery, in particular [9, 10]. Currently, a position statement on IONM for the lower cranial nerves is being finalized for publication by a cranial nerve monitoring task force appointed by the AAO-HNS.

Intraoperative nerve monitoring is now considered a core competency by the American Board of Otolaryngology – Head and Neck Surgery. A 2017 survey sent out and analyzed by the AAO-HNS Intraoperative Nerve Monitoring Task Force polled otolaryngology – head and neck surgery residency program directors regarding the state of IONM in residency training [2]. The task force found that program directors reported universal resident exposure to IONM for neurotologic and endocrine/head and neck procedures and 61% of programs had formal training on setup, utilization, troubleshooting, and interpretation of results. Formal documentation of resident competency in IONM was also reported from the majority of programs (83.3%).

Operating surgeons have arguably the highest vested interest in the appropriate use and interpretation of IONM given their ultimate medicolegal responsibility for the patient and patient safety. However, management of IONM currently can fall to a wide range of middle parties including nonsurgical staff, audiologists, and even remote monitoring companies. Currently, the ability for the operating surgeon to bill and be reimbursed for IONM by private insurers and the Centers for Medicare and Medicaid Services is extremely limited. This chapter outlines some of

W. Liddy (✉)
Department of Otolaryngology – Head and Neck Surgery, Northwestern University Feinberg School of Medicine, Chicago, IL, USA
e-mail: Whitney-Liddy@northwestern.edu

© The Author(s), under exclusive license to Springer Nature Switzerland AG 2022

J. Scharpf, G. W. Randolph (eds.), *Intraoperative Cranial Nerve Monitoring in Otolaryngology-Head and Neck Surgery*, https://doi.org/10.1007/978-3-030-84916-0_20

the current practice patterns as well as key concepts and current arguments for IONM reimbursement by the operating surgeon.

IONM as a Distinct Procedure

While IONM was developed as an adjunctive tool to aid the surgeon in procedures where cranial nerves are at risk, the argument for separate billing and reimbursement for IONM is based on its distinction as a separate procedure from the primary surgery. Guidelines for the standardization and optimization of IONM have been published in the otolaryngology literature and detail the unique requirements for IONM including specialized equipment, setup, and expertise [5, 11]. Although there are various formats for intraoperative monitoring of cranial nerves, the optimal use of IONM requires detailed knowledge of anesthesia concerns, data interpretation, and troubleshooting. The argument for IONM as a separate billable procedure has been accepted by the Centers for Medicare and Medicaid Services in its reimbursement policies, although the operating surgeon is currently not standardly included in the list of accepted reimbursable parties.

Role of the Operating Surgeon

The argument against the operating surgeon as an allowed reimbursable party for IONM has been based on the supposed inability of the surgeon to pay adequate attention to both the surgery and the intraoperative nerve monitoring equipment and data simultaneously. However, arguments presented by the cranial nerve monitoring task force endorsed by the AAO-HNS have centered on the operating surgeon as the most well-suited and well-equipped party to actively monitor nerves during surgery (Fig. 20.1).

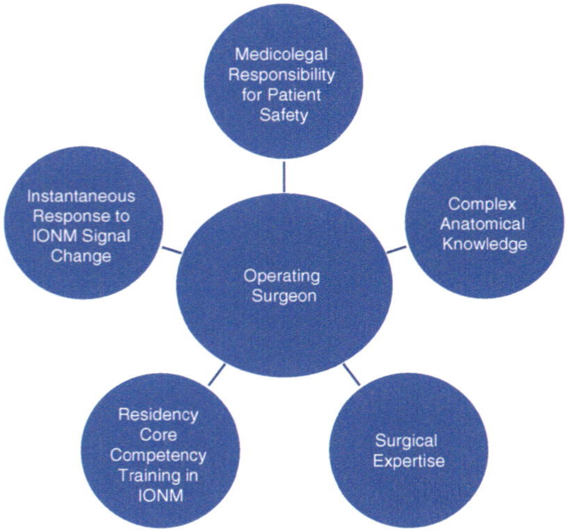
Medicolegal Responsibility for Patient Safety
Complex Anatomical Knowledge
Instantaneous Response to IONM Signal Change
Operating Surgeon
Residency Core Competency Training in IONM
Surgical Expertise

Fig. 20.1 IONM reimbursement by the operating surgeon. Key components for the argument by otolaryngologists promoting billing and reimbursement for intraoperative nerve monitoring (IONM) by the operating surgeon

As the American Board of Otolaryngology – Head and Neck Surgery now requires training in intraoperative cranial nerve monitoring as a core competency during residency and fellowship training, IONM can be considered fully within the scope of an otolaryngology – head and neck surgery practice. Position statements endorsed by the AAO-HNS and standardization guidelines regarding intraoperative cranial nerve monitoring by subspecialty interest groups, such as the International Neural Monitoring Study Group (INMSG) for thyroid surgery, further support the surgeon as the optimal manager of IONM [3, 5, 9–11]. The surgeon is uniquely positioned for this role based on a combination of comprehensive medical and anatomical knowledge, surgical technique, and training in the performance, interpretation, and strategic utilization of intraoperative cranial nerve monitoring.

Recurrent laryngeal nerve injury is the leading cause of litigation in thyroid surgery [12, 13], and facial nerve injury is second only to hearing loss for litigation in otologic surgery [14]. The operating surgeon has ultimate medicolegal responsibility for intraoperative neural injury and therefore has a particular interest in patient safety. This line of reasoning has suggested then that the party primarily responsible for patient safety would be the best choice for the optimal management of IONM. The lack of reimbursement to surgeons for performing IONM has been argued as inconsistent with the surgeon's primary role in ensuring a patient's well-being through prevention of neural injury [15].

Active participation by the surgeon in standardized IONM equipment setup, coordination with anesthesia, real-time interpretation of electrophysiologic data, and implementation of troubleshooting algorithms allows for optimal use of IONM for patient safety. In particular, the surgeon's unique ability to instantaneously respond to IONM feedback has been argued as a critical component for prevention of nerve injury [5]. Essentially, optimal performance of IONM requires instantaneous interpretation of data in order to take immediate corrective action in the setting of an impending nerve injury. The surgeon must interpret the data and correlate this data with surgical findings to decide whether to alter or adjust surgical maneuvers to maintain nerve integrity while also completing the procedure [2]. This cannot be optimally fulfilled by a middle party reading the monitor in the operating room or by monitoring from a neurophysiologist off-site, where there can be delays or failures in the communication of potential detrimental changes in electrophysiologic signal. In alignment with this argument, current intraoperative nerve monitoring systems are designed to facilitate ready accessibility by the operating surgeon with immediate and easy-to-read graphics and visual and auditory signals.

Reimbursement for IONM

Despite emerging arguments for reimbursement of the primary surgeon for IONM, there remains limited acceptance by insurance companies. In 2011, the Centers for Medicare and Medicaid Services altered the rules for reimbursement for nerve monitoring to exclude the operating physician from being able to bill. While criteria for commercial payers vary, there is a trend among private payers toward CMS rules [16], and currently these rules allow billing for IONM from the following providers: (1) a physician who is not performing the surgery, (2) an audiologist trained and certified in electrophysiologic monitoring, (3) a physical therapist trained and certified in electrophysiologic monitoring, and (4) a neurophysiologist, neurologist, or physiatrist [17]. The rules do not preclude monitoring from a remote site and even allow for simultaneous monitoring of multiple cases at one time, which is discordant with the argument that the primary surgeon cannot adequately operate and monitor the nerve simultaneously. Practice guidelines published in 2014 by the American Society of Neurophysiological Monitoring acknowledge that with off-site management of concurrent cases of IONM, "attention will be unevenly divided among cases of varying complexity and acuity" [18]. The number of concurrent cases being monitored is, therefore, up to the judgment of the IONM supervising professional. The guidelines further acknowledge the role of the primary surgeon as the supervising professional in certain areas where they hold "expert understanding," with examples given including facial nerve and recurrent laryngeal nerve monitoring by otolaryngologists [18].

Perhaps the best-case scenario within otolaryngology regarding current IONM reimbursement patterns for primary surgeons comes from the otology and neurotology literature regarding the use of intraoperative facial nerve monitoring (IOFNM) in ear and skull base surgery. IOFNM has been extensively reviewed in the literature and has been shown to be cost-effective and to reduce the rate of facial nerve injury in many otologic and skull base surgeries [1, 3, 19, 20]. In a study published in 2018, the AAO-HNS Intraoperative Nerve Monitoring Task Force evaluated survey results from members of the American Neurotology Society, American Otological Society, and American Society of Pediatric Otolaryngology regarding IOFNM practice patterns and reimbursement [2]. Results of this survey showed that most surgeons (61.1%) perform electrode placement and verification of monitoring integrity themselves, and even more (85.5%) were primarily responsible for real-time monitoring of the facial nerve during surgery. Despite this, most surgeons (64%) do not submit a bill for reimbursement. When further questioned regarding reimbursement patterns, only 20.2% of surgeons reported private insurance reimbursement, and only 4.4% of surgeons reported receiving reimbursement from Medicare.

Primary billing for IONM by the operating physician can be more cost-effective than payment to a second party or off-site nerve monitoring service. Despite a generalized lack of knowledge among surgeons regarding effective strategies for IONM billing and reimbursement, in a few local markets, surgeons have been successful in carefully negotiating fair reimbursement with local CMS representatives and private payers [2, 15]. This can be further facilitated in cases where practices have ownership of the nerve monitoring equipment. In all cases, arguments for billing for IONM as a separate procedure by the operating surgeon have been successful when the surgeon demonstrates active control of the key aspects of IONM and provides appropriate separate documentation. An example of a successful billing strategy has been the use of CPT code 95940 (monitoring oversight within the operating room, with Medicare allowable reimbursement of $37.61 per 15-minute increment) in combination with CPT code 95927–26 for evoked potentials technical setup (with modifier 26 to signify the professional component of the service with supervision, interpretation, and written report by the surgeon).

Documentation for IONM

In cases of successful reimbursement for IONM by the operating surgeon, a separate procedure report is documented in addition to the operative note. This is in alignment with the previously discussed recognition of IONM as a distinct procedure from surgery requiring separate expertise, setup, and interpretation. Based on the American Society of Neurophysiological Monitoring guidelines [18], a comprehensive IONM procedure note should include:

- Patient history
- Surgical procedure
- Modality of IONM used
- Baseline neural responses
- Any neural topographic/mapping data acquired
- Significant intraoperative changes in neural response and any interventions performed
- Closing neural responses
- Immediate postoperative findings

However, adequate documentation may be brief with the most basic information included, such as preoperative and postoperative diagnosis, basic equipment setup, baseline electrophysiologic data, and a short description of the IONM procedure.

Conclusions

Intraoperative nerve monitoring is a widely accepted and cost-effective patient safety tool for a wide variety of otolaryngologic procedures. The operating surgeon is the best equipped to primarily manage optimal utilization of IONM in real time, given the unique combination of a complex medical knowledge base, surgical expertise, and dedicated training in nerve monitoring. The ability of the surgeon to instantaneously respond to real-time IONM signals prevents the potential delays in communication that could exist with middle parties or off-site monitoring. The surgeon also maintains primary medicolegal responsibility for patient safety, garnering the most vested interest in postoperative neural outcomes. Reimbursement policies set forth by insurance companies should be adjusted to allow for billing by the primary surgeon when appropriate active control of the key aspects of IONM is clearly documented. Such policies are in alignment with recent and forthcoming position statements set forth by the cranial nerve monitoring task force endorsed by the AAO-HNS.

References

1. Wilson L, Lin E, Lalwani A. Cost-effectiveness of intraoperative facial nerve monitoring in middle ear or mastoid surgery. Laryngoscope. 2003;113:1736–45.
2. Gidley PW, Maw J, Gantz B, et al. Contemporary opinions on intraoperative facial nerve monitoring. OTO Open. 2018;2:2473974X18791803.
3. Vivas EX, Carlson ML, Neff BA, et al. Congress of neurological surgeons systematic review and evidence-based guidelines on intraoperative cranial nerve monitoring in vestibular schwannoma surgery. Neurosurgery. 2018;82:E44–6.

4. Alesina PF, Hinrichs J, Meier B, Cho EY, Bolli M, Walz MK. Intraoperative neuromonitoring for surgical training in thyroid surgery: its routine use allows a safe operation instead of lack of experienced mentoring. World J Surg. 2014;38:592–8.
5. Randolph GW, Dralle H, International Intraoperative Monitoring Study G, et al. Electrophysiologic recurrent laryngeal nerve monitoring during thyroid and parathyroid surgery: international standards guideline statement. Laryngoscope. 2011;121 Suppl 1:S1–16.
6. Lanisnik B, Zitnik L, Levart P, Zargi M, Rodi Z. The impact on post-operative shoulder function of intraoperative nerve monitoring of cranial nerve XI during modified radical neck dissection. Eur Arch Oto Rhino Laryngol. 2016;273:4445–51.
7. Birinci Y, Genc A, Ecevit MC, et al. Spinal accessory nerve monitoring and clinical outcome results of nerve-sparing neck dissections. Otolaryngol Head Neck Surg. 2014;151:253–9.
8. Lee CH, Huang NC, Chen HC, Chen MK. Minimizing shoulder syndrome with intra-operative spinal accessory nerve monitoring for neck dissection. Acta Otorhinolaryngol Ital. 2013;33:93–6.
9. Position Statement: Intraoperative Cranial Nerve Monitoring in Otolaryngology-Head and Neck Surgery: American Academy of Otolaryngology-Head and Neck Surgery (AAO-HNS/F) 2018 April.
10. Position Statement: Intraoperative Nerve Monitoring in Otologic Surgery: American Academy of Otolaryngology-Head and Neck Surgery (AAO-HNS/F) 2017 March.
11. Barczynski M, Randolph GW, Cernea CR, et al. External branch of the superior laryngeal nerve monitoring during thyroid and parathyroid surgery: International Neural Monitoring Study Group standards guideline statement. Laryngoscope. 2013;123 Suppl 4:S1–14.
12. Dralle H, Lorenz K, Machens A. Verdicts on malpractice claims after thyroid surgery: emerging trends and future directions. Head Neck. 2012;34: 1591–6.
13. Hayward NJ, Grodski S, Yeung M, Johnson WR, Serpell J. Recurrent laryngeal nerve injury in thyroid surgery: a review. ANZ J Surg. 2013;83:15–21.
14. Ruhl DS, Hong SS, Littlefield PD. Lessons learned in otologic surgery: 30 years of malpractice cases in the United States. Otol Neurotol. 2013;34:1173–9.
15. Maw J, Gidley PW. Brief Commentary on Gidley et al: "Contemporary Opinions on Intraoperative Facial Nerve Monitoring". Otolaryngol Head Neck Surg. 2018;159:601–2.
16. Cigna Medical Coverage Policy: Intraoperative Monitoring. Available at: https://static.cigna.com/assets/chcp/pdf/coveragePolicies/medical/mm_0509_coveragepositioncriteria_intraoperative-monitoring.pdf.
17. Intraoperative nerve monitoring reimbursement coding guide: Medtronic, 2016.
18. Skinner SA, Cohen BA, Morledge DE, et al. Practice guidelines for the supervising professional: intraoperative neurophysiological monitoring. J Clin Monit Comput. 2014;28:103–11.
19. Kartush JM. Electroneurography and intraoperative facial monitoring in contemporary neurotology. Otolaryngol Head Neck Surg. 1989;101:496–503.
20. Heman-Ackah SE, Gupta S, Lalwani AK. Is facial nerve integrity monitoring of value in chronic ear surgery? Laryngoscope. 2013;123:2–3.

Ethical Considerations for Nerve Monitoring

21

Peter Angelos

Introduction

In the upcoming pages, I will consider the essential issues in the ethical considerations for neuromonitoring. I will begin by considering the ethical issues in surgical informed consent in general. The issues of informed consent in thyroid and parathyroid surgery will then be considered with specific attention to nerve monitoring. The legal issues that are related to standard of care determinations in thyroid and parathyroid surgery are considered. In the final section, I will consider recommendations for the ethical use of nerve monitoring.

Informed Consent

Informed consent is central to the ethical practice of surgery. In order for a surgical procedure to be an ethically acceptable behavior, the patient has to have been provided adequate information by the surgeon. There are minimal acceptable standards for informed consent. First of all, the patient must have the capacity to make a decision. If a patient lacks the capacity to make a decision, then there is no reason for the surgeon to spend time discussing the operation with the patient. In those situations, the surgeon will seek an appropriate surrogate decision-maker. The surrogate decision-maker could be someone identified by the patient in a durable power of attorney for healthcare document. Frequently, however, patients have not filled out such documents, and surgeons must go to the next of kin for decision-making. In the case of a married patient, this would be a spouse. In the case of an elderly patient who has no spouse, an adult son or daughter would be the appropriate surrogate decision-maker. Once the determination is made that the patient or appropriate surrogate has the capacity to make a decision, surgeons must move on to discuss the risks, benefits, and alternatives of surgery with the patient or surrogate. When these conditions have been met, the patient or surrogate may agree to the procedure.

Several important aspects of surgical informed consent are worthwhile considering. First of all, the surgeon-patient relationship is somewhat different from the relationship between patients and other physicians. Most notably, there is a short time for a surgeon to obtain the confidence of a patient and educate a patient about the condition that requires surgery. Unlike internists or other primary care physicians, surgeons rarely have years to develop a relationship with patients prior to asking their patients to trust them. In that short period of time that a surgeon and a patient are

P. Angelos (✉)
Department of Surgery and MacLean Center for Clinical Medical Ethics, The University of Chicago, Chicago, IL, USA
e-mail: pangelos@surgery.bsd.uchicago.edu

© The Author(s), under exclusive license to Springer Nature Switzerland AG 2022

J. Scharpf, G. W. Randolph (eds.), *Intraoperative Cranial Nerve Monitoring in Otolaryngology-Head and Neck Surgery*, https://doi.org/10.1007/978-3-030-84916-0_21

discussing an operation, the surgeon must clarify the goals of the operation along with answering whatever questions are necessary in order for the patient to feel comfortable with proceeding. Another difference between the relationship between surgeons and patients and that of patients with other physicians is that the potential risks of surgery are frequently much higher than are the risks of other interventions such as taking medications. In addition, when considering surgery, the patient is in a particularly vulnerable situation. This vulnerability also has an impact on informed consent.

It is difficult to overstate the extent to which specific actions of surgeons impact the outcome of their patients. This is well described by Charles Bosk in his important sociological study of surgical residency, *Forgive and Remember*. Bosk describes the interactions that occur in the morbidity and mortality conference in a surgery department:

> When the patient of an internist dies, the natural question his colleagues ask is, "What happened?" When the patient of a surgeon dies his colleagues ask, "What did you do?" By the nature of his craft and his beliefs about it the surgeon is more accountable than other physicians and he also has much more to account for [1].

This description clearly identifies the difference in how surgeons feel about the responsibility that they have for their patients' outcomes.

It is sometimes valuable to consider how the quality of informed consent should be determined. Some commentators have suggested that the true measure of the quality of informed consent is whether the patient understands the risks, benefits, and alternatives of the procedure. Other commentators have suggested that, in fact, the quality of informed consent is determined by whether the patient is satisfied with the interaction and ultimately the surgical procedure. Alternatively, and somewhat skeptically, some have argued in the literature that we really should not be thinking so much about the patient but about the surgeon when determining the quality of informed consent. In this view, informed consent is really designed to protect surgeons from claims of liability. This last view is not consistent with the ethical analysis of the interaction since informed consent really should be directed toward improving the patient's experience with surgery. As one considers these alternatives of how to assess the quality of informed consent, it is helpful to briefly reflect on the experience of most surgeons. Most experienced surgeons report that patients do not remember much of the risks, benefits, and alternatives that they may have just heard about. I have actually asked patients shortly after they have signed an informed consent document whether they can repeat to me what the risks benefits and alternatives are that I just moments ago discussed with them. Few of them can repeat those issues that I discussed with them. Despite this, the vast majority of patients remain quite satisfied with the informed consent process.

This combination of facts raises an important question: "How can patients remember little and yet be so satisfied with the informed consent process?" I believe that this discrepancy can be best explained if one reconceptualizes informed consent for surgery as being less about information transfer and more about the development of trust between surgeon and patient [2].

Ethics and Neuromonitoring

What could possibly be unethical about intraoperative neuromonitoring? This question remains very important because throughout medicine, it is rare that a technology itself is either ethical or unethical. Rather, our assessment of whether something is ethical or unethical depends on how the technology is being used. In the case of nerve monitoring in thyroid and parathyroid surgery, the central ethical issues arise in the discrepancy between what is promised and what is delivered. Ethical concerns are thus limited as long as surgeons are not misleading their patients by suggesting that nerve monitoring can prevent the possibility of nerve injury [3]. This can be challenging for surgeons who may believe that use of nerve monitoring reduces the risks of nerve injury. However, it is essential that surgeons not overstate the value of nerve monitoring when the literature does not show a statistically significant reduction in nerve injury rates even when nerve monitoring is used. We know that when rates of nerve injury are very low as in the case of thyroid and parathyroid surgery, it would take with a very large number of participants to show a statistically significant reduction in nerve injury rate with the use of nerve monitoring.

Surgeons must be careful in their conversations with patients to not suggest more value from use of nerve monitoring than the data from the literature suggests is possible. It is not enough for surgeons to simply avoid stating that neuromonitoring reduces nerve injuries. Surgeons must also take great care for patients to not assume that the "new and innovative" technology is better than traditional techniques. In this context, surgeons should be quite explicit in not suggesting that nerve monitoring technology can do more than what has been shown by data in the literature. The use of intraoperative nerve monitoring in thyroid and parathyroid surgery should never be presented to patients as preventing a nerve injury. More accurately, surgeons should state that nerve monitoring technology may help the surgeon but cannot definitively prevent the possibility of a nerve injury.

Informed Consent and Neuromonitoring

As noted above, utilizing nerve monitoring technology does not necessarily result in improved safety. The technology can, however, reduce the risk that a patient might have a bilateral recurrent laryngeal nerve injury. Multiple studies have shown that loss of a vagus nerve signal is strongly predictive of the lack of recurrent laryngeal nerve function on that side of the neck [4, 5]. Thus, if a patient is scheduled for a total thyroidectomy, the patient should understand that nerve monitoring might allow the surgeon to decide not to go to the second side in order to prevent the possibility of a bilateral nerve injury if there is monitoring evidence of a nerve injury on the first side [3]. This description of stopping an operation after taking out only one side of the thyroid when a total thyroidectomy had been planned is referred to as a staged operation.

If a surgeon has plans to use nerve monitoring and would not go to the contralateral side if there was evidence of a nerve injury on the first side, then that plan should be discussed with the patient preoperatively. Although many surgeons might question how comfortable patients are with discussing the possibility of a staged operation, I have found that most patients are quite willing to accept the potential for a second operation if it makes the risks of a bilateral recurrent laryngeal nerve injury as low as possible.

Consider a few illustrative cases. If a 73-year-old patient was found to have a 3 cm right thyroid nodule with cytology consistent with a Hurthle cell neoplasm, there would be a little controversy about the recommendation for surgery. If there were no nodules on the contralateral side, then most surgeons would give the patient the option of a right thyroid lobectomy or a total thyroidectomy. In the circumstance where a patient is strongly in favor of a total thyroidectomy to avoid even the possibility of needing a second operation, consider what the surgeon should do if nerve monitoring shows loss of a vagal signal on the right side after removing that lobe. In such a circumstance, I would strongly favor not removing the left lobe and thus avoiding the potential risk of a bilateral recurrent laryngeal nerve injury.

One could make the same argument in the case of a 32-year-old patient with a 4.5 cm papillary thyroid carcinoma on the right side. Most surgeons would recommend a total thyroidectomy for such a patient so that radioactive iodine could be used postoperatively. However, if a vagus nerve signal is lost after removing the right lobe, the surgeon would be justified in planning a staged thyroidectomy because most nerve injuries are transient as long as the nerve is intact. If, however, the nerve injury is a transection injury that is not going to recover, then the decision-making regarding going to the contralateral side is more complex. Although it is beyond the scope of discussion for this chapter to catalog the optimal approach to staged thyroidectomy in every situation, it is important for the surgeon to have carefully considered and discussed with the patient what would be the plan with loss of vagal nerve signal on the first side.

Additional Ethical Considerations

If a surgeon does not use intraoperative nerve monitoring and has excellent results, it is difficult to fault the surgeon for deciding not to use the technology. However, there are potential problems with the selective use of recurrent laryngeal nerve monitoring technology. If a surgeon were to selectively use intraoperative nerve monitoring, it is important to ask why the choice is made to use the monitor on difficult cases. If the answer is that the surgeon believes there may be a marginal benefit in difficult cases, the natural follow-up question is, "Why would you not want that benefit for all of your patients?" There are answers to this question that are more ethically defensible than others. If the surgeon believes that dependence on intraoperative nerve monitoring would result in careless dissection of the nerve, then such an occurrence would be problematic. However, the natural follow-up question is why should a surgeon change his or her technique when using nerve monitoring technology? On the other hand, if nerve monitoring adds significant costs to a procedure then depending on the system and the availability of the technology, it might not be justifiable to utilize nerve monitoring in every case.

Another important consideration is the suboptimal use of the technology. If, for example, a surgeon has the nerve monitoring technology but does not know how to use it for the greatest benefit of his or her patient, then simply having the machine on in the operating room is not beneficial. If costs are added to the operation without any added benefits, such use of the nerve monitoring technology would not be ethical.

Medical-Legal Issues in Nerve Monitoring

Due to the multiple different laws that apply in different states and countries, it is difficult to make broad generalizations about the potential legal issues associated with nerve monitoring. However, some general comments can be made. At least in the USA, the fundamental legal issue is that of malpractice lawsuits. We know that there is wide latitude for patients to bring lawsuits against physicians. However, regardless of the operation, if there has been no harm to the patient, the lawsuit will rarely result in monetary damages being awarded. Thus, if the use of nerve monitoring technology can result in a reduction in rates of harm to patients, then nerve monitoring has value. However, if a surgeon is using the technology in a way that does not optimize patient benefit, simply having the machine in the operating room is of no value for the patient, nor is it protective of the surgeon against malpractice suits [6].

The central issue in malpractice lawsuits in the USA is whether the care rendered is commensurate with "the standard of care." As is evident, the standard of care becomes the most important issue to determine. It is important to note that the standard of care is not defined by an individual surgeon nor by a particular department of surgery. Rather, the standard of care is defined in most jurisdictions as care that meets the level that would be provided by other surgeons in that area. Thus, the standard of care is not defined by evidence in the surgical literature but by what surgeons actually do in their practices. It is evident that the standard of care changes over time, but only slowly as the practices of individual surgeons in an area change.

Conclusions

In my opinion, the ethical practice of thyroid and parathyroid surgery does not currently require the use of intraoperative nerve monitoring. If intraoperative nerve monitoring is to be used by a surgeon, it is unethical for the surgeon to not utilize it in a manner that provides the greatest safety benefit to patients. However, surgeons should not overstate the benefits of the technology when discussing risks of nerve injury with patients. If used correctly, intraoperative nerve monitoring should make the risks of a bilateral recurrent laryngeal nerve injury exceedingly low. If a total thyroidectomy is planned, the possibility of knowing that one nerve is injured is of tremendous benefit in deciding whether to go to the contralateral side. If a surgeon plans to use nerve monitoring in this fashion, then informed consent demands that patients be told of the possibility of a staged operation. Intraoperative nerve monitoring cannot prevent lawsuits but might prevent some nerve injuries, and without the presence of a nerve injury, the legal risks to the surgeon are reduced. Intraoperative nerve monitoring is an excellent tool, but as with any surgical tool, we must know how to use it and not exaggerate its benefits to patients. We must not depend on the technology to make sloppy technique safe.

Nerve monitoring in thyroid and parathyroid surgery, like any other medical or surgical technology, is neither inherently ethical nor unethical. The assessment of whether the technology is being used in an ethical manner or not is based on whether it is being used to provide the greatest benefit to the patient.

References

1. Bosk C. Forgive and remember. Chicago: University of Chicago Press; 1979. p. 30.
2. Skowron K, Angelos P. Surgical informed consent revisited: time to revise the routine? World J Surg. 2017;41:1–4.
3. Angelos P. Ethical and medicolegal issues in neuromonitoring during thyroid and parathyroid surgery: a review of the recent literature. Curr Opin Oncol. 2012;24:16–21.
4. Chiang FY, Lee KW, Chen HC, et al. Standardization of intraoperative neuromonitoring of recurrent laryngeal nerve in thyroid operation. World J Surg. 2010;34:223–9.
5. Randolph GW, Dralle HD, et al.; International Intraoperative Monitoring Study Group. Electrophysiologic recurrent laryngeal nerve monitoring during thyroid and parathyroid surgery: international standards guideline statement. Laryngoscope. 2011;121:S1–S16.
6. Angelos P. Recurrent laryngeal nerve monitoring: state of the art, ethical and legal concerns. Surg Clin North Am. 2009;89:1157–69.

Nerve Monitoring and Medical Malpractice

22

Allison Keane and David Goldenberg

Introduction

Malpractice claims in thyroid surgery are rare, with a reported 5.9 claims per 10,000 surgeries [1]. Many claims are settled outside of the courtroom and are not public record. Medical malpractice claims require evidence of a physician's duty to a patient, a breach of said duty, and harm or injury to the patient proven to be caused by the breach of duty. Medicolegally, a breach of duty is synonymous with substandard medical care. Medical malpractice lawsuits require proof that the medical care was below the standard of care and that substandard care resulted in harm to the patient. In malpractice claims in the arena of thyroid surgery, recurrent laryngeal nerve (RLN) injury is the most commonly cited harm to the patient [2].

Intraoperative nerve monitoring (IONM) enhances the identification of the RLN by providing a functional dynamic of evoked electromyography (EMG) generated through nerve stimulation. Visualization of the RLN is currently considered the standard of care for preventing nerve injury and reducing nerve palsy during thyroid surgery. The risk for permanent RLN injury is reported to be 1–2% in expert hands, but some authors believe that this number represents an underestimation. Studies have not shown IONM to reduce RLN injury risk and is thus not considered standard of care. However, in some instances, such as bilateral thyroid surgery or total thyroidectomy, IONM usage may preclude bilateral RLN injury.

This chapter reviews medical malpractice, specifically within the realm of thyroid surgery, and the implications of IONM on medical malpractice in thyroid surgery.

Medical Malpractice

Civil law refers to matters between two parties in which one party wronged the other. Medical malpractice falls under civil law instead of criminal law, in which one party commits criminal acts or offenses against the government. Medical malpractice lawsuits are tried in front of a jury unless settled outside court. The lawsuits are typically filed in a state trial court where the parties are located or where the event occurred; however, cases are argued in federal courts if the lawsuit involves a federally funded clinic such as a Veterans Administration facility, the parties are from different states, or a constitutional right is allegedly violated [3].

A. Keane · D. Goldenberg (✉)
The Department of Otolaryngology-Head and Neck Surgery, The Pennsylvania State University, The Milton S. Hershey Medical Center, Hershey, PA, USA
e-mail: akeane@pennstatehealth.psu.edu; dgoldenberg@pennstatehealth.psu.edu

© The Author(s), under exclusive license to Springer Nature Switzerland AG 2022
J. Scharpf, G. W. Randolph (eds.), *Intraoperative Cranial Nerve Monitoring in Otolaryngology-Head and Neck Surgery*, https://doi.org/10.1007/978-3-030-84916-0_22

Medical malpractice occurs when a physician causes harm to a patient due to an action or omission of an action outside the standard of practice. There are four elements the plaintiff must prove in a medical malpractice case: the physician's legal duty to provide treatment, occurrence of a breach of that duty, occurrence of patient injury resulting in damages, and causation between the breach of duty and injury [3, 4]. The plaintiff must prove the physician provided substandard or inadequate medical care that caused an injury to the patient for which subsequent damages can be quantified.

A physician's legal duty to provide treatment is established for any parties that had a doctor-patient interaction. Once the doctor-patient relationship is established, a physician is legally and ethically obligated to provide medical care. When a physician's legal duty to provide treatment is questioned, one party is a physician, but the relationship between the parties is outside of a doctor-patient relationship.

Proving the occurrence of a breach of duty requires establishing negligence or deviation from the standard of care. Physicians often discuss the concept of "the standard of care," but the legal definition is specific. The standard of care in each malpractice case is unique as each patient's medical case is unique. Generally, the "medical standard of care" is what another similarly trained physician would have done in the situation in question. In court, this is presented by the plaintiffs and defendants as expert witnesses and/or written documents [3, 5]. Qualified medical experts testify to the appropriate medical standard of care for the case's circumstances in question and how the defendant did or did not deviate from this standard. Expert witnesses also testify how the physician's actions did or did not attribute to the injuries in question. Clinical practice guidelines have been entered as physical exhibits to show the standard of care. However, legally, the guidelines are usually considered "hearsay" because the author is not available to testify [4, 5]. The contents of clinical practice guidelines are often referenced during expert testimony to provide or dispute witness credibility or prove a deviation from the standard of care [4, 5]. Adherence to clinical practice guidelines offers some protection from medical malpractice lawsuits. Still, it does not guarantee a failure to prove a breach of duty if the plaintiff can prove reasonable judgment would be to act outside the clinical practice guidelines [5].

The plaintiff must prove that harm occurred and that the harm occurred due to medical care outside the standard of care. A mistake during medical treatment or substandard care provided that does not result in harm or injury and subsequent damages to the patient cannot be legally proven as medical malpractice. For example, suppose a patient is admitted to the hospital and is mistakenly not provided their home hypertensive medication for the first 24 hours. In that case, this is a mistake or care outside of the norm. However, if the patient has no subsequent injury or harm resulting from 24 hours without their hypertensive medication, this is not a medical malpractice situation from a legal definition. Harm can be defined as a physical injury or need for further procedures and medical interventions. Harm can also be defined as an effect on the quality of life, psychosocial morbidities, strain on a relationship, reduced or loss of employment, and loss of compensation. Simply stated, medical malpractice must be treatment below an accepted medical standard of care that results in harm to the patient.

"Tort reform" refers to state-specific actions or regulations regarding the filing and process of medical malpractice cases. States have varying regulations regarding statute of limitations on filing a medical malpractice suit, venue locations for trials, and admission of physician apologies as evidence of negligence. Physicians should be familiar with their state-specific legislature regarding medical malpractice cases.

Recurrent Laryngeal Nerve Injury

Damage to the RLN can range from asymptomatic to emergent airway compromise depending on the severity of the injury, laterality, patient comorbidities, and ability to compensate. Injury to the unilateral RLN may occur postoperatively in paresis or decreased mobility of the unilateral vocal cord, but not complete paralysis. Dyspnea, stridor, aspiration, and hoarseness may occur. Alternately, unilateral RLN injury may be asymptomatic. Nerve function and vocal cord mobility may improve or resolve over the subsequent 12 months. Transection of the RLN results in paralysis of the unilateral vocal cord and similar presenting symptoms. Voice therapy and additional procedures such as a thyroplasty are potential interventions for unilateral dysfunction.

Iatrogenic dysphonia from unilateral RLN, while not life-threatening, impacts the quality of life and employment. Patients with unilateral vocal cord paralysis report communication difficulties, particularly on the phone and in social situations [6]. Dysphonia impacts family dynamics and can cause emotional and psychological stress [6]. Also, patients with dysphonia report decreased work productivity [6]. Cohen et al. reviewed a national database of work absences and short-term disability claims among patients with a dysphonia diagnosis and found the mean number of workdays absent to be 39.2 days and then mean wages lost in 12 months to be $4437.89 [7]. Other chronic diseases such as asthma or acute coronary syndrome have similar productivity loss as patients with a dysphonia diagnosis [7].

Bilateral vocal cord paralysis is significantly more severe than unilateral injury. It can lead to emergent airway compromise and the need for emergent tracheostomy. Patients who undergo tracheostomy for bilateral vocal cord paralysis will require additional future procedures as well as suffer from a significant lifestyle and quality of life change. A tracheostomy has psychosocial effects on a patient and is associated with increased morbidity. Both patients and caregivers report feeling self-conscious, unsupported, and isolated due to tracheostomy status [8]. A tracheostomy has been shown to have a negative impact on well-being, quality of life, and body image [8].

RLN injury, unilateral or bilateral, has physical, medical, emotional, and economic impacts on a patient. In medical malpractice, this is presented and interpreted as harm and the subsequent damages resulting from that harm.

Intraoperative Neuromonitoring in Thyroid Surgery

RLN injury and vocal cord paralysis are a feared complications of thyroid surgery due to the subsequent patient impact, as discussed above. Transient and permanent unilateral vocal cord paralysis has a reported incidence of 0.4–12% and 5–6%, respectively [9, 10]. The most feared complication due to the significant airway compromise, bilateral vocal cord paralysis, occurs at a reported incidence of 0.1–0.9% [9, 10]. Visual identification and surgical technique are the standard of care for preserving the RLN during thyroid surgery. Intraoperative neuromonitoring (IONM) has been employed as an adjunct to aid in identifying and preserving the RLN. While visual identification confirms the location of the RLN, IONM may provide information regarding the integrity and functionality of the RLN in addition to location.

Despite the anecdotal benefits and advantages of IONM, it has not been proven to have a significant impact on RLN injury during thyroidectomy. Dralle et al. prospectively analyzed 29,998 nerves at risk and evaluated RLN injury rate in patients with no RLN identification, visual RLN identification, and visual RLN identification plus IONM [11]. There was no statistically different rate of RLN injury between the visual RLN identification group and the group with IONM [11]. Shindo et al. retrospectively reviewed 1043 RLN at risk and compared the incidence of vocal cord injury between patients who underwent thyroid surgery with or without IONM [12]. An incidence of RLN injury was reported between 2% and 3% in each group, but there was no statistical difference in the incidence of RLN injury between the groups [12]. These and other similar studies are limited by the number of RLN at risk evaluated in each study, given the low incidence of RLN injury overall. It is estimated that 40,000 nerves at risk must be evaluated to show a statistical difference.

A decrease in RLN injury was seen in specific subgroups when IONM is employed, such as low-volume surgeons [11] or patients undergoing reoperation [13]. Chan et al. analyzed 1000 RLN at risk and compared postoperative, transient, and permanent RLN injury in patients who underwent thyroidectomy with and without IONM [13]. There was no significant difference in RLN injury between the groups. However, in patients undergoing a reoperation, transient RLN paresis was statistically less frequent in patients with IONM, suggesting a benefit of IONM in patients undergoing a reoperation [13]. Findings indicate that although IONM has not been shown to reduce RLN injury risk, it may be superior in specific subgroups. The American Academy of Otolaryngology-Head and Neck Surgery suggests the use of IONM for patients with preexisting RLN paralysis, and in revision thyroid procedures, and in total thyroidectomies or bilateral procedures [14]. Patients with unilateral RLN paralysis undergoing thyroid surgery on the contralateral side are at risk for bilateral vocal cord paralysis. Some patients may have RLN dysfunction preoperatively due to nodule or goiter compression of RLN. IONM, in such cases, can test RLN function after goiter resection. In revision thyroid procedures, anatomical landmarks may be altered and challenging to identify, making RLN injury a higher risk. While there is some evidence of the benefit of IONM in preventing RLN injury in certain situations, it has not been accepted as the standard of care.

In total thyroidectomy, IONM has been more readily adopted due to the significant consequence of incurring bilateral RLN injury. Intraoperative identification of the RLN remains the gold standard for preventing RLN injury. Intraoperative identification provides observation of nerve location and visualization of an intact nerve. However, IONM provides information regarding the functionality of the nerve. Total thyroidectomy is routinely started on the side with the larger nodules, more suspicious nodules, or worse malignant disease. If RLN injury is observed on the initial surgical side, surgery on the contralateral side may be postponed, but the area of more severe disease will have been resected. IONM provides the advantage of confirming the functionality of the RLN on the initial surgical side, not just by visualization, prior to proceeding to the contralateral side.

IONM may have changed the operative approach to total thyroidectomy and increased the use of a staged approach [9, 10, 15, 16]. The specificity of IONM in predicting vocal cord paralysis has been measured at >99% [9]. In a review of 716 patients, Cavicchi et al. found a negative predictive value of 99.7% for IONM in predicting an RLN injury and a positive predictive value of 78.3%, findings which were consistent with other studies [9]. IONM revealing an intact RLN signal after resection of the first side predicts a functional RLN 99.7% of the time. From a surgical perspective, an intact IONM signal after unilateral dissection provides more confidence to proceed to the contralateral side. However, the negative predictive value is not 100%. There are reports of an intact IONM signal intraoperatively but symptomatic and laryngoscopy proven vocal cord paralysis seen postoperatively. While this is rare, it is of consideration to the surgeon.

The positive predictive value for IONM is lower and more variable, ranging from 60% to 90% [9, 15, 17]. Loss of signal intraoperatively may result from RLN injury or may be secondary to equipment failure or patient positioning. Therefore, loss of signal may result in abortion of the contralateral procedure unnecessarily and leads to the need for a second procedure.

In the event of loss of signal on the initial side of resection in a total thyroidectomy, the surgeon is presented with a practical dilemma regarding proceeding with contralateral resection. The preoperative discussion with the patient, the indication for the procedure, the disease process, and surgeon skill are considerations for this decision. A staged thyroidectomy is easier to justify in patients with nonmalignant disease [9, 10, 15]. In patients with low-risk malignancy, a staged thyroidectomy is also more justifiable. A staged procedure allows for evaluation of resolved transient RLN paralysis, which typically is seen within the first few weeks to a month, or at the latest within 12 months of the initial surgery. This approach must be weighed with the risk of disease progression and metastasis. Low-risk malignancies that are not expected to progress significantly over a few months should be considered for a staged thyroidectomy when the IONM signal is lost on one side. For patients with advanced thyroid disease, the risk of bilateral vocal cord paralysis must be compared with the consequences of persistent or progressive disease.

A surgical plan in the event of a RLN injury should be determined preoperatively based on the patient's disease and preference. Discussion with the patient preoperatively about all possible scenarios and documentation on informed consent regarding options should RLN injury occur are recommended. The risks associated with bilateral RLN injury should be clearly discussed with the patient and documented to ensure the patient is fully informed during the consent discussion and before the procedure.

As stated earlier, the standard of care is the actions another comparable physician would do under similar circumstances; negligence is, therefore, failure to meet the standard of care. As evident by the studies as mentioned above, RLN injury has not been proven to be statistically lower when IONM is employed. As a result, regardless of the number of physicians using IONM, it is not considered standard of care [2]. The gold standard for identifying the RLN is meticulous dissection and operative skills. While medical research is not often accepted as an exhibit in court, expert witnesses who quote the above or similar studies and who have altered their application of IONM in specific patient subgroups based on these or similar studies can strengthen plaintiff arguments that IONM should have been utilized.

Some physicians utilize IONM solely because they feel this will decrease litigation risk in the incidence of an RLN injury. However, plaintiffs argue that a RLN injury despite the use of IONM also proves negligence [18]. Alternatively, plaintiffs argue an RLN injury may not have occurred if IONM had been utilized [18]. Dralle et al. reviewed malpractice cases in Germany, four of which surrounded IONM. Three of the cases resulted in favor of the plaintiff due to failure to use IONM or failure to use IONM according to international standards [19]. The use of IONM does not protect a physician from malpractice claims in the event of an RLN injury and may provoke further claims regarding the proper use and the use according to standards.

The International Neurol Monitoring Study group is a multidisciplinary group composed of surgeons, laryngologists, laryngeal electromyography (EMG) specialists, and anesthesiologists who developed international guidelines regarding RLN monitoring during thyroid and parathyroid surgery. The guidelines discuss equipment setup, endotracheal tube placement, and troubleshooting loss of signal [20]. The guidelines recommend preoperative laryngoscopy, a suprathreshold vagal nerve stimulation prior to dissection and post-dissection, as well as a postoperative laryngoscopy [20]. Pre-dissection stimulation confirms the functionality of the IONM circuit, and post-dissection predicts postoperative glottic dysfunction. Failure to comply with either provides support to a plaintiff who can argue that failure to perform pre-dissection stimulation lends question to the reliability of the circuit, and failure to preform post-dissection stimulation lends question to the claim that the RLN was intact.

Regarding equipment setup, the international guidelines for RLN monitoring advocate for confirmation of properly placed endotracheal tube by the anesthesiologist and surgeon [20]. Depth of insertion and degree of rotation of the endotracheal tube can affect the functionality of the IONM circuit. Single-electrode pads integrated into endotracheal tubes have historically been used but are subject to migration of the electrode pad and improper placement. Migration can result in loss of signal or decreased sensitivity of signal. The single-electrode setup also requires the anesthesiologist and/or surgeon to visualize the electrode is centered on the vocal cords during placement of the endotracheal tube. Patient positioning throughout surgery may change, which could also affect the electrode placement. In single-electrode systems, if the endotracheal tube is not checked by the anesthesiologist and surgeon at intubation or after final positioning of the patient, and there is dysfunction of the circuit or loss of signal intraoperatively, the plaintiff may argue the surgeon was negligent by not confirming proper endotracheal tube placement.

Alternatively, the malpractice claim may include the anesthesiologist.

More recently, double-electrode pads integrated into endotracheal tubes, as described by Choby et al. [21], have been widely adopted and utilized. The double-electrode system addresses the pitfalls of the single-electrode system and offers separate information for the right and left RLN. The double-electrode system doubles the electrode surface area which reduces the risk of loss of signal or signal intensity due to endotracheal tube migration. At intubation, the anesthesiologist intubates with the same process as with a standard endotracheal tube. Confirmation of correct placement is achieved by an endotracheal tube approximately 21 cm distal to the incisors, auscultation of bilateral lungs, and EMG signal presence on neuromonitoring [21]. Typical intubation procedure with a standard endotracheal tube can be utilized with the double-electrode system because the large surface area of the electrode pads ensure contact with the vocal cords [21]. This system negates the argument by the plaintiff that the surgeon is negligent if they do not verify and document endotracheal tube placement.

Medical Malpractice in Thyroid Surgery

Medical malpractice cases in thyroid surgery are rare. Based on extrapolation from the Physician Insurers Association of America data, Singer et al. reported about 5.9 claims per 10,000 surgeries [1]. The majority of malpractice cases in thyroid surgery involve RLN injury [2]. The most common claims revolved around lack of informed consent and need for additional procedures [22]. Bilateral RLN injury cases more often resulted in favor of the plaintiff than unilateral RLN injury cases [22]. Many of these claims are settled outside of court with only a few cases proceeding to a jury trial. Below is a review of medical malpractice claims in thyroid surgery.

Svider et al. analyzed medical malpractice claims in head and neck surgery from 2008 to 2012 identified from the Westlaw Legal Database [23]. Of the forty-four cases reviewed, endoscopic sinus surgery was the most litigated procedure (20.5%), and only eight (18.2%) of the cases ruled in favor of the plaintiff. Five of the cases involved thyroid surgery, three of which ruled in favor of the plaintiff and one of which was related to RLN injury [23].

Abadin et al. reviewed the LexisNexis Academic Legal Database for medical malpractice related to thyroid surgery from 1989 to 2009 with a focus on RLN injury [2]. A total of thirty-three cases were reviewed, fifteen (46%) of which involved RLN injury with five cases involving bilateral RLN injury, five cases involving unilateral RLN injury, and five cases with laterality unspecified [2]. Despite inclusion of cases involving events that occurred after the adoption of IONM, this was not discussed in any of the cases of RLN injury [2]. Seven of the fifteen cases ruled in favor of the plaintiff with an average award of $1.6 million, range of $150,000 to $3.7 million. The majority of these cases were filed and awarded due to a lack of informed consent or sufficient discussion regarding informed consent [2].

Swonke et al. reviewed fifty-five medical malpractice cases involving thyroid surgery between 1984 and 2018 from the Westlaw Legal Database [24]. Vocal cord paralysis was the most common injury for which medical malpractice was claimed accounting for twenty-eight (51%) of the cases, twelve of which were unilateral RLN injuries and eleven of which were bilateral RLN injuries. Of all the cases reviewed by Swonke et al., about two-thirds involved general surgeons, and one-third involved otolaryngologists. Six of the twelve unilateral RLN injury cases and nine of the eleven bilateral RLN injury cases involved general surgeons as the defendants. Eighteen of the vocal cord paralysis cases ruled in favor of the defendant, two were settled prior to verdict, and eight ruled in favor of the plaintiff. Lack of informed consent was again claimed in 30% of the cases that ruled in favor of the plaintiff. Damages related to tracheostomy secondary to bilateral vocal cord paralysis were also common in 40% of the cases that ruled in favor of the plaintiff. Swonke et al. also analyzed the geographic distribution of all cases reviewed, finding the South to have the highest incidence of claims and the Northeast and West regions to have the lowest, a finding that was attributed to tort reform [24].

Ta et al. reviewed the Westlaw Legal Database in 2014 for all cases involving iatrogenic dysphonia revealing one hundred and twenty-three cases between 1984 and 2013 [22]. Thyroidectomy was the most common procedure cited as cause for dysphonia in forty-two (37%) of the cases followed by intubation (18%). Of all the cases, 25% ruled in favor of the plaintiff. However, nineteen of the thyroidectomy cases (45%) ruled in favor of the plaintiff. Average settlement of $808,942 (range, $4250–$3,000,000) was awarded in cases involving RLN injury. The most common claims in iatrogenic dysphonia cases was need for additional surgery (33%) as well as inadequate informed consent (33%). General surgeon defendants were found to be at higher risk of a plaintiff verdict which the authors speculate is due to surgeon volume of thyroid related procedures [22].

Singer et al. reviewed the Physicians Insurers Association of America for all thyroid-related procedures from 1985 to 2008. This database includes malpractice claims that went to trial as well as those that were settled out of court and estimated to represent 25% of medical malpractice claims in the United States [1]. Three hundred eighty claims occurred, forty-two (11.1%) of which went to trial and seven of which resulted in favor of the plaintiff with average award $185,366 (range $363 to $2,000,000). RLN injury was reported in fifty-five of the cases, twenty-one of which resulted in favor of the plaintiff with average award of $350,357 [1].

Thyroid surgery malpractice cases are rare and commonly settled outside of the court room. RLN injury is the most frequently presented harm to the patient and lack of informed consent the most common plaintiff claim. Less than half the cases presented in court result in favor of the plaintiff. The harm from RLN injury can vary significantly from minor to severe which is reflected in the range of awards to plaintiffs in malpractice cases resulting in favor of the plaintiff. IONM is not specifically discussed in prior thyroid surgery malpractice literature. However, with the increasing adoption of IONM, themes from prior malpractice reviews, such as informed consent, can be applied to IONM cases.

Preventing Medical Malpractice

Recommendations for mitigating malpractice include attention to documentation, robust informed consent, and implementation of staged procedures. Preoperative vocal cord examination with laryngoscopy and careful documentation of findings provides comparison to postoperative findings in symptomatic patients. Careful documentation about the identification of the RLN intraoperatively as well as stimulation thresholds if IONM is utilized is important to show intact RLN function at the end of the procedure [2].

Informed consent should explicitly present the risks of thyroid surgery. Dysphonia, dysphagia, and dyspnea should be listed and reviewed with patients as risks associated with thyroid surgery due to the risk of injury to the RLN; the impact these symptoms can have on quality of life should not be diminished [22, 24]. Permanent tracheostomy, infection, bleeding, hypocalcemia, and death should be discussed with patients as potential complications of surgery [2]. In cases in which IONM will be utilized, the physician should discuss the use of the technology as well as the potential for technology malfunction and how the surgical decision-making proceeds in the event of equipment malfunction.

In situations of total thyroidectomy, a staged procedure should be discussed with the patient as an intraoperative decision dependent on findings of the RLN on the first side. Concern for RLN injury or IONM signal loss should lead the surgeon to consider a staged procedure after the function of the RLN is assessed [24]. These scenarios should be discussed preoperatively with the patient to ensure the patient's preferences regarding a staged versus single procedure are incorporated. The consensus from these preoperative conversations should be well documented.

Conclusion

Medical malpractice in thyroid surgery most commonly involves informed consent and RLN injury. Clear and comprehensive discussions with patients regarding the risks of the procedure as well as subsequent sequela should occur preoperatively and be well documented. RLN injury and the subsequent damages are the most common patient harm to result from thyroid surgery. IONM is an adjunct to thyroid surgery to assist with RLN identification and assessment of functionality. While IONM has been shown to be beneficial in certain patient situations, it has not been proven to decrease the risk of RLN injury. It has not been adopted as the standard of care, but as a surgeon adjunct. From a medicolegal perspective, IONM can be an advantage or disadvantage to the surgeon as arguments can be made for and against its use. Surgeon skill and assessment of each patient situation with regard to anatomy, disease process, IONM equipment, IONM limitations, and patient preferences are necessary to provide the best outcome for the patient during thyroid surgery.

References

1. Singer MC, Iverson KC, Terris DJ. Thyroidectomy-related malpractice claims. Otolaryngol Head Neck Surg. 2012;146:358–61.
2. Abadin SS, Kaplan EL, Angelos P. Malpractice litigation after thyroid surgery: the role of recurrent laryngeal nerve injuries, 1989–2009. Surgery. 2010;148:718–23.
3. Bal BS. An introduction to medical malpractice in the United States. Clin Orthop Relat Res. 2009;467:339–47.
4. Moffett P, Moore G. The standard of care: legal history and definitions: the bad and good news. West J Emerg Med. 2011;12:109–12.
5. Recupero PR. Clinical practice guidelines as learned treatises: understanding their use as evidence in the courtroom. J Am Acad Psychiatry Law. 2008;36:290–301.
6. Francis DO, McKiever ME, Garrett CG, Jacobson B, Penson DF. Assessment of patient experience with unilateral vocal fold immobility: a preliminary study. J Voice. 2014;28:636–43.
7. Cohen SM, Kim J, Roy N, Asche C, Courey M. The impact of laryngeal disorders on work-related dysfunction. Laryngoscope. 2012;122:1589–94.
8. Nakarada-Kordic I, Patterson N, Wrapson J, Reay SD. A systematic review of patient and caregiver experiences with a tracheostomy. Patient. 2018;11:175–91.
9. Cavicchi O, Burgio L, Cioccoloni E, Piccin O, Macrì G, Schiavon P, Dionigi G. Intraoperative intermittent neuromonitoring of inferior laryngeal nerve and staged thyroidectomy: our experience. Endocrine. 2018;62:560–5.
10. Christoforides C, Papandrikos I, Polyzois G, Roukounakis N, Dionigi G, Vamvakidis K. Two-stage thyroidectomy in the era of intraoperative neuromonitoring. Gland Surg. 2017;6:453–63.
11. Dralle H, Sekulla C, Haerting J, et al. Risk factors of paralysis and functional outcome after recurrent laryngeal nerve monitoring in thyroid surgery. Surgery. 2004;136:1310–22.
12. Shindo M, Chheda NN. Incidence of vocal cord paralysis with and without recurrent laryngeal nerve monitoring during thyroidectomy. Arch Otolaryngol Neck Surg. 2007;133:481–5.
13. Chan WF, Lang BHH, Lo CY. The role of intraoperative neuromonitoring of recurrent laryngeal nerve during thyroidectomy: a comparative study on 1000 nerves at risk. Surgery. 2006;140:866–73.
14. Chandrasekhar SS, Randolph GW, Seidman MD, et al. Clinical practice guideline: improving voice outcomes after thyroid surgery. Otolaryngol Head Neck Surg (United States). 2013; https://doi.org/10.1177/0194599813487301.
15. Wu C-W, Sun H, Zhang G, Kim HY, Catalfamo A, Portinari M, Carcoforo P, Randolph GW, Chai YJ, Dionigi G. Staged thyroidectomy: a single institution perspective. Laryngoscope Investig Otolaryngol. 2018;3:326–32.
16. Goretzki PE, Schwarz K, Brinkmann J, Wirowski D, Lammers BJ. The impact of intraoperative neuromonitoring (IONM) on surgical strategy in bilateral thyroid diseases: is it worth the effort? World J Surg. 2010;34:1274–84.
17. Gschwandtner E, Netz J, Passler C, Bobak-Wieser R, Göbl S, Tatzgern E, Schneider M, Handgriff L, Hermann M. The laryngeal twitch response – can it avoid unnecessary two-stage thyroidectomy? – a retrospective cohort study. Int J Surg. 2019;72:130–4.
18. Angelos P. Recurrent laryngeal nerve monitoring: state of the art, ethical and legal issues. Surg Clin North Am. 2009;89:1157–69.
19. Dralle H, Lorenz KMA. Verdicts on malpractice claims after thyroid surgery: emerging trends and future directions. Head Neck. 2012;34:1591–6.
20. Randolph GW, Dralle H. Electrophysiologic recurrent laryngeal nerve monitoring during thyroid and parathyroid surgery: international standards guideline statement. Laryngoscope. 2011; https://doi.org/10.1002/lary.21119.

21. Choby G, Trojanowski A, Johnson S, Goldenberg D. Use of double electrode pads for intraoperative monitoring of the recurrent laryngeal nerve. Ann Otol Rhinol Laryngol. 2010;119:233–5.
22. Ta JH, Liu YF, Krishna P. Medicolegal aspects of iatrogenic dysphonia and recurrent laryngeal nerve injury. Otolaryngol Head Neck Surg (United States). 2016;154:80–6.
23. Svider PF, Husain Q, Kovalerchik O, Mauro AC, Setzen M, Baredes S, Eloy JA. Determining legal responsibility in otolaryngology: a review of 44 trials since 2008. Am J Otolaryngol Head Neck Med Surg. 2013;34:699–705.
24. Swonke ML, Shakibai N, Chaaban MR. Medical malpractice trends in thyroidectomies among general surgeons and otolaryngologists. OTO Open. 2020;4:2473974X2092114.

Index

© The Editor(s) (if applicable) and The Author(s), under exclusive license to Springer Nature Switzerland AG 2022

J. Scharpf, G. W. Randolph (eds.), *Intraoperative Cranial Nerve Monitoring in Otolaryngology-Head and Neck Surgery*, https://doi.org/10.1007/978-3-030-84916-0